Live Longer, Live Better

Taking Care of Your Health

Peter H. Gott, M.D.

Quill Driver Books

Sanger, California

Published by Quill Driver Books/Word Dancer Press, Inc.
1831 Industrial Way #101
Sanger, California 93657
559-876-2170 • 1-800-497-4909 • FAX 559-876-2180
QuillDriverBooks.com
Info@QuillDriverBooks.com

Quill Driver Books' titles may be purchased in quantity at special discounts for educational, fund-raising, business, or promotional use. Please contact Special Markets, Quill Driver Books/Word Dancer Press, Inc. at the above address or at **1-800-497-4909**.

Quill Driver Books/Word Dancer Press, Inc. project cadre: Doris Hall, Linda Kay Hardie, Susan Klassen, Stephen Blake Mettee, Brigitte Phillips

ISBN: 1-884956-35-1

Printed in the United States of America — third printing

QUILL DRIVER BOOKS and colophon are trademarks of Quill Driver Books/Word Dancer Press, Inc.

To order another copy of this book, please call
1-800-497-4909

Library of Congress Cataloging-in-Publication Data
Gott, Peter, 1935-
  Live longer, live better : taking care of your health / by Peter H. Gott.
    p. cm.
  ISBN 1-884956-35-1
  1. Older people—Health and hygiene. 2. Middle aged persons. 3. Medicine, Popular. I. Title.

RA777.6.G68 2004
613'.0434—dc22
                                                                        2004019839

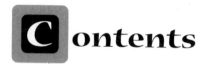

Contents

Dear Reader:

While I welcome correspondence, I don't feel comfortable making decisions about health concerns that arrive on my desk in the form of (sometimes very brief) letters from readers hundreds—even thousands—of miles away. Good medical judgement rests on a complete history (which is seldom supplied to me) and an examination (which is never possible). An analysis of the possibilities can be informative and interesting, but it will never take the place of a thorough medical history and exam.

Thus, I cannot, because of the reality detailed above and because of ethical considerations, solve the medical issues that trouble my readers. I can never take the place of a reader's primary care physician. Please do not use this book or my column as a replacement for personal, one-on-one medical advice from a qualified physician.

I can, of course, comment on my reader's concerns and wish to continue to do so. I hope that this book and my column assist people in this regard.

—Peter H. Gott, M.D.

Introduction

People often ask me about the challenges and rewards of my writing. What can I say? I have written my column, in one form or another, for most of the 40 years I have been a doctor. I love to write. I want to continue to provoke thoughtful discussion while I still have good health and a functioning brain—well, an almost-functioning brain.

I am pleased by the fact that my column is syndicated in more than 350 newspapers worldwide, but my formula for success is simple. Each day I focus on concerns which have been brought to my attention, usually in the form of one or two questions from the 2,500 letters I receive from readers weekly. I do answer as many letters in my column as I can, but, as you can imagine....

I feel fortunate that, at the time of this writing, I am engaged in a full-time solo medical practice in rural Connecticut. I don't accept the occasional criticism from other physicians that I am inexperienced. I am not writing as a "media-doc." I am a real, in-the-trenches physician. I deal with real medical problems on a very personal level with my patients. I am the only widely-syndicated columnist who maintains an active medical practice. I believe having an active practice gives me valuable insights that I try to include in what I write.

A secret: I have never admitted this in writing before, but I am also medical director of the Hotchkiss School, a prestigious coed preparatory boarding school in my community. This experience gives me a wonderful perspective on adolescent medicine, that helps counterbalance my constant exposure to elderly patients. I may see football knee injuries on Saturday and arthritic knee problems on Monday. That makes medicine far more interesting.

Like most of life's adventures, medical practice has changed dramatically in the 40 years I've been at it. Many of these changes are desirable: more powerful antibiotics, a giant leap in diagnostic technology, new life-saving surgical techniques, an improved understanding of disease processes, and—most important—an increase in the life span of people in the developed world.

However, as with any change, there are inevitable drawbacks: the astronomical increase in medical costs, the malpractice crisis, practitioners' dissatisfaction with the erosion of their autonomy, unacceptable government interference, the problems with health maintenance organizations, increasing doctor shortages, less personal physician-patient relations, and the increasing tendency of many young doctors to treat the disease instead of treating the patient as a person.

This last change reflects a dynamic alteration in the culture of the medical profession and it particularly affects senior citizens. Years ago, doctors listened to their patients and adopted a more give-and-take attitude with the elderly under their care. Patients and their families were consulted and their wishes were, as a general rule, respected.

Now, I am told, new doctors often tend to avoid eye contact, preferring instead to focus on their computers, order more lab tests, and prescribe multiple drugs. In far too many instances, physicians completely disregard their aging patients' desires, especially concerning personal choices about how best to make the remaining years of life active and enjoyable and the inevitability of death as painless and dignified as possible.

When I started practice years ago, all the doctors in my community took care of indigent, deserving patients. That, too, was my job: to serve the community. Judging from the mail I have received, this is no longer the standard. Too bad. A doctor's prime goal should be to serve the sick, and, in the past, this was considered to be part of doing one's job. But, unfortunately, I have no control over the current crop of medical doctors.

I try to cover a plethora of topics when I write, yet, now that I am pushing 70, health issues of the over-50 crowd, the core material of this book, have somehow reached a new level of importance with me.

I often write about these concerns in my column. I do this, in large part, because I am convinced that we—the elderly—need to be heard; our opinions are valid. The doctor serves us, not the other way around.

Now is the time for each of us oldies to step up to the plate. If, at a later date, we are suffering from advanced senility or an incapacitating disease, we may lose control of our lives and our futures—unless we have planned ahead.

We have an obligation to our loved ones and ourselves to become familiar with topics relating to common diseases, methods to maintain good health, and the rationale behind any proposed medical or surgical therapy.

For instance, overweight is a national crisis. It can lead to serious cardiovascular consequences. The treatment? A reasonable diet. High cholesterol levels predispose one to heart disease. The first step in therapy? A low- cholesterol diet and more exercise. Lung cancer is a leading cause of death in adults who smoke cigarettes. The best treatment is prevention: Stop smoking.

What is the common denominator in these examples? There is no surgery, medication, or therapy other than common sense. We can, in fact, be in control of much about our lives without medical assistance. People who behave sensibly usually live healthier, longer lives than those who don't. Take note.

All of us will die. (You can say that you first read this startling revelation here!) But death can be comfortable and brief or agonizing and prolonged. Each of us must decide how this difficult situation should be handled. Therefore, I urge those of us who want some say in this crucial matter to make our choices and to prepare and sign the necessary legal documents, including living wills and health care proxies, and to inform our families of our wishes.

Do I dare comment about the future of medicine? Sure. The future of medicine is—in my view—undecipherable. The profession of physician is unquestionably in crisis. We are moving at breakneck speed toward a computer-generated health system that will apportion services according to bits and bytes—unbalanced by hands-on medical contact. This, I fear, will be to the patient's great disadvantage. Maybe someday it will reach some kind of Star Trek stage: you step into a smoked-glass tube and get beamed back to good health—making medical doctors unnecessary.

Finally, I give my readers the same advice that I give myself: Find a physician who is caring, considerate and knowledgeable; maintain a living will; exercise regularly; behave appropriately; and hope that your needs will be respected when the time comes. Also, try to keep some humor in your response to life-issues. Funny is always better.

Prevention

We are all responsible for ourselves

Q. My husband is a two-pack-a-day smoker. He does not eat a healthful diet, rarely exercises, is short of breath, and complains about numbness of his hands and feet. However, he downright refuses to see a doctor, despite my urging. He stubbornly ignores my advice. What can I do?

A. Nothing, I'm afraid.

Adults have a right to ignore health issues, even when the potential consequences are dangerous. In the final analysis, each of us is responsible for his or her own health. I do not know how you can get your husband to change his behavior (unless he is willing to) except through gentle urging by you and the family (children and parents). In this context, you might remind him that numbness of the extremities could indicate a serious vascular disorder that could lead to a severe handicap if not treated. Good luck. I'm sorry that I don't have a definitive answer.

Simple blood test may prevent heart attack

Q. What is the relation between homocysteine and heart attack?

A. Homocysteine is an amino acid necessary for protein metabolism. Elevated levels of the nutrient can result from genetic factors, and a deficiency of vitamins B6, B12 and folate. Several studies have shown that excessive homocysteine in the body is associated with premature coronary artery disease and heart attacks in relatively young men and women. For example, in the Physicians' Health Study, about 15,000 male physicians without recognized heart disease were followed for five years. During that time, 270 participants had heart attacks. In *every* case, homocysteine levels were higher than in the healthy controls. Consequently, many authorities recommend routine blood tests to screen for excess homocysteine. This may constitute a valuable example of preventive care, because homocysteine levels can be brought down to normal by taking folic acid supplements (400-1,000 micrograms a day). As yet, most physicians do not include homocysteine levels in the routine testing of men and women, but I predict that soon they will.

Low-fat diet may help reverse plaque-blocked artery

Q. After experiencing chest pain and shortness of breath, my 71-year-old husband underwent heart catheterization that showed one severely blocked artery. This was followed by two angioplasties, because the first one failed.

The doctor said that blocked coronary arteries are irreversible and placed my husband on prescription medicines. Isn't there something we can do with diet and exercise?

A. Yes, there is. People with coronary artery disease usually have high blood levels of LDL (low-density lipoproteins, the "bad" cholesterol). Several studies have proven that a low-fat diet, in conjunction with cholesterol-lowering drugs (Mevacor, Zocor and others), may not only retard the progression of arteriosclerotic plaque but may also reduce deposits that have already blocked the arteries, leading to angina and other symptoms.

I don't agree with your husband's cardiologist, because—although not a universal cure by any means—a low-fat diet clearly helps many patients. Given your husband's situation, such dietary modification certainly won't hurt. In addition, a closely supervised exercise program would probably improve his health.

Here is what I suggest he do:

• Follow a strict low-fat diet. He will need a licensed dietitian to help him plan nutritious meals that are also appetizing.

• Consider taking a cholesterol-lowering drug. By using the medicine and the diet, your husband should aim to lower his LDL level to at least 130 milligrams per deciliter. If he can get the level below 110, so much the better.

• Strive to maintain appropriate control of the blood sugar. As a ball-park figure, he should try to keep his fasting value less than 120 mg/dL.

• Lose weight. Many older diabetics are overweight. This can contribute to coronary blockages, as well as making exercise too strenuous.

• Exercise regularly in a monitored program. Such a program can be devised by the doctor or by specialists in a coronary rehabilitation unit. These units are available in many hospitals, both large and small.

• Continue to take the drugs prescribed by the doctor and to follow his specific instructions, particularly with respect to taking daily aspirin.

Your husband's progress can be assessed in several ways.

First, after several weeks of therapy, he should feel better.

Second, his blood cholesterol levels should be monitored every few months. A falling LDL will be proof that this strategy is working.

Third, periodic stress tests may also indicate objective improvement. As time passes, he should be able to exercise more strenuously without the stress cardiogram showing heart malfunction.

Finally, after several months in the new program, your husband may choose to have another heart catheterization which, I hope, will prove that the blockage in his artery has regressed.

Colonoscopies indicated for family with history of colon cancer

Q. My 40-year-old son recently died from colon cancer. My mother and grandfather did, too. What would you suggest the rest of the family do?

A. In my opinion, every family member—you, your siblings and children, in particular—should undergo colonoscopy. During this test, a specialist will examine your colons to determine whether a problem exists. As you know, some forms of colon cancer are inherited and, if identified and treated early, are preventable. I urge you to work through this problem with your physician. Don't delay. Seek medical attention now.

Full-body tick search to prevent Lyme disease

Q. With the Lyme disease season rapidly approaching, I am interested in learning how adults and children can avoid contact with infected ticks. Any suggestions?

A. Ticks that carry Lyme disease are ubiquitous in many parts of the country. As you point out, prevention is crucial.

Experts advise people to avoid obvious tick habitats, such as long grass, fields and wooded areas. However, in my experience, this prohibition is largely unrealistic during the warm portions of the year. I've found two more reasonable options.

First, if a child or an adult is going to work or play in an environment where ticks are a problem, the person should be sensible about protective clothing. This means long sleeves and trousers (preferably tucked into socks). Also, the clothing should be sprayed daily with a tick repellant.

How to Accept Aging

Q. Do you have any thoughts on our youth-oriented culture?

A. Some. Here goes.

When I was in my 20s and 30s, I didn't ponder the aging process. On an intellectual level, I recognized that people grew old—I may not have been too bright, but I had eyes and could see. In contrast, on an emotional level, growing old was something that happened to other people. I really couldn't conceive of myself as ever being old. My father and I were similar in appearance and he was 24 years my senior; hence, I had sort of a mirror to the future. So, I'd periodically check him out and he was OK, same old dad, through his 50s.

My father died at 80. At the end, I saw the wear and tear; he had serious health problems with multiple myeloma. Through him, I previewed myself 20 years older. This gave me pause, as I realized that I was (and am) much more interested in (and affected by) the aging process. In short, it's happening to me.

I suppose that most adults fear old age because, in our society, it is synonymous with dependency and death. Coping with aging means that we are forced to address our own mortality. However, this is by no means universal in all cultures. In more "primitive" societies, old age brings respect, perquisites and honor. The elders in most tribes are listened to and their advice is eagerly sought; they have more prestige and power than do the young. I think we're missing something here.

Let's face it; for most of us, aging is associated with failing health, declining powers and lessening prowess. The way in which we handle these alterations is a function of elegance and style, two attributes in increasingly short supply. No blueprints are available to show us how to age gracefully.

Witness the inelegant and restless seekers of trim, buff, wrinkle-free bodies who support a multi-billion dollar industry of cosmetics, health clubs and plastic surgery, all of which are designed to make us look falsely younger. Fewer of us are allowing maturity to follow its natural course. We seem to prefer cinnamon-colored, sheen-less hair and the pretense of adolescent glow applied from makeup kits. This is wishful thinking, pure and simple: If we worship the mementos of our youth and can avoid appearing old, we can fool the grim reaper. We delude ourselves into believing we can trick nature and undo the unkind Spell of the Elderly. Our fanciful efforts are reinforced by the American cult of adolescence that bombards us daily in the media with phony assurances of youthful superiority.

To a great degree, the advances of modern medicine do, in fact, permit the elderly to lead longer, more independent lives. Successful therapies for diabetes, hypertension, heart disease, cancer and a host of serious afflictions are causing a top-heavy demographic pyramid. Aged people are commonplace. The total population over 65 has mushroomed as the baby boomers enter the mix. Despite our efforts, however, the human genetic clock has its limit, probably about 110 years. How do we oldies put up with the aging process?

I submit that for most of us, adaptation is the key. To explore and exploit each decade as it inexorably overtakes us, to use our experiences wisely, to accept the consequences of aging without the desperate pretense of ersatz youth, to maintain dignity, to enjoy as full a life as possible and to preserve a sense of humor about the whole process. If we use these tools, the gels, creams, lotions, pills, nips and tucks, silicone, collagen injections and liposuction become superfluous.

Albert Camus, the French novelist, once wrote that men over 40 are responsible for their faces. By this he meant that as people age, their faces take on character. Our skin becomes a vivid testimonial; it documents the thoughts and feelings, the pain and exuberance, the sum of our experiences. I like this perspective; it allows me to accept the inevitable wrinkles of others, as well as my own. More important, it gives me permission to reset my limits—as, for example, on my recent birthday when I changed from a 10-speed racing bicycle to a 21-gear hybrid. Although I accept the reality that most of the decisions about our world are being made increasingly by people my junior, I bless any elderly person who accepts the aging process with class, a quality that is becoming increasingly rare in our society today.

Finally, a humorous note on the definition of age. According to Gott, you know you're getting older when you suggest to your wife that you both take an afternoon nap. And you do.

Second, and most important, a tick check of the body (at the end of the day) is vital. Every inch of the body must be examined for ticks, which should be promptly removed, even if they are imbedded. While it's true that immature ticks are tiny and hard to see, a combination of visual inspection plus gentle feeling of the skin is usually successful. Remember that ticks are, in a sense, very versatile. They can easily find a host (in short grass, for instance) and will often attach to a pet animal before changing to humans. Therefore, a thorough tick check at the end of the day is a reasonable strategy for anybody who spends time outdoors in an area known to harbor ticks.

People over 50, others, should receive pneumonia vaccine

Q. My son, who is 40 and has had pneumonia twice, lives in another state. I suggested that he receive a pneumonia shot, but his doctor has never heard of it and told my son that you were "nuts" for recommending such therapy. Is there a pneumonia vaccine?

A. Indeed there is. Known as Pneumovax (Merck), the injection confers immunity to 23 of the most common types of pneumococcal bacteria. It is recommended for people over 50, persons over 2 years of age with heart/lung disease or diabetes, those over 2 without spleens, immuno-compromised patients or people in high-risk environments (such as Alaskan Natives and certain Native American populations).

A booster dose should be given about every five years.

When I administer the vaccine, I am always careful to explain that there are literally hundreds of different microorganisms that can cause pneumonia: bacteria, molds, viruses—the list goes on. The pneumonia vaccine, therefore, does not prevent all types of pneumonia, only the 23 strains that I mentioned.

Your son's doctor is long overdue for a continuing medical education course; in addition, he ought to learn some manners.

Pets are beneficial for seniors' well-being

Q. I am 77 and have a pet parakeet. I keep hearing from a family member advising me to get rid of the bird because it creates an unhealthful environment due to the feather barbs that float in the air and are inhaled, which can lead to lung disease.

My pet is confined in a cage that I keep clean. I wash my hands each time I work with the bird.

It is said that pets are good for seniors.

A. And indeed they are.

To my knowledge, healthy pets are not a threat to their owners. I have never heard that feather barbs are harmful.

On occasion, people can contract a form of pneumonia from sick birds, but healthy birds are safe.

Should you be concerned about your pet's health status, discuss your concerns with a veterinarian.

Avoid using microwaves with seal damage

Q. Your comment about microwave ovens was incorrect. Microwaves are not soundwaves but electromagnetic radiation.

Also, I offer a bit of advice. Microwave door seals are made of carefully shaped pieces of metal. The safety of the ovens depends on the continuity of the seals. Therefore, people should not use ovens with any seal damage, including deposits of foreign material and food.

A. I received many letters from readers who properly pointed out my oversimplification. I stand corrected and thank you for reminding us all of the very real hazards of microwave scatter. Such electromagnetic radiation can cause serious damage to unprotected, living tissue; a good door-seal is of paramount importance. To be on the safe side, many alert consumers stand some distance away from microwave ovens that are in operation—just in case.

Wellness and health newsletters may overpromise

Q. We just received an offer to subscribe to a wellness and health publication at a cost of $39.95. This sounds too good to be true. Because my wife and I are 65 and 67 respectively, walk five miles a day, watch our diet, avoid tobacco products and take a one-a-day vitamin, we wonder is this publication is a good investment—or if we even need it.

A. Many promoters are riding what I call the "Wellness Wave," Americans' increasing interest in maintaining good health by employing certain dietary programs and using organic food and "natural" vitamins. In most cases, the health letters sold by reputable organizations are appropriate sources of information.

In my experience, however, these promoters often make fantastically absurd claims about the benefits of their programs. Therefore, if you choose to subscribe to such resources, read them with a grain of salt. If it sounds too good to be true, it probably is.

Judging from your brief description, you and your spouse appear to be following a healthful lifestyle of exercise and moderation. Keep it up. And if the publications you mentioned suggest unusual alternatives, such as megadose vitamin therapy, check them out with your family physician before committing to an expensive program that could do more harm than good. For example, vitamin toxicity can lead to liver damage and other complications.

Communal hot tub cauldron of infection

Q. There is a hot tub in my retirement community. The rule is that you must shower before entering. However, the majority of users disregard the rule. Does the gunk washed off the bods of these clods present any medical hazards?

A. There are several recognized skin infections common in habitues of hot tubs. Some, such as staph, are serious. Others, including E. Coli, are less troublesome.

Nonetheless, there is good reason for the "shower first" rule in public spas and hot tubs, because bacteria grow abundantly and readily in the superheated water.

One patron with a healthy supply of skin bacteria can contaminate the entire facility, leading to skin infections in subsequent users.

I recommend that you stay out of this hot tub until the management can stick by their guns to force users to clean up and follow the rule.

Eat raw broccoli to avoid constipation.

Q. Realizing that constipation is a common complaint among the elderly, I would like to share my remedy: raw broccoli before the main meal. This simple cure has eliminated my chronic constipation altogether.

A. Good for you. I do not know the reason for your success, except to point out that any raw vegetable contains fiber, which is an effective bowel stimulant. If you can stand eating broccoli every day, fine; it won't hurt you.

Home remedy good for minor throat irritations

Q. Is it acceptable to gargle with vinegar water?

A. Yes. Throat irritation can often be relieved by gargling with mild antiseptic solutions, such as diluted vinegar (vinegar diluted by half with water) or saltwater (one teaspoon of salt per glass of hot water).

Antibiotics before dental cleaning sometimes called for

Q. I had my left knee replaced, and my dentist now requires me to take antibiotics on the day of my dental cleaning. Why is this?

A. Any dental procedure that causes bleeding—even minor bleeding from professional cleaning—will allow bacteria normally present in the mouth to enter the bloodstream. Under normal circumstances, these bacteria are quickly gobbled up by infection-fighting white blood cells; the germs cannot find refuge.

In contrast, people with artificial joints and certain disorders of the heart valves are susceptible to infection because, before being killed, the bacteria (which circulate throughout the body) can land on and attach to the operative sites (or valves) and set up a severe infection. Your dentist is on the money. The antibiotic on the day of your visit should prevent this serious complication from developing. I should add that prophylactic antibiotics should also be administered in preparation for other surgical procedures that are known to release bacteria into the bloodstream. Such procedures include sigmoidoscopy, colonoscopy, cystoscopy (examination of the bladder), bowel surgery and so forth.

Preventing gas attacks

Q. Please discuss the causes of foul-smelling intestinal gas and how to alleviate it. I have a family member who is a real social liability because of this problem.

A. There's not much we can do to alter the olfactory characteristics of intestinal gas, which smells bad because of the internal company it keeps. If this gas is not caused by a deficiency of intestinal enzymes (such as lactose intolerance) or by some physical ailment (such as colitis), people can usually reduce the amount of gas by following these simple suggestions:

• Eat slowly and chew thoroughly. Most intestinal flatulence is really swallowed air that is not belched up but passes through the bowel and is expelled in a considerably spicier state.

• Avoid carbonated beverages for the same reason.

• Don't consume gas-producing foods, such as beans and legumes. The starch in these edibles may not be readily digested; it passes into the colon where bacteria degrade it, causing foul-smelling gas in the process.

• Consider purchasing anti-gas medication, such as those that contain simethicone.

• Make an effort to release intestinal gas in socially acceptable situations. In this way, the problem may appear to be more diminished than it really is.

Alcohol should be part of medical history

Q. I'm a healthy male, 55, with a drinking problem. What do you advise in terms of a routine medical examination and testing?

A. First, your physician must take a medical history that concerns any symptoms you have had, pertinent family illnesses, an overview of your lifestyle and a review of the things you should—or shouldn't—do to affect your health. I urge you to be brutally frank and open about your alcohol consumption. All too often doctors gloss over the subject of alcohol abuse because they feel uncomfortable about it—and, as the old adage says, an alcoholic is someone who drinks more than his doctor does.

Next, you need a full examination, which should include a digital exam of your prostate gland—and, in your case, a careful screening of the possible consequences of your alcohol habit, such as a swollen liver.

Finally, you should have a blood count, a metabolic profile (that checks your liver function), a cholesterol level, a PSA (for prostate cancer), a urinalysis, perhaps a cardiogram (or a stress test), and—if you have not had one in more than five years—a colonoscopy (to check for bowel polyps and cancer).

I would also recommend that the physician actively counsel you about the dangers of alcohol abuse. He may encourage you to reduce your consumption or—better yet—stop drinking entirely, especially if the exam and testing indicate a potential health problem.

Although your doctor may choose to fine tune some of these suggestions, the list I provided would constitute a bare minimum for someone your age.

Caring for minor cuts, scrapes

Q. Please describe the difference between peroxide, alcohol and mercurochrome and when each would be indicated for minor injuries in the home. What about an ointment that would be good for covering a cut from a glass shard or knife?

A. Peroxide, alcohol, mercurochrome (and iodine, the old standby) are antiseptics. They kill germs. Peroxide doesn't hurt; the other three do. Mercurochrome and iodine can cause tissue damage.

A generation ago, any self-respecting family had a medicine cabinet containing one or more of these compounds, which were applied liberally (and usually painfully) to minor cuts and scrapes, thereby saving innocent victims from the ravages of infection. All this was probably unnecessary.

For a long time, people have overtreated nicks and abrasions, first with the substances you mention, later with one of the ubiquitous antibiotic creams.

This is a waste of time, money and energy. All that's really necessary is to clean superficial skin injuries with warm soap and water, pat dry and leave open to the air. Nonstick dressings may help avoid subsequent bacterial contamination (and prevent blood-spotting of clothes) if the wounds are in an area that is normally clothed. Oxygen in the air helps heal wounds, so covering them with salves and ointments may do more harm than good.

Glass and knife wounds can be "butterflied" (the edges drawn together) with Band-Aids cut in half. If the cut is too extensive, the injury probably needs suturing by a doctor.

In short, the less you do to a minor wound, the better. If you really feel you have to do something, flood the area with hydrogen peroxide.

Remember that tetanus boosters should be brought up to date every 10 years.

For motion sickness try Dramamine first

Q. You have referred to the Transderm-Scop patch as an effective antagonist to motion sickness. You have also warned patients that the patch can cause untoward and unpredictable mental changes in some people. I read—but largely disregarded—your comments, until I had a personal experience that I will relate.

In June, my wife and I took an extensive voyage on a ship. She has always had a problem with seasickness, so her doctor prescribed Transderm-Scop patches, which she religiously applied starting on our second day of the voyage. (We were basically out of the harbor.)

For 24 hours, she was normal. However, the next day, she began to hallucinate. She thought she was at home with her mother, who died 20 years ago. She believed she was in church and felt threatened. Finally, the English doctor on the cruise ship concluded that the problem was the Scop patch. After removing it, he was gratified to see that she returned to normal. Are you aware of this reaction?

A. Indeed I am. That's why I routinely caution patients who use the product to be aware of mental changes.

Scopolamine is a powerful drug, sometimes referred to as "truth serum" because recipients may unavoidably let down their defenses when given the drug. It can also cause asthma, intestinal blockage, rapid pulse, dry mouth and allergic reactions. However, despite these drawbacks, it is an incredibly effective antidote to motion sickness.

I suspect that your wife is one of the unusual patients who develops marked mental changes from the medication. Ordinarily, there is no harm done when these reactions occur. Nonetheless, your wife appears to have been unexpectedly sensitive to scopolamine. Therefore, she should avoid it in the future.

Perhaps her motion sickness can be controlled with a safer medication, such as Dramamine, which is available without a prescription. Or, as I am sure you know, repeated exposure to motion sickness does, in a majority of patients, result in immunity. Therefore, see how she responds to the next cruise, as well as to future cruises. She may even get hooked.

How to avoid ear pressure when flying

Q. What can be done to avoid the uncomfortable ear pressure of flying? I usually get so much buildup that I cannot hear, and my ears hurt. The last time I was brought to tears. Now I am anticipating (with mixed emotions) a wedding anniversary trip to Hawaii. Can I handle the trip?

A. Without a doubt.

But first, you should be aware of what is happening in your ears.

When you take off and ascend in an aircraft, the air becomes less dense. Consequently, air leaves the middle ear compartment in order to equal the ambient air pressure. This adjustment never causes problems, because air readily leaves the middle ear chamber.

In contrast, during descent, the reverse is true. The environmental air pressure increases, and air must rush into the middle ear through the two vents called the Eustachian tubes. When this happens, people usually hear a "pop" that relieves the pressure.

The problem is that air has a much more difficult time entering the middle ear compartment than it does exiting from it. This difficulty is magnified by any condition—such as allergies, colds and sinus congestion—that interferes with pressure equalization. Therefore, ear pressure symptoms are only a problem during landings.

The traditional (and usually effective) methods of allowing air to enter the middle ear chamber are: frequent (forceful) swallowing, and pressing the nose tight and straining and yawning. Unfortunately, these techniques are not always effective—in part because they must begin at the earliest sensation of descent—but also because of congestion, Eustachian tube dysfunction and other ear disorders. In such instances, including yours, I recommend the following:

• Don't fly if you have active allergies, a cold, sinus congestion or an upper respiratory infection.

• Have your doctor prescribe a non-sedating antihistamine to be taken four to six hours before your flight.

• Pay no attention to the pressure changes during ascent.

• Use Afrin nose spray one to three hours before landing.

• Make sure that, at this time, you have chewing gum or fluids handy so that you have enough lubrication to swallow forcefully.

• At the first sensation of increased ear pressure during descent, begin your forceful swallowing and yawning exercises. (If you delay, the pressure can quickly build to uncomfortable levels that may be impossible to control.)

• Try the Valsalva maneuver (straining against a pinched nose), and repeat it if appropriate. (By increasing the pressure of the air at the back of the throat, this technique may drive air into the middle ears.)

These are the acute guidelines that are, in most cases, effective. Other techniques include nasal steroid sprays and referral to an otolaryngologist.

Remember that acute aero-otitis (inability to equalize air pressure) is a common occurrence that, fortunately, rarely leads to serious consequences or ear damage. Even if you land at ground level with a pressure in your ears of 35,000 feet, the situation will resolve—usually within 24 hours. Be patient, follow the instructions I suggested, and have a wonderful anniversary in Hawaii.

Daughter's concerns about aging mother valid

Q. My mother is 75 and lives alone. I am very concerned about her health and safety. She has pain, tingling, cramping and numbness in her legs. She frequently falls; the last time, she cracked two ribs. She is forgetful; stumbles when she walks and may not consume a well-balanced diet.

Her doctor, who told my mother that I was "a fanatic" about health issues, refuses to order diagnostic testing. Shouldn't my mother have a bone density test to check for osteoporosis and other tests for her memory and nerve problems?

I believe that Mom is not getting adequate medical attention because she survives only on Social Security and Medicare. Am I wrong to be so concerned? How can I resolve this problem?

A. This all-too-common situation is complicated.

First of all, I do not believe that your mother's financial status is playing a role. Medicare will pay for appropriate professional attention, and no doctor can ethically deprive a senior citizen of needed medical care.

Second, I thoroughly agree with you that your mother needs a meticulous physical (and mental) evaluation, in addition to testing. Given her history of falling, a bone density is appropriate—as are blood tests and (probably) CT scanning to diagnose her gait disturbance and failing memory.

While the cause of her problems may be the normal aging process, I worry that a treatable condition—such as a thyroid disorder, anemia or vitamin deficiency—is being overlooked. Once a diagnosis—or diagnoses—is established, your mother would benefit from specific therapy. Her doctor should include consultations with specialists, such as neurologists and physical therapy professionals.

Third, I am extremely concerned about your mother's safety. Perhaps it is time for assisted living in a nursing facility, or maybe her home situation needs revision so that she can live on one floor, use railings, have a lifeline telephone to summon help, obtain Meals-on-Wheels, have someone do her shopping and prepare at least one nutritious meal a day, employ a certified nurse's aide to monitor her hygiene and check on her situation several times a week. Your local visiting nurse association should, on the doctor's order, be able to provide extensive assistance.

Finally, your worries about your mother do not seem to me to be fanatical. I sense your frustration and understand your need to help. I suspect that your mother's current physician is not a good choice. I advise you to search out a practitioner with whom you can work, a doctor who will address your mother's health requirements—as well as involving the family in important decisions.

2

Taking Charge of Your Health

Doctor needs lesson in humility

Q. I am 60 and have hypertension, arthritis, glaucoma and high blood fats, all of which are under treatment by my very competent doctor.

Because my triglycerides are 210 and should be less than 150, my physician recommends that I double my Lipitor from 20 milligrams to 40 milligrams a day.

However, I am aware of dose-related liver and muscle damage from the drug—especially as the levels increase. When I raised this issue with him, he said, "You are the patient. I am the doctor. Stop worrying." I don't feel comfortable with this advice.

A. Nor do I. Your doctor needs a lesson in humility. No physician worth his salt is going to take this unrealistic view, because no professional can predict the potential negative consequences of drug therapy or the problems stemming from any drug.

In my view, your physician should have taken a few minutes to discuss with you his rationale for doubling the dosage of Lipitor.

Then, armed with this information, you would be in a much sounder position, either to accept his recommendations or to have him modify them. "Trust me, I'm a doctor" is no longer a reasonable excuse for doing anything.

Educate your doctor

Q. My doctor seems too busy to sit and talk with me for more than a few moments. Is this a professional tendency?

A. I am frequently amused by television commentators who state that the program will continue "after some brief messages." These "brief messages" are more than a dozen 30-second commercials, annoyingly extensive and hardly brief. I suppose that these breaks come with the territory, but they bug me because, in my opinion, the commentators should at least be honest and say: "We'll be back after six minutes of commercials."

The same cultural phenomenon contaminates the interaction between doctors and patients. In this circumstance, the doctor honestly believes that he can discuss a problem (read: what he wants to discuss) in a 30-second sound bite—and then move on to his next patient. This problem is not so much a medical one as it is a reflection of our current obsession with instant information in the shortest possible time.

I think you need to educate your physician. Keep a written list of the topics you want him to cover. Don't let him shut you down until your questions have been answered. Make sure that you don't leave the office until he has addressed all your concerns.

Warning: This is going to make him crazy. But it is necessary and he should allow time for it. For example, I have a 99-year-old woman who sees me every four weeks (her choice, not mine), to complain that she is "growing old." After biting my nails and experiencing severe heart-burn, I realized that her enunciation of health problems (old age) was actually therapeutic. She wasn't as interested in providing relevant infor-mation as she was in complaining. Thus, her "complaining" (as opposed to "complaints") was the reason she frequented the office. Medicare won't pay for this nonsense, so I absorb the cost.

What the heck? If I ever reach 99, I'll be obligated to complain about my age, too. As long as I can help her, God bless her. But I do become somewhat nuts when I see her name in the appointment book.

"Gardening skills" worth maintaining

Q. I am 88. Thirteen years ago, I had successful open-heart surgery to bypass a blocked artery. No problems since. I play golf, walk a lot, do a little gardening, eat plenty, drink a little, get a hot temper and admire beautiful women. I'm on a bunch of medications. Why should I keep seeing doctors, have annual exams, stress tests and blood tests?

A. Duh. So you can continue to admire beautiful women. Next ques-tion, please.

Seriously, I am sure that your physician is committed to preserving your quality of life. Thank goodness. As a result, he iş eager to monitor your progress and make sure that you don't risk developing any treatable consequences of aging. Also, your "bunch" of medications may need to be adjusted periodically.

While I would advise you to question your doctor about any suggestions or recommendations, it seems to me that you are similar to an 89-year-old man (also from Florida) that I am privileged to care for. When he came to the office last year, I asked him what his primary health concerns were.

"Independence and snuggling," he replied.

"I understand the independence issue," I responded, "but tell me about the snuggling." (I questioned him about this because intimacy often produces chest pain as a result of coronary artery disease.)

"Well," he said, "I'm in a unique position. Most of the women I know are widows who need hands-on attention. While I may not be able to provide sexual fulfillment through intercourse, sometimes I can. More important, my partners value just closeness and touching. I do not want to forfeit any of my skills."

His articulate message rang a bell for me: Age itself may not be the governing factor in disease; attitude and ability may also play important roles.

So, I promised him that I'd support his wishes. And I have. He is now taking lower dosages of medication and I will see him once a year when he visits from Florida. I wish the elderly ladies in the southeastern United States good luck; this guy is a rip. But he is real. And, above all else, he has successfully maintained his "little gardening" skills (define that as you choose).

Doctors are obligated to speak clearly

Q. I find that doctors speak too rapidly (and with too much scientific jargon) when talking to elderly patients. Older folks can't comprehend as quickly as can younger ones, and sometimes they miss instructions and are too embarrassed to ask that the doctor repeat what he has said. Also, we have a lot of foreign doctors in my community who are also difficult to understand. Perhaps you could address this important issue.

A. You are not alone in your frustration and concern. Doctors often explain things in technical language that is not understandable, or they may provide overly complicated descriptions that are impossible to comprehend. This situation is made intolerable, of course, if there is a language problem or if the physician fails to enunciate and speak clearly.

When patients find themselves in these awkward circumstances, they must politely, but firmly, stop the discussion and ask for clarification. Also, written instructions are often more appropriate (providing the doctor writes legibly) when dealing with complex issues or lengthy suggestions about which medicines to take and how often.

Finally, the crucial step. Elderly patients should, in my opinion, arrange to have a patient advocate present who may help to clarify confusing issues. No one needs to be embarrassed or intimidated by physicians. It's OK to ask practitioners to back off, rephrase something or say it again. After all, the patient is purchasing a service and the doctor is ethically obligated to provide that service to the best of his or her ability. Doctors who remain unresponsive to their patients' needs will soon be looking for work or may end up in court because of a bad result stemming from improper communication.

Keep badgering your doctors until they speak to you in intelligible and understandable English.

Health matters should be private

Q. I'd like your opinion about the privacy of physical therapy. I am in the process of taking such therapy in a hospital facility where many people come for daily exercise routines not necessarily prescribed by their physician.

Frankly, I am quite uncomfortable undergoing my treatment in front of all these people, especially when the therapists comment on how I am doing and review (to all those present) my capabilities and limitations. I live in a small town and do not believe that my neighbors need to know about my impairments, medications, depression and other health problems. For this reason, I am discontinuing my therapy and will probably stop altogether because the nearest similar facility is 150 miles away.

Am I just being paranoid and picky?

A. I understand your reluctance to share personal matters with others in a therapeutic milieu. And I agree that such a "support group" atmosphere may be counterproductive. Therefore, I believe that your objections are both pertinent and appropriate.

In a situation in which motivation is crucial, some professionals will attempt to capitalize on certain patients' successes in overcoming adversity in order to encourage similar patients to try harder and adopt more positive attitudes. As an example, Lance Armstrong's remarkable recovery from the ravages of testicular cancer (enabling him to win the Tour de France) was, in large part, the result of dedicated therapists. I believe that most of us, who learned from the media of his ordeal and subsequent successes, were touched and revitalized by his heroism and commitment. However, none of this information would have been made public without Mr. Armstrong's consent.

And there, I believe, is the problem. Your therapists may be unaware of your feelings. They may simply be focusing on your success. They may not recognize your discomfort in sharing personal information with others—even neighbors and friends. I view this situation as more an issue of insensitivity than of unprofessionalism.

The answer to this dilemma seems so simple and straightforward that it hardly needs stating—and is certainly preferable to stopping treatment or traveling 300 miles round trip for resolution: Talk to your therapists and—perhaps—to the physiatrist who supervises the program. Express your feelings of embarrassment, emphasize your need for privacy, and explain your concerns. I would be surprised if your therapists failed to respond to such an open dialogue. You deserve confidentiality. Insist on it and make sure that the physical therapy department understands it. No one, regardless of the therapeutic environment, should be made to feel vulnerable.

Extensive testing can lead to problems

Q. When my uncle was tested for a trivial complaint of palpitations, his bill was astronomical. Could you address this problem with a personal experience or one of your famous metaphors?

A. I'll give it a shot.

One of my most treasured possessions is a fully restored 1954 black Jaguar XK120 roadster. Now, before you turn the page because this sounds like another boring car story, bear with me; I'm going to tie this into medical practice.

The Jag is uniquely special in ways even a non car buff can appreciate. It has gorgeous curves and the unmistakable lines of the breed; in a million years you couldn't confuse an XK120 with any modern automobile. It is also very utilitarian; a simple but reliable six-cylinder engine (with which any trained mechanic would feel comfortable), functional gauges that tell you what you need to know and a four-speed gearbox. Elementary. It rides like a truck. But I love to drive it.

Unlike the (unnamed) car I use for work, the Jag has no power windows, air-conditioning, tinted glass, fuel injection or computer. Most of this stuff on modern autos is unnecessary fluff. For example, the onboard computer in my work car tells much more than I want to know: miles per gallon, average speed driven since day one, whether the parking brake is on, the outdoor temperature, and an array of other details I won't list. My work car is better—or at least has more conveniences—than the Jag. But it looks like every other car, a mere clone. To get from point A to point B with style and pizzazz, I prefer my antique auto.

Both cars are metaphors for the medical profession.

Let me illustrate by describing the following true situation. I have a lovely patient in her 70s who suffered heartburn, despite the use of antacids. After several weeks of discomfort, she agreed to an upper GI series, a type of X-ray test for examining the esophagus, stomach and part of the small intestine.

The X-rays showed considerable irritation and spasm of the lower esophagus; no ulcer was identified. In the past, I'd have prescribed medicine for my patient, drugs such as Tagamet or Zantac to reduce stomach acid and aid healing.

However, the radiologist's report concluded that the prudent physician should order endoscopy *"just to make sure"* that no early cancer was the cause of my patient's symptom. Upper endoscopy means 1) a specialist must pass a flexible fiber-optic tube into my patient's stomach to take a look at the irritated area; and 2) the patient would need light anesthesia because endoscopy, although a useful test, is not fun, not like waiting eagerly for your tax refund check.

At this point, my patient and I passed from everyday medicine into high-tech healing, from the 1954 car to a more modern model. You see, I had no choice but to proceed because of the radiologist's comment. He covered his behind; I'd have to cover mine.

Thus, the patient was readied for endoscopy. As part of this ritual, she was required to undergo blood tests. As (bad) luck would have it, one of the routine tests was abnormal, seeming to indicate cardiac damage, maybe even a heart attack in progress.

Naturally, I immediately admitted her to the Intensive Care Unit for monitoring and further testing. Cardiograms were entirely normal. Repeat blood analyses were equivocal. Therefore, I took the next step and ordered a thallium stress test, at the time a surefire way to diagnose coronary heart disease.

The test was inconclusive. My patient's simple indigestion had mushroomed into an extravaganza of hospitalization, inconvenience, expensive testing—and still no endoscopy. I was stuck.

To resolve this issue, I referred her to a cardiologist at a teaching center elsewhere in the state. She was admitted to his hospital and had a coronary artery study that was, of course, perfectly normal. Finally, after almost two weeks of excruciating uncertainty and anguish, a double hospitalization, an uncomfortable and invasive cardiac catheterization, and heaven knows what other tests, my patient underwent endoscopy. The findings: esophageal irritation from too much stomach acid.

Like the computer in my car, medical tests often provide too much information—or data that are faulty and inconclusive. Everybody in the health care profession—and I mean everybody: doctors, nurses and hospitals—is petrified of making a mistake. So we fool ourselves into believing that high-tech testing will show us The Truth. Further, the more tests we perform, the more certain we can be about situations that are, by their very nature, uncertain. We are kidding ourselves and, sadly, don't even realize it. In the medical profession, the tail is increasingly wagging the dog.

No wonder many older physicians have difficulty abandoning this trusted principle: There are few alternatives that will improve on good medical judgment coupled with basic tests.

Please excuse me for bowing out of further discussion. I have a date to wax my Jaguar.

Less quality office time?

Q. Ever since I joined a health maintenance organization, I've been struck by the fact that my doctor spends far less time with me in the office than did my previous non-HMO physician. Is this a national trend?

A. There has been a universal perception that managed care is associated with shorter office visits. Patients often complain about not having enough time; they think that doctors are more rushed and do not attend to patients' medical needs. As you might expect, this indictment has caused many people in the health care field to complain about how impersonal HMOs and doctors have become.

Thus, considerable surprise greeted the publication of a study (New England Journal of Medicine, Jan. 18, 2001) showing that in 1998, doctors actually spent *more* office time with their patients (18.3 minutes) than was the case in 1989 (16.3 minutes). The researchers discovered

Here's to a Healthy Dose of Humor

I really like my doctor.

Part of the reason is that I don't have to see him frequently; about once every five years is enough, for a routine examination.

Let me tell you about an experience I had when I visited him a number of years ago. I had known this doctor for more than 25 years; although only slightly older than I, he was one of my mentors when I was a resident. More important, he is very bright, very dedicated, likes to bicycle and has a marvelous sense of humor. This last quality is crucial to me, and I often wish more physicians had a similar, irreverent, off-the-wall perspective. True, illness is not funny. But my doctor manages a delicate balance between seriousness and drollness; when dealing with a healthy patient, there's usually a twinkle in his eye. Let me illustrate.

Just before my 56th birthday, I took a day off and traveled to the major city where my doctor practices. I thought I was due for my mid-decade checkup.

His office seemed slightly chaotic, as I knew it would be: telephones ringing constantly, patients' charts scattered all over his desk, worn carpets, doors opening and closing…you know—the usual ambience of a deliriously busy, almost out-of-control practice. He had to examine me in the X-ray room because his associate was ensconced in the main examination area. Female technicians kept sticking their heads in at the door, exclaiming "ooops!" and soundlessly retreating.

Despite the interruptions, however, my doctor was able to question me thoroughly about the usual, trivial age-related complaints that had invaded my life: getting up a couple of times at night to go to the john, less endurance during my long bike rides, pesky muscle aches, minor skin changes from years of excessive sun exposure—all the usual stuff. I allowed as how I was in a period of some stress and turmoil because my wife and I have separated. This was written down without comment, and I didn't elaborate because I was reluctant to bore him with the details of a highly personal situation over which he had no control. Anyway, I was handling it as well as I could.

Finally, he began the examination. I don't know about you, but I always feel uncomfortably vulnerable sitting on a cold examining table in my underwear, like a kid again, helpless, knowing the drill, yet being uncontrollably apprehensive that the physician might find something…something wrong, something hidden and awful. Fortunately, everything checked out and my doctor pronounced me fit.

"Now, he concluded, "if you'll just drop your shorts, I'll finish the exam."

I complied and stood before him in all my middle-aged glory, with my boxers around my ankles.

He took a step backward in disbelief, pursed his lips, arched his eyebrows and exhaled in mock seriousness.

"Well," he intoned. "I can certainly see why your wife left you."

Of course, we both cracked up. The exam was completed without further incident.

Later, while analyzing my reaction to this unusual transaction, I reasoned—once again—that humor plays an invaluable role in medical practice. My doctor is living proof that a good doctor/patient relationship doesn't have to be—in fact, shouldn't be—based on unrelieved, self-conscious seriousness orchestrated by a practitioner who is too insecure to lighten up.

I suppose a few of my own patients may believe I am sometimes too flip in my dealings with them. Maybe my personal, twisted sense of humor is occasionally misperceived as insensitivity. I hope not but it's possible. However, I'm working hard on this. I know I'll probably never achieve the enviable balance my own doctor exhibits; that's a gift. But I'll keep trying. After all, I have a darned good model to emulate.

that this trend was observed for both primary care visits and specialty visits, for both new and established patients and for both managed-care and non-prepaid visits. An editorial in the same journal asks: "How can the facts be so at odds with the perceptions?"

How indeed.

To begin with, the editor (Edward Campion, M.D.) accurately defines physicians' discontent with the entire health care system: "There is more to do, more to think about and more that is expected." Doctors are bludgeoned by increased administrative costs, frustration with bureaucracy, complex—and sometimes unintelligible—rules and requirements. Unquestionably, the health care system is often inefficient and unfair to both physicians and patients.

Also, health care has become more complicated. Patients rightly want more of a say in it. They read print media, see drug advertisements on TV, and use the Internet. Their expectations are high, as well they should be, but such attitudes can lead to a perception that differs from reality: Time can be objective or subjective.

For example, 20 years ago, I could sit a patient down after an examination and discuss in 15 minutes a low-fat weight-loss diet. I am no longer allowed this indulgence. Now patients insist on in-depth analyses of various diets, weight reduction programs, herbal supplements, prescription diet pills and the pros and cons of cholesterol-lowering drugs. When I fail to take an hour for this discussion, the patients feel shortchanged.

Therefore, if we are to believe the results of the research, doctors actually spend more time with patients. However, for a variety of reasons, this interlude may be perceived as being less productive.

There is no easy answer to the problem. Medical care—especially preventive medicine—is changing, and doctors are hard-pressed to adapt to the new criteria for excellence, which frequently involve time-consuming authorizations for procedures and referrals, concerns about liability and malpractice, filling out forms, and being forced into gatekeeper roles. Less autonomy invariably leads to demoralization.

So, I guess the bottom line is that doctors are taking more time with their patients but are not being credited for it. In part because of personal dissatisfactions, they may have become less congenial and sensitive. Consequently, time spent in interaction with patients could have become less satisfying. End result: less quality time. Solutions: Medical teams must accommodate and address patients' medical needs; for their part, patients must learn to be more considerate and less demanding. Finally, we're all in this together. Let's be more respectful of each others' problems, be they medical or stylistic. Or, as Dr. Campion urges, "The goal should be reforms that will consolidate and simplify systems, broaden access, and help free up time physicians require to concentrate on the needs of patients."

The sign of a good doctor is to admit it when he's in over his head

Q. I believe you did your readers a great disservice when you wrote "doctors in all specialties, all over the world, share their knowledge with one another…"

I am 49, very successful and of above-average intelligence. Two and one-half years ago I was diagnosed as having malignant peritoneal mesothelioma. My internist, who had excellent credentials, told me there was no treatment and I would die. He recommended an oncologist. The oncologist said chemotherapy, radiology and surgery would not be able to help and that it wouldn't do any good to go anywhere else and that I would die in the near future.

A good friend told me not to give up and to talk to an old roommate who is a doctor at a medical center in New York City. He sent me to a doctor who recommended surgery, a port to get the chemo drugs directly into my abdomen, and chemotherapy—since it had worked with a few of his patients. It did. I'm still alive. My CT scans are still negative. The local doctors did not know of this treatment, and if I had relied on them as you suggested, I'd be dead. You were very, very wrong.

A. Thank you for describing your experience, which, I believe, is unusual. Mesothelioma is not a common cancer. Still, I cannot argue with your conclusions: If you hadn't been referred to a major medical center, you might have died.

I fault your original doctors who should have made the referral in the first place. The sign of a good doctor is his willingness to admit when he is in over his head. In my view, your doctors should have realized that your condition required the services of a superspecialist.

I don't believe that such "glitches" are commonplace. Nonetheless, I admit that they do exist. I am printing your letter to help other cancer patients who may believe they have been prematurely deprived of new, potentially curative treatments that should be generally available to cancer specialists.

Examine risks and benefits of meds

Q. Are drug companies committing murder? Every year thousands of people die from prescription drugs. You recently advised a reader with gout to use Indocin, yet my copy of "Worst Pills, Best Pills" tells me it can cause depression, mood changes, confusion, epilepsy and Parkinson's disease. Now what do you say?

A. What I have said many times before.

With this issue—as with many others in medicine—it's crucial to examine the risk/benefit ratio before taking prescription drugs. For that reason, I cannot issue a blanket condemnation of pharmaceutical companies.

True, thousands of patients die every year from prescription drugs, but many of those patients suffer from incurable diseases for which potent medicines offer the only hope. Other patients have unpredictable allergic reactions; still others use the drugs improperly.

You must remember that all medicines—both prescription and over-the-counter—have side effects. When we take these medications, we do so with the knowledge that we might be one of the few people who will experience difficulty. This is the way it is; this is one of modern life's risks. However, we also must consider the enormous potential benefits of medications.

Take, for example, penicillin. This is probably one of the most dangerous antibiotics, because allergies to the drug are fairly common, and include rash, asthma and shock. Notwithstanding, it has saved millions of lives in the 50 or so years of its existence. Are we going to deprive a child with pneumonia of the very drug that could return him or her to health? Of course not. We—the doctors and the patients—weigh the benefits vs. the risks and give the drug (or withhold it) based on a rational analysis.

Similarly, in the example you give, Indocin (an anti-inflammatory medication) has predictable side effects, primarily rash and intestinal bleeding. Yet, gout is an extremely painful condition for which patients consistently request medicine for relief. The side effects you mention are exceedingly rare. Should doctors refuse to prescribe an effective remedy if the benefits exceed the hazards? I wouldn't. I'd leave the decision to the patient after I explained the potential consequences.

Here's another example. Prednisone (synthetic cortisone) is a powerful drug for treating inflammation and acute allergic reactions. But if taken long enough, it causes pronounced side effects in *every patient* who uses it. What's more, these reactions can severely disrupt health, even cause death, and include susceptibility to infection, diabetes, cataracts, osteoporosis, adrenal insufficiency and many other problems. Despite this profile, prednisone is widely, but cautiously, prescribed for many afflictions and is, in many instances, literally lifesaving. Nonetheless, patients who need it must carefully examine the risk/benefit ratio.

I'm familiar with the book "Worst Pills, Best Pills." Because I am a patient advocate and believe that people need unlimited access to health information (including drugs' side effects), I view the book as a valuable resource. But—and this is a big "but"—I encourage its readers to see the forest as well as the trees. For most medications, serious side effects are fortunately rare, and the benefits usually override the risks.

Thus, I recommend that resource books be used for resource only. Trust your doctor to give you sound advice; at the same time, ask for—in fact, demand—a coherent description about a medicine's benefits and hazards. Then and only then will you, the consumer, be able to make an intelligent decision about which therapy is right for you.

Remember the risk/benefit ratio. It will help you decide about surgery, drugs and other treatment, a second marriage, whether to fly or drive, to be fat or thin, to use tobacco and alcohol—even, perhaps, when and where to cross the street.

Common sense does not require a prescription

Q. Prescribe this, prescribe that—every problem someone writes to you about is just another opportunity for you to recommend prescription drugs or specialists. Your American Medical Association-endorsing advice is making me sick.

A. Well, this "sickness" is certainly not one that can be helped by medication.

Your basic position is, of course, valid. Many doctors are too quick to write out prescriptions; most doctors and patients would do well with infusions of common sense, a quality in short supply these days—it does not require a prescription and does not cause side effects.

Nevertheless, it's important to establish a balance between pharmacological therapy and common sense. In my column and in my office, I try constantly to achieve that reasonable balance.

Do people with trivial injuries and illnesses need medical attention and therapy? Not on your life. When we are patient and take good care of ourselves, our bodies have a phenomenal ability to cure themselves.

But we are all familiar with people, steeped in common sense, who had dangerous ailments that they ignored, only to suffer catastrophe. Intestinal bleeding, high blood pressure, early cancer and heart pain (angina) are afflictions that need drug treatment, often by specialists.

Therefore, before rejecting my position, stand back and be objective. People are living longer (and better) today in large part because of astonishing medical advances. Don't deprive yourself or your family of proper medical care, when appropriate, simply because of a set of beliefs you call "common sense."

Remember, too, that the concept of common sense changes with each generation. What was "common sense" decades ago may now be considered simply frivolous. Again, it's the balance that counts.

Hospitals keep families in the dark

Q. When my wife was recently hospitalized, I had a devil of a time obtaining information about her condition. Is this standard policy?

A. Let me respond to your question with a personal anecdote. I dedicate this response to the nurse who refused to give me information about my father's condition after he was admitted to the hospital critical care unit.

As an insider, a practicing physician who himself takes care of hospital patients, I know that the nurse's behavior was standard, ethical and totally professional. But it was also unkind and insensitive. Because I chose to play the role of an outsider, an unsophisticated family member, I learned some valuable lessons about how family members are handled in health-care institutions. Here is what happened:

I was notified that, because of pneumonia, my elderly father had been admitted to a large hospital in an adjoining state. After making my own rounds on a Saturday, I drove an hour to the hospital, parked in the visitors' lot, presented myself at the front desk, properly obtained a pass, and took the elevator to the critical care unit on the third floor.

Like similar units in other hospitals, the CCU was geared to the care of very ill patients who could not be safely monitored in what are called "floor beds"—ordinary hospital rooms. The quiet efficiency of the nurses, the beep-beeping of the machines, the IV lines, and the appurtenances of modern high-tech medicine were familiar to me. However, I remembered how intimidating this environment could be to a medical neophyte, so I resolved to play dumb.

"How is Mr. Gott today?" I asked the nurse.

"His condition is stable," she replied.

"What are his vital signs?" I inquired, referring to the bread-and-butter data concerning temperature, respiratory rate, pulse and blood pressure.

"I can't give you that information," she answered as she briskly turned on her heel.

"How about antibiotics? What is he getting?"

"I can't discuss that with you. You'll have to check with the doctor," she stated over her shoulder.

I fought the impulse to disclose my true identity. I wasn't a mere mortal; I was a physician. In other circumstances, I'd be the one

> 66 People are living longer (and better) today in large part because of astonishing medical advances. Don't deprive yourself or your family of proper medical care, when appropriate, simply because of a set of beliefs you call 'common sense.' 99

giving orders. Seeing no easy way to change from my street disguise into my red-caped Superman outfit, I shuffled after her.

"Tell me," I persisted, "is this a hospital regulation or your own rule?"

"It's just the way it is," she snapped.

Reluctantly, I relinquished control and visited my father. After establishing, as well as I could without giving the game away, that he was sick but comfortable, I approached the unit coordinator.

"Please show me where the kitchen is so that I can get my father some juice."

"That's not permitted," she said with a smile. "You'll have to ask the nurse and she's very busy."

"OK," I responded, "may I call the doctor?"

"The pay phone is in the hall," she frostily replied. Evidently, I was taking on the appearance of a troublemaker.

After further negotiation, I was able to place the call from the nurses' station. While waiting for the answer, I glanced at an open chart on the counter. It was my father's. Without touching the papers, I was able to determine that he was receiving appropriate therapy. The doctor was off duty and unavailable. Subsequently, on Monday morning, I called him and received a full report.

This brief encounter reinforced my belief that patients' families are often sadly misinformed about what is going on. Nurses and doctors adhere to the strict rules of the profession, as well they should; such rules are necessary. Yet, at the same time, they can lead to organizational insensitivity. At any point, I could have blasted: "Look, I'm a doctor and I insist that you answer my specific questions." Then all hell would have broken loose and I would have been given the red-carpet treatment, complete with a tour of the facility. But I didn't, so I was treated like any layman: given general information that served only to distance me from the problems at hand and reassure me that suitable care was being administered.

I realized that this is the way things are done in most hospitals. I understood why. This is the system. I'm part of it. I accept it. Still, it's been said that doctors and nurses should periodically become patients in their own hospitals in order to appreciate patients' isolation—and to gain empathy. Perhaps the next best thing might be for health professionals to pay an incognito visit to a sick loved one, just to experience what it feels like to be in another world.

The balanced doctor

Q. Please settle an argument. My friend would rather see a doctor who reads novels. I prefer a physician who reads medical journals. Who is right?

A. Every patient is entitled to a physician who keeps abreast of medical advances. Remaining "current" is each practitioner's goal and duty. Therefore, it's important to choose a doctor who engages in continuing medical education, be it through lectures, seminars, conferences, video or audio tapes, journals or other methods of continuing education.

On the other hand, caring for sick patients requires a broader view than mere technological advances. The good doctor takes into account many aspects of a patient, including psychological, ethical, humanitarian, and socioeconomic factors. In dealing with people, the capable and competent physician must consider far more than the basic disease process itself.

Consequently, in answer to your question, I'd have to conclude that you and your friend are right—and wrong. What you both need to find is a doctor with balance, someone with technical skills who is more than an automaton.

Most well-rounded physicians eagerly assimilate new advances and therapies. But they will be equally committed to broadening their horizons by reading novels, seeing plays, going to concerts and the opera, and participating in other nonmedical activities that are intellectually stimulating. The "complete" doctor also values time spent with his family, in recreation and sports, in spiritual pursuits, and in community service.

In my opinion, patients are best served by a practitioner with varied interests. I am not unique in this view. Many medical school admissions committees have come to realize the value of a liberal arts education, and often give preference to applicants who have nonscientific backgrounds, in contrast to the previous emphasis on biology, physics and chemistry. In short, the pre-med who is familiar with Faust may turn into a better doctor than the young person who spends all his or her time unraveling the mysteries of DNA synthesis.

You and your friend have raised an important issue. The most skilled doctor must, of course, keep up with medical advances in journals. However, a concomitant emphasis on nonmedical topics will also serve to enrich the physician and those he serves.

Being cautious best with mysterious "mass"

Q. After a week in the hospital, four months of outpatient visits and three CT scans, I was told I had an inflamed pancreas with a "mass" associated with it. After agreeing to one more CT scan (when I was symptom-free) and having already run up a $15,000 bill, I have been told by my physician that everything is fine; the mass isn't there anymore. What do you think of this situation?

A. It's hard to know what to think. The Case of the Disappearing Mass may raise more questions than it answers. On the surface, it looks as though someone fouled up your diagnosis—at considerable expense, I might add. And many people would be unjustifiably tempted to have at the medical establishment for being inept and overpriced.

However, in my experience, pancreatic problems can be exceedingly difficult to sort out. For example, an inflamed pancreas can cause abdominal pain that resembles many conditions, including peptic ulcer, because the organ lies close to the stomach and intestine. Furthermore, pancreatitis usually leads to swelling of the gland on CT scanning. Once the inflammation has healed, the swelling (which looks like a mass in the X-ray films) regresses and—eureka!—no more mass. This is what probably happened in your case. A further possibility is that a cyst formed in your inflamed pancreas. Once your problem resolved, the cyst did, too.

The doctors were understandably concerned because pancreatic cancer is difficult to diagnose without an operation and biopsy, and such a tumor is all but impossible to treat. Therefore, I conclude that you are fortunate that the "mass" disappeared. While your recent experience with the medical profession was far from ideal and once again proves that medical testing is not 100 percent reliable, you got through the ordeal with flying colors. Congratulations.

3

Exercise

Exercise sensibly

Q. I have heard that exercise may be more harmful than beneficial. How much exercise is required for optimum health before it becomes counterproductive/

A. Exercise is beneficial to everyone, even cardiac patients. However, as you point out, the question is how much is enough. I cannot give you a specific answer.

People who are active in their younger years seem to enjoy ongoing exertion as they age. Some people continue to ski, run and play tournament tennis into their 80s and 90s. On the other hand, a backhoe couldn't move some middle-aged folks from their favorite chairs in front of the television.

Exercise is a very individual matter. In general, you may safely exercise to the point of fatigue at any age. Dangerous exercise consists of sudden strenuous exertion performed intermittently or on rare occasions. Any exercise is good if it makes you feel good, but you have to be sensible. If you are basically sedentary, take it easy at first. Work into an exercise program gradually.

Walking and swimming are safe and healthful hobbies, particularly for people who do not engage in regular sports. A brisk hour's walk, performed several days a week, can tone up any cardiovascular system.

Moderate exercise is different from training. Although training produces more striking physiological changes, it is not appropriate for the average person.

My rule for exercise is to do it, but start slowly and listen to your body when it tells you that you have had enough.

I do not believe that every person over 40 requires a special cardiac evaluation before beginning an exercise program. Since I am in the minority, you may want to ask your doctor about this. However, the only problems I have encountered are in people who impulsively begin strenuous activity without first warming up and starting with light exercise. This holds true for aerobics as well as for serious running. Your body is the best judge of how far you should extend yourself; listen to what it has to say.

Stair climbing is good exercise

Q. I walk on the stairs in my house. I am 80 years old and believe that this exercise is beneficial. However, my wife is concerned that fifteen stairs will tax my heart. I hope you can comment.

A. Climbing fifteen stairs at a brisk rate will not injure your heart, even if you have coronary blockage. If you are symptom-free, you can safely continue the practice. You might even consider performing this exercise two or three times a day.

Avoid overuse syndrome

Q. I'm 80 and have had shoulder pain for 10 years. The problem probably originated when I started lifting weights in my local fitness center. My doctor shakes his head, suggests ibuprofen and forbids me from continuing my weight program. Predictably, my shoulder muscles are becoming atrophied, and I have noticed a significant loss of strength. Can I get cortisone shots for this condition? The inactivity is driving me batty.

A. Strenuous exercise can lead to overuse syndrome, in the young as well as in the old. Running is commonly associated with knee, ankle and hip pain, for example, and weight training is a notorious culprit for upper body stiffness and pain.

The obvious answer to the problem: Stop the offending activity. However, for many sportsmen and sportswomen, this is an unacceptable option.

In similar situations, I ordinarily advise my patients to modify their workouts. If, for example, running causes pain, stop this activity and turn to biking or swimming. Or, if your shoulders are painful during bench presses or curls, switch to other upper-body exercise that is not painful. Experiment. Alter your program. Hire a trainer.

In my opinion, cortisone injections may relieve the pain of irritated tendons and muscles, but are not a cure; the shots treat only the symptom (albeit at some risk) without addressing the cause. Choose a program that is not painful (or is associated with only minimal discomfort).

The currently available weight machines offer an almost inexhaustible menu for conditioning. You can work on your arms, shoulders and chest in a variety of exercises. You can use free weights. You also have the option to emphasize cardiovascular fitness (stationary running, and so forth).

Remember that despite any sort of training, you are unlikely to achieve the "buff" appearance that you may have enjoyed as a younger man. Aging does take its toll on joints, tendons and muscles.

> 66 *Exercise is beneficial to everyone, even cardiac patients.* 99

Therefore, I suggest that you adopt a prudent approach. Exercise regularly. Engage in activity that is not significantly painful. Define your goals. Work with a trainer or physical therapist to achieve those goals. Be (mentally) flexible about your program. Use ibuprofen as needed. Avoid steroid injections if possible. Check with your doctor about specific recommendations.

Hypertension and weight training

Q. I am taking medicine for hypertension. I've been lifting weights for the past 12 years with my doctor's approval. However, recent media reports emphasize that straining can worsen high blood pressure and should be avoided by hypertensives. Must I forgo my workouts?

A. No, but you may need to alter them.

Straining raises the blood pressure. Therefore, most authorities agree that power-lifting or the strenuous use of weights is inadvisable for patients with hypertension.

On the other hand, if you use relatively light weights and engage in repetitions, you're probably not harming yourself. In addition, when you lift, exhale; this maneuver will prevent you from straining too hard.

Be sure to describe your weight-lifting workout to your doctor. Depending on the seriousness of your hypertension, he or she may advise you to modify your training program or engage in alternative conditioning pursuits, such as running, swimming and bicycling.

According to an article in the Wall Street Journal, March 13, 2003, the weight-lifting fitness craze in the United States may have produced negative consequences, such as strokes and aneurysms, in people who overdo it. For example, medical authorities at Yale University School of

Medicine and the Stanford University Medical Center recommend that people over 40 should bench press no more than half their body weights.

For most hypertensives, exercise is beneficial. Also, blood pressure can be lowered by maintaining an ideal body weight and limiting salt consumption.

Rehab may lead to muscle pain

Q. After having had open-heart surgery three years ago, I joined a local wellness group for rehabilitation. Everything went well until about a year ago when, while lifting weights, I suffered severe upper-arm pain, making it impossible for me to continue curls or any upper-body conditioning. My cardiologist prescribed physical therapy, which I enthusiastically followed—without benefit. My arms are still a problem. Why would the pain remain and what can I do?

A. Weight lifting often leads to tendon inflammation (and other muscle abnormalities) that can be chronic, distressing and difficult to cure. Such a scenario is especially common in older adults whose muscles may easily be injured, stretched or inflamed by an aggressive rehab program.

For example, I know several cardiac patients who developed bicipital tendonitis (inflammation of the arms' biceps tendons) from weight training and, in some cases, the pain lasted more than a year despite physical therapy. In such instances, I worry that the tendons may have been torn.

Therefore, I suggest that you be checked by an orthopedic surgeon; you need a diagnosis and advice. If you have torn tendons, intensive therapy (perhaps surgery) may be necessary. On the other hand, if the tendons have merely been overused and are inflamed, the specialist may prescribe untrasound therapy with cortisone cream, a method that I have found to be enormously successful in treating bicipital tendonitis.

While you await resolution of your arm problem, don't forget to continue a regular exercise program. Lower-body weight training, swimming, brisk walking and cycling are excellent substitutes for an upper-body workout.

4

Heart & Things Circulatory

Circulatory problems often affect us oldies

Q. My internist has prescribed several different medications to control my dizziness, which he believes is caused by hypoglycemia. Despite the therapy, I am still dizzy, extremely fatigued, have blurred vision, insomnia, staggering, anxiety and forgetfulness. I'm 77 and realize that some of my symptoms may be related to aging—but all of them?

A Hypoglycemia (low blood sugar) is diagnosed by a blood sugar level below 45 milligrams per deciliter in the presence of faintness, lightheadedness, hunger and lassitude. Treatment consists of a low-sugar diet with frequent feedings and occasional snacks of fruit when symptoms appear. To my knowledge, there is no medicine to treat this condition.

Given your age, I'm more concerned that your symptoms could reflect a circulatory deficiency. For example, temporary interruptions os blood flow to the brain related to small blood clots (transient ischemic attacks) are a common cause of fatigue, visual disturbances, poor coordination and forgetfulness in the elderly. Also, heartbeat irregularities and arteriosclerotic blockages in the brain's arteries may contribute to these symptoms.

I suggest that you seek a second opinion from another internist or, preferably, a neurologist. In my opinion, you need further testing—such as blood analyses and imaging studies of your brain and its circulation—to determine the cause of your problem. If, indeed, you do have hypoglycemia, your doctors, working in concert, should be able to offer suggestions about diet and additional therapy.

Alcohol may be cause of enlarged blood cells

Q. Does a low RBC count and a high MCV need to be treated? My only symptom is fatigue.

A. A low red blood cell count is diagnostic of anemia. However, in your case, the mean corpuscular volume is high, indicating that your red cells are larger than normal. This could be due to a vitamin deficiency, or, most commonly, regular consumption of alcohol. In my opinion, these abnormalities should be investigated. Check back with the physician who ordered the blood count and see what he says. Meanwhile, if you drink alcohol, stop. The cause of your anemia should be addressed so that you can receive proper treatment.

Chronic lymphatic leukemia usually benign

Q. I have been diagnosed with lymphatic leukemia. My white blood cell count is 35,000. My doctor told me that treatment is not necessary at this point, but may be necessary in the future as my white count rises. I've had multiple blood tests, a CT scan and a bone marrow analysis. I feel perfectly normal. Is my doctor on the right track?

A. Chronic lymphatic leukemia is, in most instances, a relatively benign condition. Marked by an increase in certain blood cells (called lymphocytes), CLL does not usually affect health until the white blood cells exceed 75,000.

At that point, antimetabolic drugs, such as Myleran, are prescribed to lower the WBC count. (A high count is associated with excess thickening of the blood, which causes complications, such as blood clots.)

I believe that your doctor is on the right track. You need periodic blood counts (every six months or so) to monitor your lymphocytes. No therapy is indicated until the count increases to about 75,000.

Bruit: swooshing sound in blood vessel

Q. I'm 60, in good health, abstain from cigarettes and alcohol, walk two miles, and eat a healthful diet. I'm puzzled because I have a very noticeable wheeze in a blood vessel in my head (or neck) when I bend over to pet my cat or pick something up. Could this noise be the result of arteriosclerosis?

A. An audible swooshing sound in a blood vessel is called a bruit. This often results when an artery is partially blocked or kinked, and the blood flow undergoes turbulence.

Bruits in the neck may indicate the presence of arteriosclerotic plaque in the walls of the carotid arteries. Many experts believe that such plaque can be a source of blood clots that may break off, be carried to the brain, and cause stroke.

Although many bruits cause no symptoms and can be ignored, others reflect a critical degree of obstruction that must be addressed. Therefore, I recommend that you bring this issue to your doctor's attention. If you do have plaque in one or both of your carotid arteries (as determined by a Doppler ultrasound examination), the physician might advise you to take an aspirin a day (to discourage clot formation) or refer you to a vascular surgeon for possible operative intervention.

May need to live with pulse-swishing

Q. I have a constant pulse-swishing in my head. To date, I have had the following normal tests: CT scan of the head, CT scan of the adrenal glands, ultrasound of the thyroid gland and carotid arteries, MRI of the head, MRA of the neck, upper GI and small bowel series, barium enema, echocardiogram and stress test.

My doctors have advised me to live with the sensation. But it surely gets on my nerves. What do you advise?

A. Live with it.

You have had a truckload of tests performed, all of which were normal. Your doctor should be congratulated; he investigated every potentially serious cause of your symptom. Now that he has confirmed that you don't have a significant problem, such as a cancer or an arterial blockage, you can relax. Perfectly normal people often experience an awareness of the pulse beat in the head and ears. In such instances, physicians may come up short with a diagnosis; their primary goal is to rule out a serious medical condition. In your case, this was—thankfully—the result. As an ancillary suggestion, I recommend that you check with an ear-nose-and-throat specialist who, perhaps, can advise you about methods to control your symptom.

Anemia may cause weakness, fatigue

Q. I'm a male, age 81, with arthritis in my neck. I feel so weak at times that I can't get out of my chair. Recently, I had bronchitis. Blood tests show anemia. Why do I feel so bad?

A. Although your problem is complicated by a variety of symptoms, I cannot help but conclude that your ill health may be related to your anemia. Such a condition, which is marked by too few red blood

Angina

Angina is a brief but recurring discomfort in the chest, arms or shoulders caused by a temporary reduction in the blood flow to the heart. The full name of the condition is angina pectoris, which means "chest pain." The sensation is most evident during exercise or emotional stress, when the heart beats faster and the demand for oxygen is increased. Angina is a sign that the heart muscle has been deprived of oxygen, a condition called ischemia.

The feeling of angina has been described as pain, heaviness, tightness, pressure, squeezing, burning or numbness. The sensation, which generally lasts no more than a few minutes, usually starts behind the breastbone and may spread to the shoulders, arms, wrists, neck or jaw.

Although the condition can be frightening, especially the first time it is felt, angina is not a heart attack. Since the reduction in the blood flow to the heart that produces angina is only temporary, it causes no permanent damage. By contrast, with a heart attack, the interruption is permanent and sudden, and the resulting pain is usually much more severe. The two conditions do, however, share the same cause: atherosclerosis, a narrowing of the coronary arteries caused by a buildup of cholesterol and other fatty deposits. Because the blood vessels are partially blocked, less blood (which carries needed oxygen and nutrients) can reach the heart muscle. Coronary heart disease due to atherosclerosis is the leading cause of death in the United States for both men and women.

According to recent statistics compiled by the American Heart Association, more than six million Americans suffer from angina, and more women are affected than are men. Several million more people have silent ischemia, which means they have the same underlying arterial blockage but have no symptoms. These people may remain unaware of their problem until they suffer a heart attack. Therefore, the pain of angina is an important warning signal.

Sometimes the body can compensate for partially occluded coronary arteries. In a process called collateral circulation, the surrounding arteries may expand and produce new branches, thereby permitting more blood to reach the affected area. If the collateral circulation becomes well-developed, the symptoms of angina may disappear. Usually, however, angina and heart disease are considered to be irreversible conditions, and angina often heralds a future heart attack.

Prevention

The goal is to prevent them from inexorably progressing. This may be accomplished in the following ways:

- Eating right
- Stopping smoking
- Controlling blood pressure
- Exercising regularly
- Taking certain prescription drugs

Risk factors of angina and atherosclerosis

The following factors increase the risk of angina, atherosclerosis and heart disease in general:

- Elevated blood pressure
- High blood cholesterol
- Smoking
- Diabetes
- Obesity
- Lack of exercise
- Heavy drinking
- Family history of early heart attack in parent or sibling
- Aging. The older we get, the greater the risk of heart disease for men and women.
- Stress. Highly stressed, impatient Type A personalities are at increased risk.

cells, can result in weakness, lassitude and fatigue—all of which could have been accentuated by your bronchial infection. Arthritis is probably not a factor in your illness.

In particular, I'd be interested in the cause of your anemia. Could you have hidden intestinal bleeding? A vitamin or iron deficiency? Bone marrow failure?

Return to your doctor. You need further testing, such as a chest X-ray (to determine if you have ongoing pulmonary infection) and a fecal analysis for blood. Once the cause of your anemia is diagnosed, your physician should be able to treat the condition and restore you to normal.

Numbness in mouth may be circulatory

Q. I've recently been experiencing spells of light-headedness followed by a numb sensation in my mouth, as though I'd received a shot of Novocaine. What's the cause?

A. Based on the sparse information you supplied, I cannot diagnose your condition without more data. Is there, for example, a pattern to your "spells"? How long do they last? Do you have significant health problems? Any other symptoms?

The symptoms you described suggest a circulatory disturbance. Often, when inadequate amounts of blood reach the brain, numbness and tingling may result due to depressed oxygen supply to nerves. For instance, a sudden drop in blood pressure can cause light-headedness, so if you're taking medication for hypertension, your doctor may wish to reduce the dose.

Also, cardiac irregularities (such as fast or slow pulse) can cause faintness.

Finally, little blood clots in the brain, termed "transient ischemic attacks," will cause similar symptoms that disappear completely in minutes or hours.

You should bring your "spells" to your doctor's attention. In my opinion, you need a checkup and, probably blood tests and cardiac monitoring.

Got cryoglobulinemia? Head to Florida

Q. I've been diagnosed with cryoglobulinemia. Do you have any information regarding this disorder?

A. For unknown reasons, as they age, some people develop abnormal proteins in their bloodstreams. One such protein, called cryoglobulin, is especially sensitive to cold. When chilled—even in the body—it tends to gel, especially if the extremities and skin are cool. This can cause damage to small blood vessels (capillaries), leading to bruising.

Therefore, while the cryoglobulin is itself not harmful, it can cause damage when it cools and changes its physical characteristics. As a result, patients with this condition must make every effort to remain warm and avoid cold environments. No other therapy is necessary.

Warfarin kills rats, helps people

Q. While sitting at a wedding reception, a bunch of us oldies were discussing—what else?—our various health problems. The minister interjected that he will never take "statin" drugs for excess cholesterol because they are basically rat poison. Is this true? I hope not.

A. In the past, I have been criticized for overstepping my training by addressing issues having to do with evolution and religion. Perhaps my critics are justified, but I remain fascinated by the interaction between faith and medicine.

Your brief experience is an example of the reverse: an inaccurate medical conclusion by a well-meaning man of the cloth. To my knowledge, statin drugs do not contain rat poison.

The minister was probably referring to warfarin (Coumadin), an anticoagulant that is commonly prescribed to prevent harmful blood clots from forming in the vascular system. Such clots often lead to stroke, heart attack and lung damage. Because it is so effective, warfarin is also included in many brands of rodenticide, bait that causes vermin to bleed to death when they feed on it.

Millions of people enjoy the beneficial effects of Coumadin; the fact that the drug has other uses should not deter patients from taking it. Controlled anticoagulation is a necessary medical intervention. It is appropriate therapy for a host of potentially serious disorders, including heart irregularities, such as atrial fibrillation and venous disorders, such as deep vein thrombosis.

While my immediate reaction to your question was to suggest that the minister confine his comments to theological subjects, I chose a different tack—one of non-judgmental explanation that, I hope, will give me the privilege to continue addressing occasional topics that are not strictly medical. If my column is not somewhat provocative and fun to write, then I've been missing out on something for more than 20 years.

Deficient circulation linked to fainting

Q. What is vasovagal syncope? I've passed out four times in restaurants. What makes my blood pressure drop so precipitously? Glucose tolerance tests are negative.

A. The pulse rate is under partial control of the vagus nerves. Stimulation of these nerves causes the pulse rate to slow; this, plus an associated tendency to low pressure, can temporarily deprive the brain of circulation and oxygen, leading to syncope (fainting). No one knows why some people exhibit accentuated responses to vagal stimulation, but the phenomenon is real and can result in periodic loss of consciousness.

Vasovagal syncope is often caused by intense physical or mental stimulation, such as pain, fright or the sight of blood. In fact, patients who feel light-headed or pass out during routine blood tests usually do so because of low blood pressure and the slow pulse that follows stimulation of the vagus nerves by the brain.

This fainting is almost always preceded by symptoms, such as nausea, weakness and sweating; therefore, patients with vasovagal syncope can prevent fainting by lying down or sitting with the head bowed between the knees. Also, these patients readily discover what kinds of stimulation cause the syncope, so they learn to avoid such situations.

I do not know why you experience symptoms in restaurants. Persons with hypoglycemia (low blood sugar) may experience light-headedness and weakness a couple of hours after eating sugar and high calorie foods. Evidently, your glucose levels were normal. Therefore, you need to see a cardiologist or circulatory specialist to determine the cause of your symptom.

Remember that with vasovagal syncope, as with any cause of fainting due to deficient circulation, you can prevent serious injury (from falling) by getting your head down. This maneuver allows gravity to maintain adequate blood supply to the brain. Therefore, when you're light-headed, don't tough it out; bend over or lie down before you faint.

Arteriosclerosis inevitable but may be slowed

Q. What can be done to help hardening of the arteries? Medication doesn't seem to work and I exercise as much as possible by walking.

A. If anyone had an answer to this question, he or she could retire to a private island in the Caribbean.

Arteriosclerosis (hardening of the arteries) is an inevitable consequence of the aging process. True, some people—chiefly diabetics—have accelerated arteriosclerosis, but all of us will get it sooner or later. There is no cure for it and no medicine to slow its inexorable progression.

Nonetheless, people can do much to compensate for it. Stop smoking. Pay attention to your cholesterol and eat a balanced, low fat diet. Keep as physically active as possible. Take care of yourself by getting adequate rest, moderating alcohol consumption and treating illnesses (such as hypertension) as they arise, also, listen to what your body is telling you and get an annual checkup from your family physician.

Other than following these suggestions, there's not much else you can do. Aging is built into our genes and, until scientists can rearrange these genes, we have to accept the hands we have been dealt.

One last thought: Don't forget to keep a sense of humor.

Low white blood cell count requires evaluation

Q. Does a low white blood cell count reflect a serious disease?

A. White blood cells are the body's infection fighters; therefore, any reduction in their number is cause for concern. There is a day-to-day variation in white cell counts, and some innocuous viral infections, such as mononucleosis, are associated with a temporary deficiency in the count. Nonetheless, physicians take very seriously any severe or long-standing low white cell count, because such a reduction can make the patient extremely vulnerable to any and all infections. In my opinion, a persistently low cell count requires medical evaluation.

Chalk craving may be iron-deficiency anemia

Q. I crave chalk. I eat one stick a day. My favorite is the large sidewalk chalk in red, white and blue. I am also anemic. Is the chalk harming me?

A. Pica is the craving to eat indigestible substances, such as chalk, laundry starch, clay and similar compounds. The condition may be primary—meaning that it has an emotional basis that should be addressed by a physician, who may recommend counseling. Or the pica may be secondary to iron-deficiency anemia. The basis of this relation is not understood, but once the anemia has been corrected with iron supplements, the pica disappears.

In either case, you need medical attention. Chalk, dirt and other substances can lead to nutritional deficiencies if consumed regularly and in sufficient quantity. In addition, pica may cause intestinal upset. See a doctor and, during the interview please be honest about your craving for chalk.

Varicose veins often genetic

Q. Are varicose veins inherited? My mother had them (after delivering eight children), I have them (after delivering five) and my sister has them (after delivering four).

A. The tendency to varicose veins is probably genetically determined. However, such swollen veins normally tend to accompany the aging process and are certainly more common in women after multiple pregnancies— and in both men and women who stand for extended periods.

Regardless of cause, varicose veins can easily be treated with leg elevation and the use of elasticized support hose. More advanced conditions respond to surgery. In most people, the decision about how to treat varicose veins depends on the severity, the cosmetic implications and whether the dilated veins tend to form blood clots. Your doctor can advise you about appropriate therapy.

Varicose veins: treatment varies from stockings to surgery

Q. I'm 71 and have suddenly developed varicose veins in my legs. Is there a healing salve that I can use?

A. There is no effective topical treatment, such as creams or salves, for varicose veins. As we age, the veins in the legs tend to dilate, leading to the unsightly varicose veins with which we're all familiar. In severe cases, blood clots may form in such veins or the varices can affect circulation, resulting in troublesome skin ulcer.

As a general rule, mild/moderate, uncomplicated varicose veins in the legs are best treated with elastic support stockings, elevation of the legs when sitting and avoidance of prolonged standing. More severe varices, especially those associated with skin damage, usually have to be surgically removed.

Ask your doctor about this. I am sure that he can give you some pertinent tips about your condition—or he can refer you to a surgeon for a second opinion.

Alternatives to surgery available for varicose veins

Q. I have had varicose veins since age 37. My doctor is reluctant to refer me to a surgeon for vein stripping but is not specific about the reason for his reluctance. Is this procedure dangerous?

A. Any surgical procedure carries risks. However, I do not know why your doctor is reluctant to refer you for a surgical opinion. Insist on an explanation. The slight risks of venous stripping, such as infection and scarring, may be outweighed by the potential benefits. You also might want to look into alternative treatments—for example, sclerosing (injection) or laser therapy. Just because you obtain a second—or even a third—opinion doesn't mean

> 66 *Stop smoking. Pay attention to your cholesterol and eat a balanced, low fat diet. Keep as physically active as possible. Take care of yourself by getting adequate rest, moderating alcohol consumption and treating illnesses (such as hypertension) as they arise, also, listen to what your body is telling you and get an annual checkup from your family physician.* 99

that you are obligated to a particular course of treatment. Additional opinions will simply give you more information on which to base your decision about what to do.

Cholesterol

Causes of increased blood fats

Q. What is hyperlipidemia? Is there a cure for this disease or can it be controlled?

A. There are two major blood fats—cholesterol and triglycerides. Hyperlipidemia simply means that the blood level of these fats is elevated. Experts recommend that cholesterol not exceed about 200 milligrams per deciliter; the upper limit for triglycerides is 150 mg/dL.

Hyperlipidemia has many causes; the most common is a genetic predisposition. Diet also plays a large role, and diseases such as diabetes can raise the blood fats.

A high cholesterol level is associated with an increased risk of cardiovascular disease, including heart attack. Excess triglycerides can cause inflammation of the pancreas, as well as contribute to cardiovascular damage.

In general, most people can lower their blood-fat levels by adhering to a prudent diet that contains less fat than Americans are in the habit of eating. Regular, strenuous exercise will also reduce fat levels, as will moderation in alcohol consumption.

For people whose blood fats continue to be excessive despite dietary modifications and lifestyle changes, physicians ordinarily prescribe the fat-lowering drugs (Lipitor, Zetia and others).

Because hyperlipidemia may lead to serious health consequences, it should not be ignored; individuals with this disorder should be under medical supervision.

Addressing high cholesterol

Q. The Johns Hopkins Medical Letter recently published information about high cholesterol levels, based on updates of the National Cholesterol Education Program's recommendations. How does this affect the average consumer?

A. The NCEP is an initiative of the National Institutes of Health, the leading arbiter of standards of cholesterol screening and treatment. In a recent report, the organization revised and updated its recommendations. These findings were widely reported in several medical schools' health letters, including the Johns Hopkins that you kindly sent me.

To begin with, the NCEP calls for more widespread screening (and aggressive treatment) of elevated blood fats, both cholesterol and triglycerides. Experts estimate that about 65 million people should be taking medication.

The normal accepted blood-fat levels are as follows: total cholesterol, 200 milligrams per deciliter; LDL (low density lipoproteins, the "bad" cholesterol) 130 mg/dL; HDL (high density lipoproteins, the "good" cholesterol) greater than 40 mg/dL. (Patients with known heart disease need stricter control of cholesterol levels); triglycerides less than 150 mg/dL.

The first plan of therapy included appropriate dietary restriction of products containing animal fat, such as red meat, whole milk, cheese, eggs, mayonnaise and other high-cholesterol foods. Next medication may be appropriate, including niacin and "statin" drugs such as Lipitor, Zetia and others.

What does a high triglycerides level mean?

Q. I'm 77 and healthy. My cholesterol is normal (210), but my triglycerides are 258. How can I lower them?

A. Your cholesterol level is, indeed, normal for a person your age. (Patients with coronary artery disease, on the other hand, should have cholesterol levels below 200 milligrams per deciliter.)

The role of triglycerides, the other major blood fat, is less clear. While the range of normal is up to 150 mg/dL, many elderly patients run levels somewhat higher—without apparent health consequences. Therefore, whether you should take a prescription drug to reduce your triglycerides is a decision best left to you and your physician. If you are physically active, follow a prudent low-fat diet and don't smoke, I believe that you can safely monitor your triglycerides level and take no additional action for now. As a general rule, triglyceride and cholesterol counts can be lowered by limiting saturated (animal) fats in the diet. Such fats include butterfat (in whole milk, cheese and ice cream), as well as eggs and the fat in red meat.

Remember that diabetes is often associated with excess triglycerides, so you'll want to keep an eye on your blood sugar. Triglyceride levels, in this instance, can usually be reduced by maintaining a blood glucose in the normal range, through diet and/or medication.

Same diet, different cholesterol levels

Q. I'd like some information on cholesterol. My reading is 275, yet my husband's is 190. We both eat the same foods, so I am at a loss to explain the difference.

A. Cholesterol is one of two major fats in the blood. (The other is triglycerides.) These fats are necessary for normal metabolism. Excess cholesterol (above about 200 milligrams per deciliter) or triglycerides (above 150 milligrams) increase the statistical risk for heart attacks and cardiovascular ailments.

The level of blood fats appears, in the main, to be genetically determined. Therefore, even though you and your husband have identical diets, your cholesterol is higher than his because of your genetics.

You may be interested to learn that a cholesterol of 275 mg/dL would be cause for alarm in a person under 40, the basis for concern in a woman in her 50s and 60s, of no special consequence in a female in her 70s, and probably normal for an adult over 80. Thus, age plays a crucial role in defining an abnormal cholesterol level. The reasons the elderly, in most instances, seem to be protected against the ill effects of cholesterol are not known.

Despite your apparent genetic predisposition to high cholesterol, you could probably lower the level through diet: Reduce your consumption of cheese, change from butter to corn oil margarine, use skim milk, avoid luncheon meats/bacon/sausage, limit your eggs to no more than two a week (this includes "hidden" egg products, such as Hollandaise, Bernaise and mayonnaise), buy lean cuts of meat and trim any excess fat before you broil it.

Also, eat more fiber, especially psyllium. Exercise regularly. And, finally, consider prescription drugs to lower your cholesterol; your doctor can advise you about this.

I've given you a mere thumbnail sketch of the problem. For example, I purposely omitted consideration of the types of cholesterol in your system: High-density lipoproteins (HDLs) are good; low-density lipoproteins (LDLs) are bad. Your physician should discuss with you the components of your cholesterol panel, your triglyceride level (if elevated) and other issues pertaining to your situation.

Combination cholesterol-lowering medication

Q. I recently read conflicting advice. One source stated that niacin should not be taken with "statin" drugs, such as Zocor or Lipitor. Another equally reliable source said that the combination is a good idea. How should I resolve this disagreement?

A. I am not aware of any prohibition concerning the simultaneous use of niacin and statin drugs to lower cholesterol levels. In fact, this has always seemed to me to be a good idea. My position was recently confirmed by the introduction of a new medicine, called Advicor, which is a combination of niacin and lovastatin. Whether this medicine will be a success and has a favorable safety profile has yet to be determined.

> 66 *Age plays a crucial role in defining an abnormal cholesterol level. The reasons the elderly, in most instances, seem to be protected against the ill effects of cholesterol are not known.* 99

The risks of statin drugs must be considered

Q. At age 60, when my cholesterol level was 218, despite a low-fat diet, my physician insisted that I begin a statin drug. Since then, I've felt terrible: headache, muscle pain, stiffness and soreness. My liver and blood tests are normal, and my cholesterol is 128. What should I do?

A. Stop the medication.

Therapy is supposed to make patients feel better, not worse.

More important, I'm not at all sure that you need drugs to lower your cholesterol . A cholesterol of 218 at age 60 would be, to me, relatively normal. I'm concerned that the risks of therapy exceed the benefits. For example, were your cholesterol 418, I'd endorse therapeutic intervention (translation: drug therapy). However, your level of 218 is minimally elevated. In such an instance, I'd stop the medication, put you on a strict low-cholesterol diet, recheck your level in two months and then decide how to proceed. A cholesterol of 128 is very, very low—appropriate if you have documented coronary artery disease but not needing attention if you are in good health. In all medical situations, the benefits of treatment must exceed the risks. Review this issue with your physician.

The risk versus the benefit of Lopid

Q. Because my cholesterol level is very high (570), my doctor prescribed Lopid. However, I note that this drug can cause acute appendicitis and gallstones, so I am reluctant to use it. On the other hand, I can't afford premature heart disease. Do I have other options?

A. A good question that once again brings into play the risk/benefit ratio of medication. The incidence of appendicitis and gallstones from Lopid therapy is truly small, probably in the range of less than 1 percent of the patients.

In contrast, your cholesterol is very significant and places you at an unacceptably high risk for heart disease and vascular problems. Thus, in my view, the hazards of the medication are exceeded by the negative consequences of high cholesterol. (Authorities have concluded that cholesterol levels should be 200 mg or less.)

Niacin to lower cholesterol

Q. I am taking 1,000 milligrams of Niaspan because of my high cholesterol count. So far, I've had no side effects, such as flushing, so my doctor wants me to increase the dosage to 2,000 milligrams a day.

Will this damage my liver? I had triple bypass surgery in 1998 and don't want to risk unnecessary health consequences from the medication. What's your advice?

A. High doses of niacin, a vitamin that lowers serum cholesterol levels, is an ideal solution for some patients who cannot tolerate "statin" drugs, the more traditional solution. While it's true that niacin can cause uncomfortable flushing and sweating, this complication can be solved by taking an aspirin tablet with the Niaspan.

However, like other cholesterol-lowering medications, niacin can cause liver inflammation in some patients.

In my opinion, this fact should not deter people from following their doctors' recommendations on this issue. As long as you have periodic blood tests of liver function, you should not suffer any "unnecessary health consequences" from the therapy.

If your physician has prescribed high-dose niacin, I'd go ahead and try it. But I also believe that your should have blood tests for liver function about once a month for three or four months. If everything is stable and you tolerate the niacin, the testing schedule can be appropriately changed to once or twice a year.

No-cholesterol diet is often effective

Q. I'm a 70-year-old widow whose cholesterol was above 360 milligrams for 20 years, despite a diet that was low in cholesterol-rich foods, such as meat, eggs and dairy products. It wasn't until I completely eliminated these foods that my cholesterol fell to 200 mg, where it has stayed. I maintain that a low- cholesterol diet is useless; a no-cholesterol diet is the way to go.

A. Your experience is not unique. In fact, Dr. Dean Ornish (a physician, nutrition expert and bestselling author) has proven that the lower the dietary cholesterol, the lower the serum cholesterol. However, many patients have complained that such a restrictive diet is difficult to follow year after year. So the issue is compliance, not effectiveness. If you are comfortable with such a diet and it is working for you, bravo. Stick with it. However, for most patients who have trouble committing to such rigid restrictions, the judicious use of prescription drugs to lower serum cholesterol levels is an appropriate option.

A possible alternative to treating high cholesterol

Q. I've had success in lowering my cholesterol— not with expensive "statin" drugs, but by using a combination of other foods and a dietary supplement.

At age 65, my cholesterol was 288 despite an alteration in my diet. My doctor prescribed Lipitor, but after 90 days stopped it because of adverse liver enzyme readings. So, we agreed to try an alternative therapy.

I now use a dietary supplement called red yeast rice, a staple for centuries in the traditional Chinese diet. Instead of using margarine, I've substituted Take Control, a soybean extract that contains sterol plant esters. Also, I sprinkle a packet of instant oatmeal over my usual bowl of breakfast cereal. Within two months, my cholesterol level dropped to 195, my "bad" LDL level to 120; my "good" cholesterol has remained normal.

There are no side effects and these products are much less expensive than prescription drugs.

I wanted to share this with you and your readers.

A. Your response to alternative therapy is certainly significant, and I agree with you that "natural" products are preferable to expensive medications that carry the risk of side effects, such as liver inflammation. However, your experience is not universal; your program does not work for everyone.

Nonetheless, it is certainly worth trying, and I am publishing it for general public interest. I endorse any safe diet plan that can reduce serum cholesterol levels below 200 milligrams per deciliter, and drop LDL levels below 130 mg/dL.

I would appreciate follow-up comments, both pro and con, from readers who choose to try your suggestions.

6

Hypertension

New criteria for hypertension

Q. What are your thoughts on the new criteria for high blood pressure? I'm 75, active and take three medications for hypertension. My blood pressure consistently runs about 150/70. Frankly, I'm reluctant to increase my meds for fear of side effects.

A. This is an important issue that has recently been in the news because authorities reduced the level of normal blood pressure to 120/80; formerly, the limit was about 140/90.

You should review this problem with your primary care physician.

In my practice, I pay a good deal of attention to the relation between age and blood pressure. While a level of 140/90 would be absolutely abnormal for a teenager or a young adult, I'd accept it in an 85-year-old under treatment. Am I saying that the new guideline is unrealistic or unnecessary? No, but I believe that age has to be factored in.

Also, doctors have to be careful in interpreting blood pressure readings obtained in the office, because many patients will show a stress-related elevation when, at home, their pressures are completely normal. Therefore, my policy is to follow up on patients with higher-than-normal blood pressure, treated or untreated, but part of that follow-up includes home BP readings—and, as I mentioned—age is a definite consideration.

Here is a brief example of this.

Last week, I rechecked an 88-year-old healthy woman whose only medical problem had been hypertension. She was taking two drugs to lower her blood pressure, which was maintained at 150/80.

Based on the recent recommendations, I increased one of her medications. Three days later she telephoned me to complain that she was dizzy, light-headed and had terrible balance problems. Her BP in the office was 115/60, well within the new normal range but, obviously, too low for her. Therefore, I revised her medication dosages and told her to return to the former pattern, which she did. Three days later, her BP was 150/85 at home and her symptoms had entirely disappeared. Based on this experience, it would take an act of Congress for me to increase her medication again. She is stable and the quality of her life is (by her own reckoning) much improved. In this instance, her "elevated" blood pressure is appropriate, even necessary.

By the way, there is no one number that satisfies the definition of low blood pressure. Some oldies tolerate pressures in the 90/60 range; others feel faint at 120/75. Therefore, a blood pressure that is too low is one at which people have symptoms of weakness, loss of energy, light-headedness, unsteadiness and fainting. In the absence of symptoms, the lower the blood pressure, the better.

My long-winded answer to your question is for information only, not for guidance. This, as I mentioned above, is something you should discuss with your own physician.

High blood pressure is a "red flag"

Q. What would cause a sudden elevation in blood pressure? At 73, my reading has been around 114/74. Suddenly, it's changed to 180/105. My doctor put me on medication for control, but I want to know what has caused the increase since I've had no change in diet and no stress in my life.

A. A sudden and unexplained increase in blood pressure is always a "red flag" to physicians. This could reflect a problem with kidney function or some other physical abnormality that should be addressed. For example, a "silent" (non-painful) kidney stone could elevate your blood pressure.

In your case, your doctor should closely monitor your blood pressure without increasing the dose of medicine. If the blood pressure remains high for a week or two, you need special X-rays and blood tests to discover the cause, which—if corrected—will allow your blood pressure to return to normal.

Know the limits of hypertension

Q. I'm a male with borderline hypertension. My last reading was 150/82. I always thought it was the bottom number that made you have high blood pressure. What can I do to bring the reading down, and what does my salt intake have to do with the condition?

A. The blood pressure is expressed as two numbers: systolic and diastolic. Systolic pressure (the top number) is measured when the heart contracts; diastolic (the bottom number) when the heart relaxes and fills with blood in preparation for the next contraction.

New guidelines suggest that the normal blood pressure for an adult should not exceed 120/80 millimeters of mercury. (A child's blood pressure should be much lower.)

In the past, doctors believed that the diastolic blood pressure was more important than the systolic; that is, a consistent diastolic elevation was more apt to cause stroke and heart disease than was a high systolic pressure.

However, studies have shown that both components are equally important and, when elevated, should be seriously addressed.

It's not always necessary for hypertensive patients to take prescription drugs. Alterations in lifestyle will often reduce high blood pressure to normal levels.

For instance, hypertension is frequently associated with obesity, smoking, excess dietary salt, lack of exercise and alcohol consumption. Thus, hypertensive patients may substantially lower their blood pressures by losing weight, stopping smoking, cutting back on salt, exercising regularly, and imbibing less alcohol.

Many people with high blood pressure suffer from a kidney abnormality, such as renal artery stenosis, that prevents them from excreting unnecessary salt. When such patients consume too much salt, the body retains the excess (along with fluid), which increases the blood volume and leads to hypertension.

Consequently, these patients should reduce their intake of salt by shunning salty foods and avoiding the salt shaker. A well-balanced diet will provide adequate salt without the necessity of adding extra amounts to the food.

With your doctor's approval, follow the suggestions I made. You may be quite surprised at how effective they are in lowering your blood pressure—which really isn't that high to begin with but will probably increase as you grow older unless you take steps now to correct it.

Home blood pressure monitoring

Q. I am aware that one should rest 15 minutes in advance (or wait 30 minutes after eating) before measuring the blood pressure. What is the best time of day to get the most accurate reading?

A. Our blood pressure readings constantly change, minute by minute, during the day. As a general rule, readings are lower early in the morning, when we awaken, and tend to rise with activity and stress. In the main, these fluctuations are unimportant. True, were you to measure your blood pressure directly following a period of strenuous exertion, it would be higher (but not necessarily abnormal), because the body adapts to exercise by increasing the blood pressure to drive oxygen and nutrients into exercising muscles. On the other hand, I do not believe that eating will significantly alter blood pressure readings.

If you are monitoring your blood pressure outside of a doctor's office, I suggest that you record the date and time of day, along with your readings. In this manner, you will be able to detect any important variations in the pattern of your recordings. When your physician review your diary, he will be able to identify significant fluctuations that are present.

In my practice, I ask my hypertensive patients to record blood pressure measurements two or three times a week (with date and time of day). I am mainly interested in the general pattern. If, for example, a reading is low (120/70) in the morning, but high (160/90) in the late afternoon, I am much less concerned than I would be if the BP were 180/110 morning and afternoon, irrespective of work, play or naps.

Whether to treat a blood pressure level, ignore it or consider altering therapy is a personal decision that every doctor (and patient) must make on an individual basis.

Let me add two further observations. First, many perfectly normal, non-hypertensive people crank up their pressures in the doctor's office. Known as "white-coat hypertension," this disorder was, in the past, considered to be a common, anxiety-induced, flight-or-fight phenomenon. It was ordinarily not treated, unless severe.

Modern hypertension experts caution that this form of "labile hypertension" may, over time, progress to dangerous levels needing treatment. So, the home readings become increasingly important in ferreting out such patients.

Second, hypertension is a major killer in our society. Therefore, it must be taken seriously and treated in its earliest stages. Few patients have a normal blood pressure on Tuesday and develop significant hypertension on Thursday. The process is subtler than that. Hence, the reason that I ask my hypertensive patients to monitor their BPs at home is to identify pattern changes. Last year, John had a blood pressure of 130/85 in the afternoon, considered to be high. This year, he was 150/95 in the morning, 165/100 in the afternoon. John needs close attention and probably therapy. I say "probably" because he may be able to lower his BP by losing weight, reducing salt intake, exercising regularly, cutting back on alcohol, dealing with stress and stopping smoking—a challenging adventure.

Therefore, my message is: For people who have hypertension (or may be in the early stages of it), home BP monitoring is appropriate (much as diabetics check their blood sugars periodically). Treatment is indicated for persons whose blood pressures remain elevated. This therapy should include personal responsibility for lifestyle changes, as well as medication. Treatment and follow-up are the responsibility of the primary care physician AND THE PATIENT, working as a team.

Proper technique to measure blood pressure

Q. Please settle a family disagreement.

When my wife and I go to the doctor, the nurse takes our blood pressures over whatever garment covers the arm. I maintain that a true reading cannot be obtained in this manner. My wife believes otherwise.

A. You and your wife are both correct.

When the blood pressure is taken, the cuff is wrapped around the upper arm and inflated to a level that stops blood flow in the arm. Then the pressure is slowly reduced until the examiner hears the thud-thud sound of the blood flow returning. That is the systolic pressure. As the pressure in the cuff is further reduced, the sound disappears; that is the diastolic reading.

A thick garment, such as a sweater or flannel shirt, will invariably muffle the systolic and diastolic sound-changes, making the reading imprecise. More important, in order to shut off the blood flow at the beginning of the maneuver, the garment (as well as the arm) must be compressed. Because more force is required to compress a heavy garment, the systolic pressure will be incorrectly elevated. The advantage of a bare-arm blood pressure determination is that it avoids these two pitfalls. So, as a general rule, most practitioners use this technique.

However, a thin garment, such as a cotton shirt or a silk blouse, will rarely interfere with the transmission of systolic/diastolic sounds. And these fabrics are not really compressible, so they don't alter the accuracy of the measurement.

Thus, the issue depends on what kind of clothing is involved. In my practice, especially during the cold winter months, I ask patients to remove thick garments (without rolling them up) but allow thin sleeves for reasons of comfort. The bottom line is that blood pressure can be most accurately determined by cuffing a bare arm, but thin sleeves should not appreciably alter the reading.

Stress can elevate blood pressure

Q. What would cause extreme differences in blood pressure readings? One day, my wife is at 148/90, the next 118/70. Her doctor is not concerned.

A. Many people show enormous variations in their blood pressures; most of us exhibit modest fluctuations, depending on what we're doing or how we're feeling.

To doctors, concerned about the danger of sustained hypertension, it's not the degree of fluctuation that matters. Rather, it's the overall pattern.

For example, a person can run a consistently elevated blood pressure of, say, 160/95 millimeters of mercury. Unless this pressure regularly drops into the normal range (below 150/90 or lower, depending on age), such a patient is at risk for a plethora of medical complications, ranging from stroke to heart failure.

In contrast, another adult can exhibit blood pressure readings of 170/100, alternating with normal values. Such a patient is said to have "labile" hypertension, which does not need treatment.

Similarly, an individual can have high readings, at times of stress, for several days a week. However, he or she need not worry if the blood pressure falls to normal even one or two days a week.

Stress, genetic factors, obesity, a sedentary lifestyle, kidney disease, and a diet high in salt are common factors leading to hypertension. Appropriate attention to any (or all) of these factors will reduce blood pressure levels, without the need for medication.

Although your wife may occasionally have a mildly elevated blood pressure (148/90), she then falls to 118/70, a normal value. Thus, she does not have hypertension. Perhaps her high readings are caused by anxiety—the apprehension of being in a doctor's office, for example.

She can investigate such a pattern by taking her own blood pressure. This exercise may enable her to identify environmental (or personal) issues that cause her blood pressure to rise. Her doctor is not concerned because she does not have a serous problem with hypertension.

Nonetheless, he is obligated to discuss this situation with your wife, to put the readings into perspective. Also, he should probably reassure he, thereby lessening her anxiety and, I hope, reducing her pattern of high readings.

Exercise and hypertension

Q. If exercise raises the blood pressure, should hypertensive patients avoid it? Once the high blood pressure is treated, does any organ damage regress?

A. Increased blood pressure is a normal physiologic response to stress or exercise—the old "fight or flight" phenomenon—and, as such, is appropriate and unavoidable. Problems develop when the blood pressure constantly remains high, irrespective of a person's activities.

For example, regular exercise raises the blood pressure, which, however, should return to normal during periods of rest and relaxation. In addition, the more a person exercises, the more blunted the blood pressure rise.

Also, it's well known that regular exercise actually lowers the blood pressure during times of inactivity. Therefore, exercise is good for everyone—in moderation. Those who anticipate a rigorous exercise program would be prudent to consult first with their physicians.

One of the most dangerous consequences of persistent hypertension is damage to vital organs, such as the heart and kidneys. If a hypertensive receives effective drug therapy before this damage occurs, the potential harm is avoidable or, if mild, reversible.

However, once structural alterations—such as heart enlargement—have appeared, the changes remain. The kidneys, in particular, are quite susceptible to blood pressure injury; renal function may diminish and remain inefficient long after the blood pressure is brought under control. Moreover, abnormal kidney efficiency can itself contribute to hypertension and an array of other medical problems, including anemia.

Thus, in answer to your question, the degree of remedy depends on the severity of the high blood pressure, the extent of the organ damage and the length of time the untreated hypertension has been present.

Using drugs from the astonishing spectrum of modern anti-hypertension medicines, physicians can effectively treat virtually 100 percent of hypertensive patients. In this day and age, there is no compelling reason why every person with high blood pressure cannot be treated appropriately. The problem, of course, is the cost of the medicines for uninsured, financially strapped patients. More on that in another column.

Curious symptoms need specialists

Q. My husband takes Capoten twice daily for hypertension. However, every day, usually within a half hour of waking, his tongue, throat and lips go numb and he salivates to the point of drooling. His face becomes flushed, he gags and shudders. This lasts several minutes. Our family isn't concerned and attributes it to the medicine. Can you shed some light on this?

A. I can't for the life of me figure out what is affecting your husband. If it's a strange reaction to Capoten (ordinarily a safe drug), the medicine should be changed. If, however, he is suffering from some kind of circulatory disturbance, such as mini-strokes, he needs further testing and treatment. In particular, he should be examined at precisely the moment he experiences his symptoms. Perhaps your family physician would be willing to make a morning house call to see for himself what is going on.

As a second option, I recommend a consultation with a neurologist. Such a specialist should be able to sort things out and, I hope, give your family doctor some guidance and continuing medical education.

Low blood pressure may have consequences

Q. What can you tell me about POTS—postural orthostatic tachycardia syndrome?

A. Sometimes, in the presence of heart disease and drug therapy for cardiovascular ailments, people experience a sudden and substantial drop in blood pressure when they quickly sit up or stand. This causes weakness, light-headedness or fainting that is associated with tachycardia (rapid pulse, as the heart tries to compensate by pumping more blood, against gravity, to the brain).

The causes of this affliction are legion, but the end result is the same: postural low blood pressure with secondary tachycardia, causing far more pronounced symptoms than the mild light-headedness we all may occasionally experience upon rapid standing.

In patients taking medicine to lower blood pressure, the drug may be to blame. Thus, the syndrome can be prevented with a simple reduction in the drug's dosage, under medical supervision. For those who are not medicated, the therapy is somewhat more complicated. Regular exercise will help by toning up the cardiovascular system. (POTS is much more frequent in sedentary individuals and is common in people who have been confined to bed.)

Also, doctors may encourage more dietary salt (to increase blood volume and blood pressure), or prescribe elastic support stockings (to stabilize the circulation and prevent pooling of blood in the lower extremities).

In my experience, however, patients with non-drug-induced POTS should be examined by cardiologists and have further evaluation, such as Holter monitors and stress tests.

> 66 It's well known that regular exercise actually lowers the blood pressure during times of inactivity. Therefore, exercise is good for everyone
> —in moderation. 99

Hypertension in any form needs therapy

Q. I'm an elderly woman with primary pulmonary hypertension. My blood pressure consistently hovers around 160/90. I'm on Vasotec, but my doctor has not explained my illness. What's my prognosis?

A. Pulmonary hypertension is somewhat different from arterial hypertension, the high blood pressure that is diagnosed with a familiar device applied to the upper arm.

Pulmonary hypertension is increased pressure in the blood circulating through the lungs. It has many causes, including blood clots in the lungs, lung surgery, chronic pulmonary disease and cardiac disorders. An uncommon form is of unknown cause.

Ordinarily, the condition can be diagnosed with a cardiac echo or ultrasound test. Sometimes, a cardiac catheterization is necessary to directly measure the pressures in the heart's chambers and in the lungs.

As the pressure in the lungs increases, patients experience difficulty breathing during exercise, fainting and weakness. Their hearts may enlarge. Thus, any cause of pulmonary hypertension must be identified and treated. In addition, most patients require therapy for the hypertension itself. Vasotec, for example, lowers arterial resistance and thereby reduces pressure in the lungs.

I am somewhat concerned that, despite treatment, your blood pressure remains elevated; in such a situation, your lung pressure is probably high as well. This combination is exceedingly dangerous and should be addressed immediately with an increase in your medication or a drastic change in therapy.

Perhaps this would be a suitable opportunity for you to suggest that your primary care physician refer you to a cardiologist or pulmonary specialist for a second opinion. First, there should be an effort to discover the cause of your pulmonary problem. Second, your blood pressure needs to be lowered into the 120/80 range.

Once these goals have been accomplished, your prognosis should be favorable. Until that time, however, you are at risk for complications such as heart failure, so don't delay.

Symptoms of overmedication

Q. I'm on medication for high blood pressure. Two years ago, I had triple-bypass surgery and didn't take my blood pressure medication for several months. Then my doctor insisted on placing me on Lopressor, based on my blood pressure reading in his office.

For the past six months, I've notice light-headedness; my hearing and eyesight are failing; I'm forgetful and have no energy. Although I've mentioned these symptoms to my doctor several times, he hasn't done anything about them. Memory loss is what bothers me the most. I don't know what to do next.

A. I cannot diagnose your condition without examining you. However, you should consider the possibility that you are overmedicated. Your blood pressure may actually be too low. This situation is far from rare. In fact, many patients consistently show higher blood pressures in doctors' offices than they do at other times. Allow me to share a vignette with you that I think proves my point.

A few years ago, I had a hypertensive patient on medication and I was certain that the medicines were working perfectly, because every time I checked her blood pressure it was 130/80 in the office, what I considered to be an ideal reading.

While I was congratulating myself on being so knowledgeable and efficient, she was falling down at home because she felt so faint.

Eventually, in desperation, we agreed that she would check her own blood pressure at home. Lo and behold, it consistently ran about 100/50, an extremely low reading for an elderly adult. This observation solved the mystery. Her blood pressure in the office was predictably higher than at home. This was a classic case of hubris: I was aggressively treating the hypertension without regard for the patient as a whole. I was treating only what I could see, with the result being that she was overmedicated.

I halved her medication, her blood pressure stabilized at 130/75 (160/90 in the office), she felt much better, and I learned an important lesson.

She is active and alert in her early 90s and is one of my most loyal patients and friends.

Show your doctor my response to your question and ask him to authorize a home blood pressure monitoring device. These units are readily available at reasonable prices in many pharmacies. Once you learn how to take your own blood pressure, you'll be amazed at how easy the procedure is. This way, you will be more in control of your health—and you can help your doctor in the bargain.

If he is unsympathetic to your plight, ask for a second opinion—or change physicians.

"Fainting spell" must be treated

Q. I've had five spells where I pass out with no warning. The first time it happened, my pressure dropped to 100/50 and my pulse to 48. I was diagnosed with vasovagal syncope. I don't understand what this is.

A. The walls of arteries contain muscles. When these muscles contract, the arteries become smaller, compressing the blood within them. This raises the pressure of the blood. When the arteries remain constricted, the pressure stays high and a person is said to have hypertension. Conversely, when the arterial muscles relax, the diameter of the blood vessel enlarges and the blood pressure falls, leading to hypotension.

Ordinarily, there is a constant balance between arterial constriction and dilation. The blood pressure remains normal.

However, as we age, this delicate balance is often upset. As I mentioned, hypertension results from inappropriate, sustained arterial constriction. But the reverse can also occur.

For unknown reasons, some older persons may suddenly experience a drop in blood pressure and a fall in pulse rate, which leads to arterial dilation and a slowing of the heart rate.

This phenomenon produces symptoms of light-headedness, weakness and faintness, similar to the feelings we may all normally experience from time to time upon standing suddenly from a sitting position. The disorder is called vaso (blood vessel) vagal (coming from the vagus nerves) syncope (faintness).

Your case is not unusual. During each of your five "spells" the blood pressure and pulse fell, no enough blood reached your brain, and you passed out. Because of the obvious dangers associated with this condition, such as the risks to yourself and others, vasovagal syncope must be treated.

Along with diagnosing vasovagal syncope, your physician must attempt to discover why these events are happening. Vasovagal syncope usually signifies a form of heart disease, so you need special testing, such as a stress test and cardiac ultrasound.

If heart disease is present, your doctor will probably prescribe medicine, such as nitroglycerine and others, to improve blood flow to the heart muscle and prevent reflex hypotension. However, in severe cases, an artificial pacemaker (to drive the pulse at a higher rate) may have to be implanted. Or you might be helped by consuming extra quantities of fluids and salt, which will increase your blood volume.

In any case, you need further testing—and, I hope, a detailed description from your doctor about what is happening. If your family physician is not inclined to press the issue, ask for a referral to a cardiologist.

7

Memory Loss, Alzheimer's, Senility & Dementia

Flawed recall mechanism

Q. I'm a 75-year-old man with what I term a flawed "recall mechanism." I have problems remembering names, but if I think of something else, the situation eventually corrects itself.

A. According to some authorities, once we reach age 25, we begin to lose brain cells at a rate of 50,000 per day.

Although I question this figure, there is no doubt that memory fades as we age. Called the "benign forgetfulness of old age," the syndrome is virtually universal and is caused by what I term "shrinking brain." As we get older, the brain literally diminishes in size because neurons shrivel and die. This eventually leads to poor memory and various cognitive disabilities.

Of course, such mental alterations can also be caused by Alzheimer's disease and mini-strokes; therefore, I urge you to be examined by your primary care physician—or perhaps a neurologist. Once your diagnosis has been established, the doctors should be able to offer appropriate therapy.

Vitamins for memory?

Q. I am 77 and forgetful. Is there a vitamin, supplement, food or medication that I could take to regain my memory?

A. Memory loss normally accompanies the aging process. However, it may also reflect early dementia. Therefore, I urge you to have a full neurological evaluation, imaging studies and blood tests to make sure that you don't have a vitamin deficiency, an underactive thyroid gland or some other treatable cause for your problem. To my knowledge, there is no diet, supplement or herbal remedy to help you regain memory. Some patients have had beneficial effects from the prescription drug Aricept, but—in my experience—such improvement is inconsistent and disappointing. I believe that your best option is to see a neurologist.

Senility, dementia, and Alzheimer's defined

Q. What is the difference between senility, dementia and Alzheimer's disease?

A. As we age, our brains age as well. They don't work as well as they did when we were younger. This is one reason elderly people are more forgetful than the young, sleep less soundly, and learn less readily. Like failing vision and diminishing coordination, these mental changes simply come with the territory.

Senility merely describes these changes in the very old. Such people may forget names and recent events; they seem to live in the past.

Dementia, on the other hand, is a progressive failure of cognitive function that exceeds senility. It occurs at an earlier age—sometimes in the 50s—and is more pronounced than age-related senility.

For example, a senile patient in his 80s may not remember how to get home from the supermarket. He may be frustrated and short-tempered, because he realizes that his mental efficiency is waning.

In contrast, the demented patient shows unmistakable disintegration of personality and intellect. Along with forgetfulness, he may have speech disturbances, misperception of his environment, obsessions, rigidity, and periods of violent anger. He is not aware that these changes are occurring. Depression and the blunting of feelings are common—all at a relatively young age.

Dementia can have many causes, including hypothyroidism, vitamin deficiency of B12 and folic acid, small strokes—and Alzheimer's disease. Therefore, Alzheimer's disease is just one cause—albeit an important one—of dementia. The various factors that form the basis of this tragic ailment are diagnosed using blood tests and special X-ray studies, although there is no definite test for Alzheimer's disease.

In short, some degree of senility will affect us all as we enter our 80s and 90s. Dementia, which generally strikes at an earlier age, is associated with more widespread mental abnormalities. Many types of dementia are correctable—or, at least, treatable—except for Alzheimer's disease, whose victims usually need eventual institutional care.

Is it Alzheimer's or dementia?

Q. What is the difference between senile dementia and Alzheimer's disease?

A. The term "dementia" refers to the progressive decline of mental functioning. Patients with the disorder exhibit forgetfulness, confusion, poor judgment, and diminished cognitive ability.

There are many causes of dementia, including alcohol abuse, hypothyroidism, Parkinson's disease, vitamin B12 deficiency, stroke, and Alzheimer's disease. Often, very old people experience an age-related ("senile") dementia, the cause of which is unknown but may be the consequence of "mini-strokes."

As a general rule, Alzheimer's disease strikes at an earlier age than does senility, progresses more rapidly and is more profound.

Identifying the cause of dementia can be a difficult task. For example, Alzheimer's patients frequently have normal CT or MRI scans, whereas senile patients show merely "cortical atrophy" (brain shrinkage).

In my opinion, patients with declining mental ability should be examined and tested by neurologists, especially if such patients have symptoms at a relatively early age—say, younger than 80 years. Although there is no definitive test for Alzheimer's disease, some forms of dementia are both preventable and curable.

Causes of dementia

Q. Please give me a thumbnail review of dementia.

A. Of all the serious diseases that can affect humans, none is so devastating as dementia, the progressive and inexorable decline in memory and intellectual function. Judging from the comments made by many of my patients, dementia is the most feared disorder—more frightening even than heart attack or cancer—because victims gradually lose the very qualities that make them human. As memory, judgment and emotional control wane, dementia patients become burdens on their families, loved ones and caregivers. Eventually, institutional living is required, which can completely absorb a nest egg, life savings and insurance coverage, while such patients continue to live for decades as mere shadows of their former shelves, not knowing or caring. Nothing.

Experts now recognize three general classes of dementia: those associated with other neurological diseases, those seen in conjunction with general medical afflictions, and those defined as primary disorders.

Alzheimer's Disease

Alzheimer's disease is the major and most severe form of "senility" in old age. Although we sometimes label the occasional forgetfulness and memory loss associated with old age as senility, Alzheimer's disease is a much more severe disorder. It can be catastrophic—and, at present, there is no prevention or cure.

The initial symptoms of confusion and forgetfulness, especially about recent events, are minor and often attributed to emotional upsets, physical illness or aging itself. As the disease progresses, changes in personality and behavior become more marked and alarming. Victims may do such things as forget how to make coffee, not remember where they live or fail to recognize a spouse. Writing, reading, speech and naming of objects may also be affected. Victims eventually lose control over motor behavior and bodily functions and are likely to spend their last days in a nursing home or long-term-care facility.

Who gets Alzheimer's?

Alzheimer's disease is a disorder that affects the brain cells, but it is not a normal consequence of aging, so not everyone is at risk. However, it is regarded as the major form of old-age senility. The National Institute of Aging estimates that it is the cause of serious confusion and forgetfulness in about two million elderly Americans and is a probably contributor to the institutionalization of as many as half of the more than one million elderly Americans in long-term-care facilities.

Alois Alzheimer, a German neurologist, first described this disease in 1906 in a 51-year-old patient. Since that time, the disorder Alzheimer described has become divided into two diagnoses: Alzheimer's disease if the onset of illness is before age 65; and senile dementia for onset after age 65. Some experts believe that Alzheimer's disease and senile dementia are the same thing, regardless of the age of onset, because the basic disease process and pathological findings are the same. In scientific publications, researchers are increasingly adopting the term "dementia of the Alzheimer type" to refer to the disorder in a person of any age.

The onset of Alzheimer's disease is most frequent in the age group 65-69. When the illness occurs in younger patients, it tends to be more severe, and consequently of shorter duration. When the onset occurs before age 44, the average survival is 4.5 years. When the disease first appears at ages 65-69, the average survival is 8.5 years.

Treatment approaches

Because one of the most consistent changes in Alzheimer's disease involves a decrease in the activity of the chemicals comprising the brain's cholinergic system, scientists have attempted to find out what causes this decline and ways to compensate for it to treat the serious symptoms of Alzheimer's disease.

Early attempts to increase acetylcholine production in the brain by ingesting some of the precursor substance from which it is made did not show any marked or consistent benefit. Research has subsequently turned to investigation of substances that block the otherwise-fast breakdown of acetylcholine in the brain.

Several studies of the aging brain have indicated that calcium activity decreases with aging, and acetylcholine is one of several neurotransmitters partially influenced by calcium. In laboratory studies, investigators are attempting to stimulate calcium concentrations, thereby increasing the synthesis and release of acetylcholine.

Another approach is based on the possibility that aluminum may play some role in the disease. This approach is focusing on whether removing this metal from the body has any effect on the disease. Czechoslovakian investigators suggested that aluminum interacts with fluoride ions and is thus excreted from the body. Following this lead, scientists at the National Institute of Mental Health are conducting a long-term study of the effects of sodium fluoride on the course and outcome of Alzheimer's disease.

In the first category, patients suffer profound personality alterations that result from conditions such as mini-strokes (multi-infarct dementia) and Parkinson's disease. If these afflictions can be diagnosed early, treatment often slows—or even halts—the progression of cognitive malfunction.

In the second category, the dementia is a consequence of a medical disorder. The most common are AIDS, vitamin B12 (or folic acid) deficiency, syphilis and hypothyroidism. AIDS dementia is probably caused by viral invasion of the brain. It may be treatable with anti-HIV drugs; however, the final word is not yet in. Vitamin B12/folic acid deficiency can be reversed by vitamin injections or supplements; syphilis can be cured with antibiotics; and thyroid function can be restored with inexpensive thyroid hormone pills. In short, such therapy can reverse the mental changes if given early in the course of the disease.

The third category, primary dementia (which are usually irreversible, includes alcohol dementia syndrome (common in heavy drinkers as alcohol poisons their brains), Pick's disease (a rare disorder marked by brain deterioration) and Alzheimer's disease.

Primary dementia is incurable and, at the present time, are treatable only with powerful drugs that control a demented person's aberrant behavior without affecting the dementia itself.

Alzheimer's disease has been estimated to affect almost 50 percent of people over 85 years of age. The cause is unknown, but a genetic tendency seems to exist.

The diagnosis of the different types of dementia depends on a thorough neurological examination, blood tests and special scanning techniques, such as MRI.

I should interject that many medications (including digoxin, antidepressants, anticonvulsants, and—in rare cases—antibiotics) may cause reversible mental changes that resemble dementia.

Therefore, all patients with dementia should be examined and thoroughly tested by neurologists, in an attempt to identify causes that can be treated, as well as to give family members more realistic expectations about the future and to allow them to develop a comprehensive care plan.

Loss of short term memory may be sign of early dementia

Q. Could the medications captopril and furosemide, used for hypertension, cause memory loss in an 85-year-old man?

A. Elderly people universally experience short-term memory loss. As we age, for example, we become less facile with names and other everyday events. I find myself more forgetful than I was previously and have to make lists. I know several dear old friends who can clearly remember childhood occurrences, but throw up their hands when questioned about what they had for lunch yesterday.

Unfortunately, not all memory loss can be classified as "benign forgetfulness of the elderly." I recently had the pleasure of meeting a new patient, a charming and articulate gentleman, who was referred by his family doctor for memory loss. The patient and I carried on a lengthy discussion about his medical history, diseases and operations (all negative). He was quite clear about his good health. He had never really had to see a doctor and, despite his age of 76, professed no particular urge to see one now. He was well shaven, well groomed and impeccably dressed. He appeared confident and strode purposefully into the examining room, a big smile on his face, with handshake extended.

On a hunch, before beginning the exam, I decided to ask him a few current-events questions, the kind most people could answer without thinking.

"Who is the governor?" I inquired.

He paused and grinned. "Oh," he replied, "I don't much like him. Say, that's a handsome tie you're wearing."

With my interest piqued, I thanked him. "Seriously," I continued, "what's the governor's name?"

"Doc, what a silly question! Are you serious?"

"Just asking."

"Well, I don't really remember. Can you give me a clue?"

I mentioned several recent governors' names. At each one, he shook his head. When I gave him the present governor's name, he brightened up and proudly exclaimed: "Yep, that's the one!"

I wouldn't let him off the hook. "Who's the vice president?" I queried. He had no idea.

"OK, what's the president's name?" I asked.

"Gosh, Doc, everyone knows that. He sure is doing a great job. Whatta guy. I'd certainly vote for him again." He turned and began removing his coat, still smiling, affable and unconcerned.

I persisted but, again, he need "a clue." He knew it wasn't Eisenhower

("Heck, Doc, I'm not an idiot!"), Kennedy, Johnson, Nixon, Ford, Carter or Clinton. When I mentioned "Bush," he said: "He's the one! Good old George," folded his coat and placed it carefully on a chair. I didn't choose to stress him further about which George.

That was the extent of the mental examination, because I'd learned what I needed to know. He had an early dementia for which I ordered a truckload of blood tests and a CT scan of his brain, in an attempt to discover a treatable cause (such as anemia, folic acid deficiency, thyroid disorders or a stroke) for his problem. Everything turned out normal, so I ended up referring him to a gero-psychiatrist, a specialist in brain malfunction in the elderly, who diagnosed Alzheimer's disease.

I digressed with my anecdote to point out that a phenomenal amount of memory loss may occur before a clever patient with a severe mental condition can be diagnosed. This is usually more than simple age-related memory deficiency. It is a big-time problem, often a consequence of alcohol abuse, Alzheimer's disease or mini-strokes.

The 85-year-old man in your question needs a thorough mental evaluation. Captopril and furosemide, two drugs used to treat hypertension and heart disease, do not ordinarily cause significant loss of memory. But, obviously, any drug has the potential for affecting mental function in an elderly person whose memory may already be borderline or—in the case of my patient—significantly impaired. A doctor is the logical resource to sort out the various factors that can cause poor memory; and such a practitioner can also recommend therapy or referral to an appropriate specialist.

Do vitamins affect dementia?

Q. Is it true that some types of dementia are caused by a vitamin deficiency? If so, which ones?

A. A deficiency in folic acid or vitamin B12 can lead to the profound mental changes called dementia. This is why doctors usually check folate and B12 blood levels when testing a patient with disordered thinking. Moreover, many authorities advise folate and B12 supplements for elderly patients whose diets may, for one reason or another, lack necessary nutrients. For most adults, however, a well-balanced diet will supply all the required vitamins and minerals.

Don't assume forgetfulness means Alzheimer's

Q. We are not sure if my 78-year-old mother is in the beginning stages of Alzheimer's disease. She admits to having trouble remembering names and words, but her disability goes beyond that. For example, she could not figure out how to operate the windshield wipers in her new car or how to get the lint tray back into her new dryer.

Her doctor put her on medication that merely worsened the situation. She is currently off all medicine. She has had no testing. How should we proceed?

A. When I first read you letter, I was rushed and concluded that your mother probably has Alzheimer's disease. But on a second reading (is this a symptom of my own dementia?), I noted the phrases "new car" and "new dryer." Given the fact that I am a grouchy old technophobe who has great difficulty dealing with the "bells and whistles" of new gadgetry, I found myself sympathizing with your mom. Today's machines and devices may give us oldies more information than we need or can handle. Also, I find that all this crap is distracting. For example, do I really need a satellite navigation system to commute the two miles to my office? No. But these systems are basically standard in new vehicles— and we pay for them, believe me, we pay dearly. And how do we follow them when the car is in motion? In addition, I cannot remember names, either. Or, more accurately, it takes me several minutes (or hours) to retrieve such information from my computer/brain.

Now that I have had some fun sharing my own views and defects, let me address the serious problem with your mother.

First of all, she needs testing. And I fault her physician for not ordering it before he prescribed medication. Dementia has many causes. Alcoholism, mini-strokes, thyroid disease and vitamin deficiencies are four of the most common, treatable conditions.

Therefore, I urge you to have your mother examined by a neurologist, who will, I am sure, order additional scanning studies and blood tests. Then, based on his evaluation of the situation, the specialist can diagnose your mother's condition and suggest therapy. For example, alcohol prohibition, medicine to reduce blood clotting, thyroid supplements and additional vitamins may "cure" certain forms of dementia. In contrast, if she does have early Alzheimer's disease, there are prescription drugs, such as Aricept and others, that may slow progression of the disease.

Therefore, my position is: let's get more data and then proceed with appropriate therapy.

With respect to my own mental problems, I subscribe to the traditional medical dictum that doctors aren't supposed to get sick or suffer the infirmities common to the aging process. In other words, we're different. Yeah. And you say this guy isn't nuts?

Blocked blood flow may cause forgetfulness, other symptoms

Q. I have been told that I have "cerebral vascular insufficiency." What is this? I am 79 years old, forgetful, and sometimes have difficulty saying the word I want to speak.

A. As we age and arteriosclerotic plaque builds up on our arterial linings, we often develop symptoms, depending on which organ is affected by the deficient blood supply.

For example, coronary artery blockage frequently results in angina or heart attack, renal artery occlusion can lead to hypertension, and occlusions in the leg arteries may cause muscle cramps.

When such blockages affect the cerebral (brain) circulation, the patient is said to have cerebral vascular insufficiency. This can lead to forgetfulness, confusion, periodic weakness, difficulty speaking, and a wide variety of other symptoms. The basic problem is twofold: how to improve blood flow to the brain and how to prevent blood clots from forming on the arteriosclerotic plaque, because such clots may be carried to the brain and cause a stroke.

The task of improving circulation is really tough. No medication has been shown to be effective. Therefore, in selected cases, surgeons may have to try to remove the blockages, especially if the plaque affects the blood vessels (such as the carotid arteries) in the neck.

The challenge of preventing blood clots is, surprisingly, relatively easy and is now standard practice. Patients with cerebral vascular deficiency are advised to take one aspirin a day to retard clotting. In advanced cases (or in instances where the heart beats erratically), prescription anticoagulants, such as Coumadin, are used.

Exactly which method of treatment is appropriate for you I cannot say. This is a decision best left to your doctor, with the help of a neurologist, perhaps. But I can say that, at the least, you should be taking aspirin therapy. Ask your doctor about this.

New blood test to predict Alzheimer's disease

Q. My friend swears that there is a blood test for Alzheimer's disease. Is this true?

A. There appears to be a newly discovered relation between the level of homocysteine in the blood and Alzheimer's disease, as reported in the New England Journal of Medicine (Feb. 14, 2002).

For years, homocysteine has been known to have a direct toxic effect on cells lining the body's arteries. The compound is clearly related to coronary artery disease, stroke, peripheral vascular disease and the aging of the brain.

The new study indicates that the higher the homocysteine level, the more likely a person will develop Alzheimer's. This finding is doubly important because homocysteine blood levels can be significantly reduced by supplemental folic acid, a vitamin, in dosages of one to two milligrams a day. The relation of homocysteine to vascular diseases is so compelling that the United States government now mandates folic acid fortification of the food supply.

High homocysteine levels precede the development of Alzheimer's disease by several years. Therefore, early detection coupled with folic acid therapy could, in theory, prevent the disastrous consequences of homocysteine-induced vascular disorders. Here is an instance where inexpensive treatment can be truly useful.

The case of the shrinking brain

Q. My husband, 69, is very forgetful and testy. He is also quite confused. An MRI scan showed "cortical atrophy." What is this? Could it be the cause of his problems? Is it treatable?

A. As we age, our brains shrink. The current theory is that this inescapable situation is related to death of neurons (brain cells), probably caused by tiny blood clots that deprive the nerve tissue of oxygen and nutrients. Doctors believe that such clots form in cycles over a period of decades. Each event is so tiny that we fail to notice anything is amiss; however, the cumulative effect eventually leads to a significant loss of cognitive function, memory and judgment. No one knows why this process if accelerated in certain people. For instance, many adults in their 80s (and beyond) continue to function at relatively high levels of cognition; they may forget names and have to make lists, but their reasoning, judgment and personality characteristics are not dramatically affected. On the other hand, some men and women in their 60s and 70s suffer definite and progressive difficulty with thinking; they often exhibit early disability that quickly progresses to senility and dementia. On a positive note, many authorities are convinced that these neurological abnormalities can be arrested—or at least minimized—if older people continue to stimulate their brains with intellectual projects, such as learning, reading, problem-solving and working. The theory is that new neurons may form and begin to function (to compensate for the shrunken tissue) as a consequence of intellectual challenge.

Because your husband had an MRI, I assume that he has seen a doctor who ordered the scan. Therefore, I believe that this physician is the logical resource to answer your specific questions about treatment. He may choose to refer your spouse to a neurologist—my preferred option. Or he may suggest that your husband take an aspirin a day (to reduce the formation of tiny clots) or have further testing (such as a carotid ultrasound to examine the arteries in the neck for sources of clots); he may prescribe Aricept (a medication that improves memory in some patients) or involve your husband in a program of intellectual stimulation designed for patients with cortical atrophy and other causes of dementia, such as Alzheimer's disease.

I suspect that the major thrust of therapy will be to retard the speed of intellectual deterioration; that is, your husband may not improve but even arresting the process at this point would be a worthy goal. Remember that the physician can also prescribe medicine to combat the rage, frustration and belligerency that commonly accompany the process of brain cell malfunction. Such therapy may permit your husband to remain at home for several years, rather than having to be cared for in a nursing facility.

Treatment for organic brain syndrome

Q. My 80-year-old sister has been diagnosed with organic brain syndrome and was admitted to our local psychiatric unit. She imagines she has hair growing all over her body and stands by the sink for hours, scrubbing her skin until it is raw. Is there any help for her?

A. Organic brain syndrome, complete mental deterioration, is a catastrophe for patients who have it and a tragedy for their families. The causes of this malady, which commonly affects the elderly, are legion and include Alzheimer's disease, stroke, brain tumors, Parkinson's disease, infections and idiosyncratic reactions to drugs. Your sister has developed a serious mental disability, the cause of which—I hope—has been thoroughly investigated by her doctors, using imaging studies and blood tests.

Even so, the situation is probably beyond remedy. Apparently, all you can hope for now is that the psychiatrists will prescribe appropriate medication to lessen her agitation, delusions and tendency to self-abuse. These drugs also relieve the bizarre behavior, confusion, belligerency and panic of organic brain syndrome. Still, I suspect that your sister will need permanent 24-hour care: This could be provided at home (expensive and difficult for most families), in a psychiatric hospital (should not be necessary if drug therapy is successful) or in a skilled nursing facility (probably your best option).

In my opinion, you should follow a step-wise approach to this problem.

First, make sure that the basis of your sister's brain syndrome has been diagnosed and that treatable/curable causes (such as hypothyroidism and vitamin deficiency) have been ruled out. Second, see how she responds to her new environment. I'd be particularly interested in whether antipsychotic drugs help her to feel more comfortable and able to carry out the activities of daily living, such as unassisted eating, elimination and personal hygiene. Third, depending on the success of her therapy, you can make a sensible decision regarding her future. While I lean toward admission to a skilled nursing facility, your sister's reaction to her medications may well calm her down enough to allow her to return home with only minimal supervision. The important consideration here is—as I know you are fully aware—her safety and quality of life. Nonetheless, the emotional health of the family is also crucial, so some level of institutional care may be the best long-term solution.

Wellbutrin may be behind "loss for words"

Q. I'm a healthy mother, age 40, who sometimes struggles to find words when I am speaking. I'll be talking and suddenly some normal word will be at the tip of my tongue, but I just can't get it out! I'll tell my children to go upstairs and shower, but the word "shower" just won't come out, and I'm left saying: "Go take a…a…a… ." Or I'll be trying to say: "I've got to run to the store to pick up some bread" and I'll get stuck on the words "store" or "bread," trying desperately to dig them out of my mind. While I do eventually get it out, it's only after a lengthy pause during which my mind races through a number of connections before I can pull it out. I also find myself regularly walking into a room—and suddenly, not remembering why I went there.

Sure, all these things are normal and happen to everyone occasionally, but they are happening to me more frequently. I "lose" words several times a day and forget why I went downstairs or into the kitchen at least a few times a week. This tendency is becoming more evident to other people; I struggle so often for words that my family and friends comment on it and are concerned.

I've been taking Wellbutrin for about eight months. The medicine has certainly helped my depression, put me in better control of my emotions and enabled me to deal more effectively with life stresses. Could my word problem be a side effect of the Wellbutrin? Confusion is among the listed potential side effects, but I'm not sure that I could be characterized as being confused. Could this be an early sign of a neurological disorder, such as Alzheimer's disease? Should I see a doctor and, if so, what kind?

A. The last time I was struck by the side effects of Wellbutrin was a year or two ago when a patient on Zyban (which is Wellbutrin used for smoking cessation) ran his car off the road because he became confused. Since that event (which, fortunately, did not injure him), I have had a renewed respect for the complications of antidepressant medications.

So, in answer to your question, yes, the medicine may be affecting your memory and powers of recall. However, your symptoms could also be secondary to an unrelated neurological disorder. Therefore, my advice to you is to make an appointment to see a neurologist.

In my community, the neurologists are so busy that they cannot see non-emergency patients right away; there is a four to six week waiting period. If this is true in your town, it may work in your favor and save you a lot of money. When you make the appointment, immediately taper your Wellbutrin; go to alternate day therapy for a week, then one dose every three days for one week, followed by one dose twice a week and then stop. If your word problems disappear, you've got your answer: The Wellbutrin is the culprit. You should stay off it and work with your primary care physician or psychiatrist to find an appropriate substitute.

If, on the other hand, your symptoms persist after stopping the drug, keep your appointment with the neurologist. Hint: I doubt this will be necessary. I put my money on the Wellbutrin.

Help for a relative with senility

Q. My 92-year-old mother has had three strokes that appear to have spared her movements and motor function. However, she has become impossible. She is mean to my sister and me, won't cooperate, squeezes our hands and pulls our hair, is constantly furious, won't listen to anything we tell her, demands the car keys, and makes life miserable for all those around her. What can we do?

A. Sounds like a normal parent to me, paying you guys back for all the discomfort you put her through as adolescents.

I'm just pulling your chain. Your situation is, quite clearly, a serious problem that needs to be addressed.

I gather from your brief comments that your mother lives with you or your sister and that her care is rapidly becoming more than a 24-hour job. Now you have to deal with her anger, lack of cooperation and wish to drive. Let's keep it simple.

At your mother's age, three strokes could be catastrophic. They surely affected her judgment and cognitive ability. In medical parlance, she probably has multi-infarct dementia. In everyday English, she is becoming increasingly senile because of damage to her brain from the strokes. The situation is further complicated by her belligerency, obsessiveness and oppositional behavior—all of which, I might add, are predictable given the overwhelming apprehension and fear she must feel as a consequence of her vascular events.

Nonetheless, let's not lose sight of the crucial goals: 1) Your mother's safety and happiness; 2) The stress level of her caregivers. You and your sister are about to run out of steam.

In terms of help, you have several options.

First, you should consider a skilled nursing facility. Your mother's physician (with whom you must discuss your concerns) would be an appropriate resource. Perhaps a brief hospitalization (to initiate drug therapy) is in order. During this time, arrangements can be made to transfer your mother to a long-term facility (or, once she is medicated, she may be suitably manageable to return home. But I doubt she will.)

Second, consider additional help at home, either courtesy of family members (not a good choice) or by hiring caretakers. This will remove much of the pressure that you now experience.

Third, you may substitute the home care option for the hospitalization, but in either case, I think your mother needs appropriate medication to improve the quality of her life. In my practice, I prefer to enlist the services of a psychopharmacologist—a psychiatrist who is an expert in the use of the many medicines use to treat mental problems. He or she could easily consult with your mother in the hospital; if she is at home, an office visit is appropriate. Once your mother's behavior and attitude have been improved with medication, she should be a different person.

Fourth, consider permanent placement, even with medicine, in an appropriate facility. This may be your best option, because your mother will receive the hands-on care she needs, and you—as medical nonprofessionals—will no longer be stretched beyond reasonable limits.

Fifth, if—once on medication—your mother's attitude improves, you may be able to put off institutionalization and keep her at home with the support I mentioned above.

Sixth, she should not be allowed to operate a motor vehicle. Even though your description of her behavior and attitude is sparse, I believe that even under the most favorable circumstances, your mother would be a candidate for road rage. So take the car keys.

In all likelihood, you and your sister have become the objects of your mother's frustration. This is understandable. Many people tend to take out their grudges on those closest to them; that's human nature. However, remember that help is available. You don't have to compromise your commitment to your mother; you simply need to find the best solution to the problem.

Let me close by saying that my comments are the result of how I handle similar situations in my own private practice. Therefore, while my suggestions may not be perfect solutions for you, they are still valid. Specifically, I am advising professional intervention by caregivers, social workers, physicians and psychiatrists. I believe that this approach is appropriate.

When to take charge

Q. During the last few years before my father's death from Alzheimer's disease, the family was in a quandary. When did he become so incompetent that legal intervention should have become mandatory? Is there some magical time that doctors can identify?

A. This is a decision based on what physicians term "clinical judgment." Some forms of dementia—regardless of cause—develop slowly, and it may be difficult to ascertain what you call the "magic time." For example, many patients with neurological diseases lose recent memory early on. They can't remember names and may forget where they are and why. Usually, this progresses to the point where they cannot balance their checkbooks, are unable to make appropriate purchases, become consistently confused and exhibit inappropriate behavior. The next stage is ordinarily marked by difficulty in carrying out the activities of daily living—such as bathing, eating, dressing and/or driving—that may take years to develop. Eventually, severely demented patients often become combative, uncooperative and totally dependent on caregivers.

On the other hand, other neurological disorders, such as repeated mini-strokes or brain damage from alcohol abuse, progress rapidly, within a matter of months.

> 66 *The new study indicates that the higher the homocysteine level, the more likely a person will develop Alzheimer's. This finding is doubly important because homocysteine blood levels can be significantly reduced by supplemental folic acid, a vitamin, in dosages of one to two milligrams a day.* 99

Consequently, function—more than time—is the important consideration. When family members and health professionals become concerned about significant cognitive loss, associated with loss of independence, the prudent family should step up to the plate and begin the legal process of declaring the patient incompetent. This action, although painful, is truly in the patient's best interests.

Here is how the system works—at least in my state. The family chooses one member to have power of attorney (which permits the signing of checks and general financial responsibility), as well as a health care proxy or conservatorship (which enables that person to make binding decisions about health matters, including Do Not Resuscitate orders). This petition is then submitted to the local probate court. Immediately thereafter, the attending physician or psychiatrist is required to provide an opinion about the patient's mental competence. This process is ordinarily successful and will save the family untold frustrations and stress, along with enabling the patient to receive necessary supervision and medical care.

In my practice, I tend to speed up the process, because I do not believe that the patient's best interests are served by waiting until advanced dementia is present. Consequently, I ordinarily encourage a probate petition at the point where the patient is too confused to carry out normal, everyday functions—if, for example, his driving is erratic, the unpaid bills mount up or he is unjustifiably uncooperative. Again, this is a "clinical" decision and depends, in large part, upon the home environment, the degree of dementia and the willingness of the family to become active in the solution to a problem that is guaranteed to worsen.

Thus, in summary, an early legal decision is probably advisable in situations where loved ones suffer from dementia. There is no consistent timetable for such intervention, which should be made by the patient's family and health care providers.

The tragedy of Alzheimer's

Q. My grandmother has Alzheimer's disease, and it is heartbreaking to watch the withdrawal of this active, life-loving woman into a world we cannot enter. Although she no longer responds to questions, I notice some of her former personality and facial expressions seem to return when she is gently touched. Is this a common phenomenon? If so, why?

A. If your grandmother truly has Alzheimer's disease and not some other form of dementia, she may still—at times—respond to touching and caressing. But these interludes will become increasingly rare as the disease envelopes her. Recognition of and reaction to loved ones are attributes of most dementia. Unfortunately, Alzheimer's patients inexorably retreat into private, withdrawn worlds of their own. Enjoy your grandmother while you can and give her as much kindness as you can muster. Soon it will be too late.

8

Anxiety & Depression

Anxiety and depression aren't always permanent

Q. Do depression and chronic anxiety ever correct themselves? If not, what effect is produced by the long-term use of antidepressant and antianxiety drugs? What's the answer for people like me?

A. Certain forms of depression—such as those caused by normal reactions to divorce, the death of a loved one, or loss of a job—will, over time, improve. The temporary use of prescription medication may be of help in these situations.

There are, however, some depressions that bear little relation to external factors and will not self-correct; in such cases antidepressant drugs may be a godsend and are safe for long-term treatment.

Anxiety, too, often improves with time. As I'm sure you are aware, anxiety tends to appear in cycles anyway. An anxious person typically experiences repeated periods of hyper-anxiety, superimposed on a more-or-less constant background of low-grade apprehension. Antianxiety medicine should not be used for indefinite intervals, in my view; most of these drugs do have a potential for abuse and habituation.

The answer for people like you, who may not be incapacitated by anxiety/depression and do not wish to take medication, may be counseling. Anxiety and depression, providing the combination is not too severe, can often be helped by "talking it out" with a health professional, such as a psychiatrist, psychologist, mental health counselor, minister or rabbi.

Depression in the elderly: a primer

Q. At 87, I suffer from angina and arthritis. These conditions I can handle with medicine prescribed by my very caring doctor. What I can't deal with is depression. I constantly contemplate suicide but always conclude this would be a cop-out. What I'd really like is a good belly laugh, a smile from some of my acquaintances in the nursing home and the privilege of seeing my great-grandchildren more than once a year at Christmas. Do I need an antidepressant?

A. Excellent question. Depression in the elderly is a major concern of health professionals. Symptoms of hopelessness, insomnia, loss of self-esteem and dread may reflect a hidden epidemic that devastates the over-65 age group, members of which are often too afraid, confused or embarrassed to ask for help.

In the past, depression was considered to be a purely emotional maladjustment, and little effective therapy was available. Today, however, there are dozens of medications that reverse what we now know is the cause of depression: an imbalance of serotonin in the brain.

The situation is further complicated by two very real influences: a loss of loved ones and the inescapable reality of physical diseases (such as angina and arthritis) simply confirm the depressive's perception that the future is bleak and life is not worth living. Consequently, help with a grieving process and effective therapy for physical ailments may help lift the numbing mantle of depression. Control of physical symptoms will usually provide benefit, as will effective therapy for heart disease that may simply limit a person's activities and independence.

Remember, too, that elderly patients in nursing homes have even more to deal with. In addition to the boarding-school schedules concerning activities, meals and sleep, such residents are often literally abandoned by the very family members they most cherish.

In my experience, it is a rare nursing home resident who doesn't have a phenomenally intriguing history. My most enjoyable and notable patient was Margaret Hamilton, who played the wicked witch in the classic *Wizard of Oz* movie. I'll never forget her—or her characteristic cackling laughter, which resonated frequently around the nurses' station. We professionals need to remember our clients' successes.

Finally consider that elderly people can easily become depressed because they are in the final stage of life, experience incurable ill health and discover that their friends and acquaintances have either died—or, almost worse—have themselves required nursing home care. As one of my brightest and most upbeat patients told me: "You bet I often get depressed. There's nobody my age left who isn't confused or senile. My family is preoccupied with other interests, as well they should be. I'm lonely. And I don't have a helluva lot to look forward to."

As might be predicted, fear (of the present or future) can be a substantial component of depression.

Drug therapy can literally make the difference between death and life. In the elderly, such treatment can produce truly astounding results. I urge any elderly person, whether at home or in a nursing facility, to be evaluated for depression. If this affliction is present, appropriate medication is advisable.

In addition to drug therapy, several other resources are available. Clergy can often help. Counseling is sometimes beneficial. Family members, once they appreciate the reality of the situation, can offer support. Outside interests—such as church get-togethers, cards, bingo, concerts, discussion groups and hobbies—may assist the depressed to "get out of themselves." There is nothing like a new great-grandchild or a holiday reunion to help old people feel needed and to refocus their attention on life around them. Laughter is certainly beneficial.

I think it's fair to say that depression in the elderly comes in many forms and in varying degrees of severity. Each case must be considered individually. Thus, my comments are purposefully general.

Thus, I respectfully refer you back to your primary care physician, who can prescribe—with the help of specialists, as needed—appropriate medication to treat your depression. Also, your doctor may choose to involve your family in a more "hands-on" approach. Frequent visits, trips home and holiday get-togethers could well fill a void in your life and make your growing older a more positive experience.

Depression may have physical cause

Q. In many of your columns, you seem to favor medication for physical problems but not for mental problems, such as depression.

Are you aware that many types of depression have a physical cause? In such instances, antidepressant drugs can make an enormous difference in the quality of life.

A. Many types of depressions are indeed related to the imbalance of brain chemicals. This is, as you pointed out, a physical disorder that can be helped by appropriate drugs. I am sorry if I gave the wrong impression. I take depression seriously and agree that affected patients are usually helped by drug therapy.

Of course, it's a matter of degree. People who suffer an acute and profound sense of loss—from a divorce, death of a loved one, or financial reversal, for example—usually become depressed, but can work through the difficulty without supporting the pharmaceutical industry. On the other hand, chronic depression that is not caused by situations in the environment almost always responds to the judicious use of antidepressant drugs. In such instances, medical attention and prescriptions are in order.

Nonetheless, we—as a society—rely too heavily on drugs. Many of us incorrectly believe that there is an antidote for every ailment, that happiness comes in a pill bottle, and that you can feel good simply by taking the right medication. We forget about the very real—and sometimes dangerous—side effects that any drug can produce.

> 66 I think it's fair to say that depression in the elderly comes in many forms and in varying degrees of severity. Each case must be considered individually. 99

Therefore, in my columns, I tend to harp about harmony and balance. It's all right to stop whining and get on with your life—and all of us know people who could profit by this type of tough-love advice. It's all right to exercise more (because exercise can relieve mild depression), drink less alcohol (a depressant) and rely on our gargantuan capacity to heal ourselves without medication. Each of us feels blue now and then. We get over it.

My comments are not meant to malign the very real problem of depression that millions of people experience. Such patients, after a thorough medical examination (to rule out hypothyroidism, anemia and other causes of depression), can lead happier and more productive lives if given antidepressant drugs. Depression is real; it can be incapacitating, but it is treatable. Yet, as is true with any medication, we must carefully weigh the risk-benefit ratio.

Anxiety shouldn't always be avoided

Q. Please discuss the medication Xanax. What are the specific symptoms of addiction? How can I be certain that the sensations I feel are due to underlying anxiety and not a need for the drug? I confess that I have taken a generous daily amount of Xanax for several years, but I would really like to cut back or discontinue the drug, a decision that, in and of itself, makes me terribly anxious!

A. Xanax (alprazolam) is used to treat excessive anxiety. Although it may cause drowsiness and light-headedness, it is surprisingly safe and free of side effects, when used appropriately under medical supervision. Nonetheless, like many similar pharmaceuticals (such as Valium and Librium), Xanax does have a potential for addiction if taken regularly, in high doses and for extended periods. This is the reason that most responsible physicians prescribe it only for brief courses of therapy or for low-dose, long-term treatment of disorders such as insomnia. If you have taken the drug regularly and constantly for more than a few weeks, your body may have become habituated to the compound. In this instance, were you to discontinue Xanax suddenly, you might suffer from insomnia, nervousness, vomiting, sweating, tremors and muscle cramps. Thus, any effort to reduce the dose of medicine should involve a health care professional.

Unfortunately, the symptoms of anxiety (which led to the Xanax in the first place) may mimic the symptoms of withdrawal. This is the reason I suggest a gradual reduction in dosage. Be sure to check with your doctor about this if you choose to discontinue the Xanax.

I'd like to close my answer in a somewhat extended and nonconformist manner. I want to give a locomotive cheer and a standing ovation for anxiety. Yes, you read this correctly: I'm pro-anxiety. Here's why.

There's a modern, troubling tendency among well-informed adults to view any degree of anxiety or emotional discomfort as something bad—worse, un-American. More and more folks express the mistaken conviction that freedom from anxiety and worry is an inherent right, for which instant relief is mandatory. If you believe these people, you'll get into trouble sooner or later by treating (normal) anxiety with a couple of drinks, a marijuana joint or a little tranquilizer pill.

Anxiety, like an annoying case of hemorrhoids, is often misperceived as something abnormal, a feeling to be got rid of as quickly as possible. (I'm not referring to debilitating anxiety of the sort caused by terrorism. That needs to be addressed professionally and realistically.)

It's all too easy, in our headlong rush toward Nirvana, to forget the trade-offs: The very drugs (licit and illicit) that we use may have terrible consequences, such as addiction. Thus, many people trade in their anxiety for a lifetime of drug servitude. This lousy deal is one of the reasons that alcoholism and drug addiction are such enormous public health concerns today.

Therefore, I'm eager to go on record as saying that most anxiety is normal. It's part of the human condition. Rather than burying it in a pharmacological mulch pile, we need to use it constructively. Very often, it's nature's way of telling us to look sharp, make changes, alter our attitudes, cope, grow—not to self medicate into a state of somnambulistic indifference. It's not the anxiety that matters; it's the way we handle it that counts.

Alcoholics often whine: "If you had my problems, you'd be a heavy drinker, too." Bull. That's just an excuse, not a reason. Years ago, Valium was the most briskly sold tranquilizer in the world. Its misuse led to a generation of sedated, addicted victims who floated through life without touching ground. These people chose to avoid the perfectly normal experience of living—with all its attendant grief, emotional pain, frustration, discouragement and anxiety. By tranquilizing themselves, they also avoided the happiness and satisfaction that are part of the human existence and may, at least in some of us, overshadow the negative, unavoidable aspects.

So, valued reader, revel in your anxiety. Use it to make needed alterations in your life. Instead of relying on medicine or drugs to relieve your emotional discomfort, talk it out with a friend or counselor. Don't cave in to the liquor/pharmaceutical lobby. Slowly discontinue the Xanax under medical supervision. Begin to feel and don't be afraid of those feelings. Get help if you think you need it but, above all, let go of the conviction that anxiety is something to be avoided at all costs. This approach works. In fact, I feel less anxious just having written this column.

Anxiety attacks aren't abnormal

Q. I've heard more and more people say they have anxiety attacks. What are they talking about?

A. Anxiety attacks are episodes of nervousness and apprehension. They are milder than panic attacks. Anxiety is a universal, unpleasant sensation of tension, fearfulness and irritability. We all experience some type of anxiety on a regular basis. Most forms of anxiety need no treatment; the person copes with an uncomfortable situation and the anxiety goes away.

Many people believe that tension and anxiety are "unnatural," and they try to eliminate them by using tranquilizers or other medications, "recreational" drugs and/or alcohol. This belief is wrong—and the "cures" can be damaging. Anxiety is a normal human emotion. If people accept it as such, they will deal more effectively with stress and not have to rely on drugs or alcohol. In most cases, these simply cover up the anxiety, prevent people from finding satisfactory solutions to problems—and also can lead to habituation or abuse.

In short: Pain or distress, whether physical or emotional, mean that something's wrong and must be treated or resolved. This isn't done by covering up the symptoms.

Battling the terror of panic attacks

Q. What information can you provide on panic attacks? I've had several and medication doesn't seem to help. Can they be chemically caused?

A. No one knows if panic attacks have a biochemical basis, but the possibility exists.

In many cases, panic disorder can be quite disabling. The patient suddenly (and for no reason) experiences periods of nameless terror, haunting dread and fear of imminent catastrophe, often associated with trembling, shaking, rapid pulse, sweating, dizziness, nausea, hyperventilation, and other symptoms.

Psychological counseling is usually required if the panic attacks are severe. Antianxiety prescription drugs, such as Ativan or Xanax, often reduce—or even eliminate—the severity of the panic disorder and are used for short periods in conjunction with counseling.

If you have continuing attacks despite therapy, you should seek the services of a psychiatrist, who may prescribe stronger medication, such as major tranquilizers.

Excessive anxiety is treatable

Q. Please discuss chronic anxiety. My doctor hasn't been much help.

A. Chronic anxiety, the vague feeling that something's not right (coupled with the diffuse fear of unidentified future catastrophes), is a common disorder that has, unfortunately, been enormously (and understandably) magnified by the events of September 11, 2001. Anxiety can be truly disabling. The worry about death, divorce, one's children and new challenges—you know what I mean if you're over the age of 10—can disrupt a life and lead to serious depression and health consequences (such as alcohol and drug abuse).

However, a mild/moderate degree of anxiety is normal. We all experience it as a result of life and the world at large. Unlike people who rant about every little uncertainty, I believe that some anxiety is a healthful part of the human condition.

Nonetheless, severe anxiety can be a terrible handicap. In such cases, counseling and prescription drugs (such as Ativan and Xanax) may be enormously helpful. Medicine is appropriate for short-term treatment of chronic anxiety, while psychiatrists, psychologists, social workers or experienced clergy try to put issues into better perspective. This enables patients to cope more effectively and achieve a better balance in their lives.

Some forms of anxiety are caused by metabolic imbalances in the brain. These need to be addressed with appropriate prescription medications. In other instances, anxiety in one person may be routine for another. Consequently, most individuals will feel relieved once they realize that they don't have to be victims of their worries and apprehensions. In short, they truly have a choice about whether or not to be anxious. This is where counseling is really important.

If your doctor has been unable to assist you with your anxiety, I suggest that you investigate the resources I mentioned. With the judicious use of antianxiety medicines and counseling, I'm sure you can be helped.

Valium may not be appropriate treatment for anxiety

Q. I disagree with your conclusions in a recent column that people with severe anxiety do not need Valium. I suffer from this condition, and without the drug, my life would be in shambles. You advised the reader to put up with the anxiety or seek alternative treatment. Obviously, you have not experienced anxiety disorder. I have tried herbal remedies, massage, yoga and psychotherapy, to no avail. Please print a retraction.

A. What is needed here is not a retraction but a clarification.

Valium used to be the drug of choice for treating anxiety disorders. However, the medication has a high potential for habituation and abuse. Therefore, I discourage its use—except on occasion—for this affliction.

By alternative therapy, I was suggesting a safer and more suitable option—Xanax or Ativan. Both these medications are marketed specifically for anxiety and can appropriately be used, in small doses, for extended periods. For those patients with depression-related anxiety, Paxil is a good choice.

I am sorry for any confusion. I was merely attempting to inform my anxious reader of newer treatments for the condition rather than having him rely solely on a medicine that could lead to long-term problems.

Treatment of anxiety

Q. I have experienced recurring anxiety attacks for more than 10 years, for which I take Xanax. Now my doctor wants to switch me to Librium, yet my pharmacist assures me that one or two Xanax tablets a day will not harm me. What's your opinion?

A. I believe that people should avoid medicine whenever possible. No matter how safe a drug is supposed to be, unusual and unexpected side effects may occur, in addition to the predictable complications that come with the territory.

For example, Xanax (alprazolam, an antianxiety agent) is generally considered to be a safe medication to control excess tension. The manufacturer lists drowsiness, depression, dry mouth, headache, constipation (or diarrhea) and nausea as the most common side effects.

However, the medicine can also cause irritability, poor concentration, addiction, amnesia, loss of coordination, fatigue, slurred speech, jaundice, weakness, double vision, incontinence and menstrual irregularities. Furthermore, "paradoxical" reactions can appear: agitation, rage, muscle spasms, sleep disturbances and hallucinations.

Despite the low incidence of these serious reactions, a patient must weigh the benefits of therapy against the potential risks. Incidentally, Librium is related to Xanax: The side effects of the two drugs are similar.

Here is your quandary: Do you put up with the occasional anxiety attacks or treat them with medicine that can be habit-forming and cause additional, unwanted problems? In my opinion, doctors and patients have been too willing to take the path of least resistance: drug treatment.

I suggest that you consider non-drug therapy in the form of counseling, stress management, transcendental meditation, prayer and other methods to reduce your level of apprehension. Some degree of anxiety is a normal ingredient in human living. It's wrong to assume that all anxiety is abnormal, unhealthful and must be eliminated.

You can probably learn ways of relieving tension without drugs. In

Mental Health Professionals

A number of health care professionals are trained to treat mental and emotional illnesses. Only a psychiatrist, however, can prescribe drugs, which may be necessary for serious mental illness. "Psychotherapist" and "counselor" are general terms sometimes used to refer to all these professionals. Here is a list of mental health professionals who treat adults and a brief description of their training.

Psychiatrists

These are medical doctors who have taken a three-year residency in the field. (Legally, any physician with a medical license can practice psychiatry, so inquire about specialized training.) After completing a residency and practicing for two years, the psychiatrist is eligible for certification by the American Board of Psychiatry and Neurology.

Psychologists

Clinical or counseling psychologists may perform psychotherapy in a clinic setting or private practice. To be licensed or certified to practice independently, most states require a doctoral degree and one to two years of practice under supervision in an approved setting. Psychologists with the proper training and experience are eligible to become diplomates of the American Board of Professional Psychologists.

Psychiatric social workers

These professionals have master's degrees in social work, including clinical training. They may work in clinics or in private practice. They can be certified by the Academy of Certified Social Workers after two years of practice and an exam.

Psychoanalysts

These are psychologists, psychiatrists or social workers who have had specialized training in psychoanalysis, in addition to the training for their primary degrees.

Psychiatric nurses

They are registered professional nurses who have received a master's or more advanced degree that qualifies them to do certain types of mental health counseling. They usually work in community programs or hospitals rather than in private practice.

a sense, changing form Xanax to Librium is like changing deck chairs on the Titanic. I advise you to use medicine only when absolutely necessary.

Varied types of emotional illness

Q. How can you tell if you've had a nervous breakdown?

A. The term "nervous breakdown" is often used to describe a mental or emotional crisis that make normal life impossible or requires hospitalization. However, "nervous breakdown" isn't a medical term or a diagnosis; this type of crisis can be caused by a variety of disorders.

A "breakdown" may be triggered by an overload of stress, anxiety or depression; it can also occur with such disorders as schizophrenia, manic depression or endogenous depression, and thus be unrelated to outside events.

A person who is heading for this type of emotional crisis may detect some warning signs: ill temper, a feeling of loss of control, exhaustion or hyperactivity, a distortion of reality, the development of certain irrational or eccentric opinions and convictions, and antisocial behavior (such as becoming isolated, developing obsessive or self-destructive habits, or becoming verbally abusive or violent). He or she also might begin to use mind-altering substances to escape overwhelming anxiety or depression.

Drugs themselves can cause a "nervous breakdown." The mental alterations caused by alcohol, crack, heroin, cocaine, marijuana and hallucinogens are indistinguishable from those seen in deeply disturbed patients—and these changes can occur with so-called "recreational use."

Treatment depends on the problem's severity. Counseling, or counseling and medication, are helpful in many cases. However, hospitalization is necessary if the patient can't manage daily life or poses a danger to himself or others.

As a general rule, anyone who begins to question or fear for his or her sanity should get professional help. Psychiatrists (M.D.s), psychologists, therapists and other mental health professionals either can help patients with their emotional problems or can refer them to specialists if necessary. In addition to private help, most communities offer mental health services for little or no fee.

People with drug or alcohol problems usually need medical intervention because of physical dependence. Help is available for a concerned friend or a distraught spouse, as well as for the patient.

9

Lungs & Things Respiratory

What is emphysema?

Q. My 58-year-old cousin has emphysema, and I am his sole care-taker. What is emphysema, and what can I expect in the future?

A. Emphysema is a chronic lung disease marked by destruction of the alveolar air sacs, the tiny compartments where oxygen and carbon dioxide exchange takes place.

The lungs are really a huge, thin membrane that permits gases to pass between the air and the blood. By dividing this membrane into innumerable, microscopic pockets, Nature has provided far more surface area for gas exchange than would be possible with a single membranous sheet. Thus, the lungs are a natural marvel because they contain square yards of active membrane, compressed into a relatively small space. This results in an extremely efficient system of gas exchange within a limited area.

Emphysema destroys this efficiency. The disease is the result of genetic factors, infection and/or pulmonary irritants that break down the walls of the alveolar sacs, causing them to collapse and coalesce, which reduces breathing ability.

In the presence of emphysema, the lungs become overfilled with stale air, which is trapped in large, inefficient pouches called bullae. These bullae prevent oxygen from diffusing into the bloodstream; as they expand over time, they also press on surrounding lung tissue, further reducing breathing capacity.

Therefore, emphysema patients are usually breathless at rest because they cannot obtain enough oxygen or expel enough carbon dioxide waste. Exercise, of course, merely aggravates the situation, so, severe emphysema is invariably associated with marked pulmonary disability.

Emphysema patients also tend to have "barrel chests" because the rib cage expands to accommodate the accumulation of trapped, stale air. Eventually, emphysema leads to the consequences of low blood-oxygen, such as heart failure, mental deterioration and, at the end, respiratory failure.

Although the damage from emphysema is permanent and incurable, the destruction of lung tissue can be arrested and treated. Patients must stop smoking (the major cause of emphysema) and avoid air pollution (which can further damage the lungs). In my experience, people who adopt these measures often experience a significant improvement in breathing, probably because avoidance of tobacco smoke and other pollutants reduces mucus production and plugging in the remaining functional pulmonary tissue.

Further, treatment of emphysema itself is beneficial. This includes special breathing exercises, antibiotics to eradicate infection, steroids to reduce inflammation and supplemental oxygen delivered through a plastic hose to prongs placed in the nostrils. In some patients with advanced disease, doctors can surgically deflate and remove large bullae (which serve no useful purpose), thereby allowing more normal pulmonary tissue to expand and function. This operation, which is relatively new, shows great promise.

Although I have made smoking cessation the cornerstone of emphysema therapy, it may be a difficult choice for some smokers—even with modern antismoking strategies, such as nicotine gum, patches and inhalers. A personal note: I completed part of my residency training at New York City's Bellevue Hospital. We had, at that time, an emphysema patient whose disease was so severe that he required the use of an iron lung for survival. He was placed in this device, which virtually breathed for him, for 23 hours a day. For one hour a day, he was taken out of the tubular machine and wheeled out of the ward—for a cigarette!

In caring for your cousin, you can expect that he will need a lot of help in coping with the disease. He should follow my suggestions and his doctor's instructions. Respiratory therapy, medications and possible surgery are certainly reasonable options. By the way, his environment should be free of pollution. That means no smoking in the house; also, visitors or family members with colds or upper respiratory infections should avoid contact with your cousin, unless they wear suitable protective masks.

Emphysema is treatable

Q. I just lost a close relative to emphysema, and I'm very hurt and angry. This person never smoked. How come we have space shuttles, space stations, nuclear bombs and men walking on the moon—but no cure for this lung disease? Is it that people just don't care?

A. You raise several pertinent questions.

First, the occurrence of emphysema in nonsmokers. While tobacco smoke is the leading cause of lung disease in the United States, emphysema is also associated with other factors, such as air pollution (including chemical fumes, hazardous dust, occupational exposure to silica and others), chronic airway hyperreactivity (such as asthma) and alpha-1 antitrypsin deficiency (an inherited disorder that can be diagnosed by blood tests and treated with a variety of medications and general health measures). Perhaps your relative worked in a high-risk environment or had a genetic disposition to emphysema.

> 66 *If a person with chronic bronchitis stops smoking, avoids air pollution and obtains antibiotics for infection, the condition can be cured, mucus secretions lessen, cough disappears and breathing becomes more normal.* 99

Second, during the grieving period following a loss, people feel hurt, angry and frustrated, which is normal. With time—I hope—you will be able to put your relative's death behind you and accept what happened. In the meantime, trying to place responsibility on society, the government or the medical profession will be counterproductive and lead to more frustration. For example, you don't mention in your letter whether your relative's emphysema was diagnosed early on, how it was treated and why the death occurred. (With modern treatment—including surgery, drugs and oxygen therapy—most emphysema patients can have normal—albeit restrictive—existences.) Perhaps you should question your relative's doctors about these issues. If your concerns can be answered clearly and honestly, your rage and grief may be ameliorated.

Third, the public and our legislators are often more intrigued by "sexy" issues, such as space travel and weapons, than they are by diseases. Nevertheless, there is considerable ongoing research being carried out on pulmonary disorders and their treatment. Sometimes, in medicine, answers to such issues take time and patience. Is's not so much a question of "caring"—after all, we all care—as it is a problem of resources and focus. In a sense, despite the extraordinary medical advances in the past few decades, medical professionals are still at a very primitive stage. As I have written before, diseases will eventually be shown to have genetic bases—so effective therapy will undoubtedly involve gene splicing, but that reality is still many years away. A walk on the moon is a simple challenge in comparison to the discovery of a vaccine, for example, that will prevent cancer and heart disease.

Please examine your expectations. Are they realistic and appropriate? And, by all means, attempt to discover the medical details of your relative's disease.

Smoking and COPD

Q. I'm a 51-year-old widow who recently had to switch to a new doctor who seems to be about the age of my grandson. After examining me and performing routine blood tests (and a cardiogram), he indicated that all were fine. He had formerly asked if I used tobacco and I told him I smoke a pack a day. I didn't read my receipt until I got home. Rather than listing hypertension that I know I have, he diagnosed me with COPD. I returned to his office for clarification and was told that he lists this diagnosis for anyone who has smoked for more than a year. I'm furious and would appreciate your comments.

A. Chronic obstructive pulmonary disease is most commonly caused by cigarette smoking, but is also associated with the inhalation of other pulmonary irritants, such as smog and dust. Basically, COPD is the consequence of both bronchitis (inflammation of the breathing passages) and emphysema (enlargement of the air spaces within the lungs). COPD is associated with chronic cough, breathlessness on exertion, recurring respiratory infections, weakness and weight loss.

The disease is diagnosed by a battery of tests, including X-rays and analysis of breathing efficiency (pulmonary function studies). Treatment includes antibiotics, drugs to dilate the bronchial passageways, special breathing exercises, and supplemental oxygen in advanced cases. Tobacco products are, for obvious reasons, prohibited.

I believe that your new doctor was premature in his assessment. I am particularly concerned that he labeled you with COPD solely on the basis of your smoking history, without the testing I mentioned. This is a bit like claiming someone is an alcoholic merely because he has a couple of cocktails a day. In my opinion, your doctor was in error and I can well understand why you are upset.

Rather than acting impulsively, you physician may actually be trying to "generate" a list of diagnoses so that your insurance company would more readily pay his bill. For instance, some health plans will refuse to reimburse the doctor for office visits due to trivial complaints, such as colds, but will promptly pay for chronic disorders, such as COPD.

In any case, I agree that his Pavlovian stance (stimulus/response; smoking/COPD) was imprudent.

Raise this issue with him and demand a referral to a pulmonary specialist for definitive testing. In our strange new world of medical insurance and HMOs, a diagnosis of COPD that goes unchallenged could come back to haunt you; you could conceivably lose your insurance, pay more in premiums or be unable to obtain any health coverage. (Insurance companies do not welcome clients with chronic diseases.)

Finally, I believe that this experience should be a wake-up call. Perhaps your physician noted certain features during your exam that suggested early COPD. In any case, it's probably time for you to discontinue cigarettes; if you're not in trouble now, you almost certainly will be in the future.

More on COPD

Q. I'm interested in obtaining information about obstructive pulmonary disease and other lung disorders. My father is handicapped because of this affliction and requires around-the-clock oxygen therapy. Is there any hope for him?

A. Chronic obstructive pulmonary disease is an exceptionally serious lung ailment, marked by low levels of oxygen in the blood and high levels of carbon dioxide retention. These abnormalities are the direct result of alterations in lung function, notably loss of alveolar air sacs (where oxygen is normally exchanged for carbon dioxide), pulmonary scarring and increased mucus secretions. COPD is a common consequence of smoking, air pollution and many lung disorders, including chronic bronchitis and asthma.

Treatment consists of drugs to release bronchial spasm, reduce mucus discharge, eliminate infection and improve ventilation. Such drugs often include steroids and supplemental oxygen therapy. Special breathing exercises may help.

In my opinion, your father should be under the care of a pulmonologist, who can prescribe the necessary medications, monitor his progress and offer suggestions about further therapy (such as surgery, if your father has certain forms of emphysema).

Also you may wish to contact the local chapter of your lung association for brochures and other written material.

COPD responds to oxygen therapy

Q. I'm a 62-year-old woman with COPD (chronic obstructive pulmonary disease), have little stamina, and get short-winded when I perform minimal exercise. I'm sure that smoking cigarettes for 40 years hasn't helped the situation. I live in a community at 6,000 feet and my doctor has suggested that I move to another area. Where in the United States is the air oxygen-rich? I really need to investigate this thoroughly because I hate to move away from my friends, daughter and grandson.

A. Patients who suffer from chronic obstructive pulmonary disease are unable to get enough oxygen into their blood streams, leading to shortness of breath and diminished stamina. For this reason, such patients are helped by breathing supplemental oxygen, delivered through nasal prongs from a tank of oxygen or an oxygen concentrator.

Because supplemental oxygen is so readily available, most physicians simply prescribe it rather than insisting that their patients move to other parts of the country.

Remember that the higher the altitude, the thinner the air and the less oxygen. Thus, if a change in residence is the option you choose, you'll have to consider communities at or near sea level, such as the Midwest or along the coasts. Even so, you will probably have to consider supplemental oxygen. Nonetheless, the lower the altitude, the richer the oxygen supply in the air.

As part of your decision, you will want to consider other factors as well, the primary one being air pollution. Therefore, I'd recommend avoiding dense, urban, industrial areas, such as New York City or Los Angeles, where air pollution can be much more dangerous than high altitudes.

Frankly, I'd stay where you are and use supplemental oxygen, an option that would be far less drastic and expensive than leaving friends and family for a faraway residence. Let me know what you decide to do—and, by all means, get a boost from supplemental oxygen.

Ways to stop smoking

Q. My husband has always been a slim man, but now he is as thin as a rail, coughs constantly and has no appetite. He has smoked one or two packs of cigarettes a day since he was a teenager. Could the cigarette smoke affect his taste buds?

A. It certainly could—as well as significantly diminishing his appetite. However, I'm less concerned about these consequences than I am about the potential damage to his lungs. Weight loss and chronic cough in an adult smoker always should raise suspicion that an undiagnosed, serious ailment is present. For instance, lung cancer and chronic obstructive pulmonary disease are common manifestations of the life-threatening price smokers may have to pay. In my opinion, your husband should be examined (and X-rayed) by his doctor. At the same time, the physician should appropriately insist that your husband give up cigarettes. While I'm certain that your spouse has significant nicotine addiction, he can be helped by a variety of products, including nicotine gum, patches and a nicotine inhaler. In addition, the drug Zyban may help some people overcome the initial symptoms of nicotine withdrawal. A doctor is the place to start the healing process.

Bronchitis can lead to serious consequences

Q. I have chronic bronchitis. You say it can be cured, my doctors say it can't. Please advise.

A. Chronic bronchitis is curable. With all respect to your doctors, this may be a semantic issue, not a medical disagreement.

To a large degree, the question of cure depends on the definition of the disease. In England, for example, chronic bronchitis is often lumped together with emphysema, an incurable, chronic pulmonary disorder. In the United States, however, chronic bronchitis is defined as a lung disease associated with bronchial irritants (such as infection and air pollutants), marked by excess mucus secretions and bronchial inflammation, leading to thickened bronchial walls and a persisting, productive cough.

In most cases, chronic bronchitis is almost always the consequence of bronchial irritation from tobacco smoke and other compounds, including infection, smog, smoke and soot. If a person with chronic bronchitis stops smoking, avoids air pollution and obtains antibiotics for infection, the condition can be cured, mucus secretions lessen, cough disappears and breathing becomes more normal.

Obviously, as untreated bronchitis progresses, structural lung damage—which is incurable—results. This includes airway obstruction from permanently thickened bronchial walls and, in advanced cases, actual destruction of lung tissue.

At this point, patients are said to suffer from chronic obstructive pulmonary disease (COPD).

I assume from your comments that your long-standing chronic bronchitis may have progressed to COPD. Therefore, your doctors may be correct. Your condition, although treatable, is incurable. On the other hand, if your disease is still at the level of bronchitis, it may be curable— providing you and your doctor take aggressive steps in that direction. This would include cessation of smoking, avoidance of air pollution and "secondhand" smoke, antibiotics for infection, steroids for bronchial inflammation and anti-asthma inhalers to prevent bronchial constriction.

Given the unclear medical opinion regarding your affliction, you should probably be referred to a pulmonologist, who will question and examine you, obtain additional testing (such as chest X-rays and pulmonary function assessments) and advise you about therapy. The specialist can also resolve the issue of whether your problem is curable or incurable.

Asthma may respond to antibiotics

Q. For the past 10 years, I've suffered from attacks of bronchial asthma. I use an albuterol inhaler, but experience stomach upset from cephalexin and doxycycline. What is the best substitute antibiotic?

A. Asthma is often complicated (and may even be triggered) by low-grade bronchial infection. Thus, antibiotics frequently improve the breathing difficulties of asthma. Of course, other drugs—such as albuterol and prednisone—are also used.

If you experience abdominal distress from cephalexin and doxycycline, your doctor might want to try ampicillin, amoxicillin or plain penicillin. Such antibiotics, when used to treat bronchial infection, would work well with your inhaler.

Steroids for asthma

Q. In a recent column, you advised asthmatics to use an inhaler for relief of symptoms, yet you failed to recommend steroid inhalers for prevention. As an asthmatic, I am now on Singulair and Serevent. Should I consider an inhaled steroid as well?

A. This is a question more properly directed to your primary care physician or pulmonologist.

In my experience, however, Singulair (a pill) and Serevent (an inhaler) are particularly helpful in preventing asthma. Nonetheless, steroid inhalers could also be considered. To a large degree, my answer to your question depends on your response to the nonsteroidal therapy: If the Singulair and Serevent are doing the job, stick with them. If, on the other hand, your asthma is breaking through, consider the addition of a steroid inhaler.

Pulmonary blood clots usually originate elsewhere

Q. I suffered two episodes of pulmonary blood clots in the past, one in 1987 and another in 1991, both of which were near-death experiences. Were I to experience another episode, is there newer treatment for my condition? I was originally prescribed heparin and Coumadin.

A. Pulmonary emboli (blood clots in the lungs) are usually the result of clots that break off from veins in the legs or pelvis. Anticoagulation drugs, such as heparin and Coumadin, remain the mainstay of therapy.

Nevertheless, you and your doctor might consider a meticulous investigation to discover if you have clots in the veins I mentioned. A Doppler ultrasound examination or venogram (X-ray of the veins) should indicate whether the veins in your legs and pelvis are free of clots. If they are, fine; you're in no danger. If they're blocked, however, you may have to consider a caval filter, a metal sieve that is surgically implanted in the vena cava (major abdominal vein) to prevent pieces of the clots from migrating to your lungs. Ask your doctor about this.

Asbestosis is permanent

Q. I'm a man, 75, with asbestosis. Although I'm in good health and don't smoke, I tire easily and become winded during the slightest exertion. Can you suggest exercises or medications that might help me?

A. I'm afraid not.

Asbestosis is a serious, chronic lung disease resulting from the long-term inhalation of asbestos fibers in the mining, milling and manufacturing occupations—or in jobs related to the use of asbestos insulation, such as contracting and plumbing. Also, asbestos-related pulmonary problems may be seen in auto repair shops because brake drums are often lined with asbestos.

Once inhaled, these microscopic crystal fibers embed in lung tissue, leading—over time—to pronounced scarring and inflammation, breathlessness and exercise intolerance. Asbestos is also associated with two forms of pulmonary malignancy: primary lung cancer and mesothelioma.

Asbestosis is easily prevented by the use of appropriate breathing filters and masks. The federal government has taken an aggressive position vis-a-vis prevention. Consequently, asbestos-related lung disease is primarily a problem in people who years ago worked in high-risk environments—such as ship building—before the hazards of the compound were fully appreciated and addressed.

Unfortunately, once present, asbestosis is incurable and leads to progressive lung malfunction. Nonetheless, treatment of symptoms—with special breathing exercises, supplemental oxygen and the services of a respiratory specialist—often help these patients to lead relatively independent lives.

Radiation pneumonia is not pneumonia

Q. Please explain the cause and symptoms of radiation pneumonia.

A. Radiation does not cause pneumonia, a lung infection; it causes pneumonitis, lung inflammation. This distinction is important because pneumonia, being an infection, is usually cured by antibiotics, whereas pneumonitis is ordinarily helped by cortisone drugs.

Large doses of radiation, such as those required to treat cancer, produce inflamed tissues, much the same way that strong sunlight causes sunburn. The X-ray therapy may lead to pneumonitis, cough, excess mucus secretion, short windedness, and shadows on the chest X-ray—in short, all the symptoms and signs of pneumonia, without microorganisms being present.

Untreated radiation pneumonitis often progresses to pulmonary fibrosis, permanent and severe scarring of the lungs. Because steroid drugs reduce inflammation, they are often useful in alleviating the pulmonary changes of pneumonitis.

Excessive doses of whole-body radiation of the type that follows nuclear disasters, such as the Chernobyl incident, cause eventual death because vital tissues, notably the bone marrow, are damaged, leading to diseases such as leukemia.

Therefore, in this country, the most common cause of radiation pneumonitis is cancer therapy; in these instances, the lung inflammation is merely the price one has to pay for receiving the treatment for cancer. The judicious use of cortisone is the accepted antidote for this unavoidable complication.

Inhalers usually safe

Q. I am 79 and have asthma. I've had inhalers for about 10 years, yet recently saw on television that such inhalers are dangerous and could kill. Do I have any other options?

A. Don't be sandbagged by the media. It's true that overuse of asthma inhalers may worsen the disorder and lead to fatal consequences, such as heart irregularities. But, in most instances, these products are a godsend for patients and should not be discarded on the basis of incomplete information.

Several of my asthmatic patients have asked me similar questions. My answer is the same: As long as an asthmatic is not overusing the sprays and has no known contraindications—such as uncontrolled hypertension or unstable heart disease—I see no reason to discontinue this very effective asthma therapy.

On the other hand, doctors for years have recognized that the overuse of asthma inhalers may worsen breathing and lead to fatalities. What can I say? Each consumer must carefully balance the benefits versus the risks of any therapy. In my experience as a child who suffered regular, severe nocturnal attacks of asthma (before inhalers were available), the inhalers have been a breakthrough. The devices really do help. I advise you to continue your inhaler on an as-needed basis, check with your family doctor about newer remedies to prevent and treat asthma and forget about the media hype.

Breathlessness may indicate heart disease

Q. My 65-year-old wife suffers from recurring attacks of breathlessness at night in bed. When this happens, it scares both of us, but my wife can overcome the problem by getting out of bed, then standing or sitting. She has recently seen her primary care physician, who isn't concerned and said, "Maybe I'll speak to a pulmonary specialist," but he never has. We're at our wit's end and hope you can tell us what to do.

A. The causes of breathlessness at night are varied. Perhaps your wife has an undiagnosed lung disorder, such as asthma, that could be easily treated with an inhaler to release the pulmonary spasms and aid breathing. Or she could—at least in theory—be suffering from a type of panic attack.

However, I am most concerned about the possibility of a heart disorder. In such instances, the cardiac contractions are weak and allow fluid form the bloodstream to leak from the pulmonary capillaries and invade lung tissue. Called paroxysmal nocturnal dyspnea (PND), the fluid buildup occurs only at night when a person is lying flat and gravity does not force fluid into the lower parts of the body.

If your wife does, indeed, have PND, the situation can readily be diagnosed by heart tests, including a cardiac ultrasound, and easily treated with medication. Therefore, I think she should be examined by a cardiologist, either before or after she sees a pulmonary specialist.

While I'm not second-guessing your wife's doctor—and not assuming that her symptom is frightfully serious—I would feel relieved (as would she) to know that a heart condition is not the cause.

Tuberculosis again on the rise

Q. My Mexican friend was diagnosed with tuberculosis. Is it contagious?

A. Without a doubt. And this is what makes it such a serious public health menace. Travelers to (or immigrants from) third world countries may be unknowingly infected, and bring the disease to the United States.

Tuberculosis, or TB, is primarily a lung infection, spread by water droplets (breathing and coughing) from an infected person.

After several years of declining prevalence, TB is once again on the rise. Most significant is that up to 20 percent of cases are resistant to antimicrobial therapy.

Consequently, TB is rapidly becoming a major public health problem. You and any individuals who came into contact with the infected person should be tested for TB. This can be done by skin tests. Ask your doctor about this.

10

Allergies

Treatment of common allergies

Q. I have a terrible time with allergies, especially during the spring and summer months. What causes them, and what can I do for relief?

A. Experts estimate that more than 40 million Americans suffer from inhalational allergies of one kind or another, and more than 16 million people rely on over-the-counter allergy medications for relief.

The most common allergies are pollens, molds, dust, feathers (in pillows), industrial fumes, insect skins and animal dander (skin scales shed by most species). Once an allergen enters the body, it stimulates the immune system to produce protective antibodies against the foreign substance. When formed, these antibodies—complex protein molecules—are more or less permanent.

When the allergen again reenters the body days, weeks or months later, it reacts with the antibodies, leading to the release of naturally occurring chemical mediators, of which histamine is a prime example. Actually, it's the histamine, not the allergen itself, that causes the inflammation and irritation leading to congestion, excess mucous secretion and the other symptoms so familiar to allergy sufferers.

Consequently, antihistamine medications are the time-honored treatment for acute inhalational allergies. Many—such as diphenhydramine, Chlortrimeton and (recently) Claritin—are available without a prescription. The new prescription antihistamines—Allegra, Zyrtec, Clarinex and others—have revolutionized the treatment of allergies because these products do not cause sedation and have very low side-effect profiles. Moreover, they are marketed in time-release, once-a-day formulations, making dosing convenient.

Nonetheless, patients with severe or incapacitating allergies may have to consider desensitization injections, compounded by allergists, administered at regular intervals and tailor-made to a person's specific allergy pattern. Such injections are extremely effective because they reprogram the immune system to diminish the allergen/antibody reaction and reduce the production of histamine and other mediators.

However, the shots are expensive and require a long-term commitment by the patient. Further, in rare cases, the recipient may experience a life-threatening allergic reaction, such as asthma or shock, to the injections themselves. (These unpredictable consequences can be avoided by careful attention to dosage; the shots should be administered in a doctor's office where anti-shock epinephrine injections are instantly available.)

By far and away, the safest and most satisfactory solution to allergies is avoidance of allergens. Here are 15 tips.

1) Avoid outdoor activities in the spring and summer between 5 A.M. and 10 A.M., when pollen levels are at their highest.

2) Keep car and home windows closed during allergy season.

3) Avoid super cooling the insides of home or auto. Ten degrees cooler than outside is ideal; lower temperatures may aggravate allergy symptoms.

4) Keep air conditioners and humidifiers scrupulously clean to prevent mold or pollen buildup in the machinery and filters.

5) Wear sunglasses or other eye protection when outdoors to protect eyes from pollen.

6) Wear a face mask over the nose and mouth when gardening or lawn mowing. Keep the lawn trimmed short because clipped grass is far less likely to bloom and pollinate.

7) Shower and shampoo following pollen exposure to wash away material that could cause a reaction hours later.

8) Don't hang clothes outside to dry. Use an indoor dryer where the fabrics cannot collect pollen.

9) Use hypo-allergenic mattresses and pillows—or cover such articles with special allergen-proof casings.

10) Vacuum box springs and upholstery frequently to reduce dust.

11) Minimize the use of rugs and carpets in the house. Hard floor coverings (or no coverings at all) are less likely to harbor allergy-producing dusts and pollens.

12) Restrict pets to certain rooms—never the bedroom—or keep them outside. If possible, people with dander allergies should refrain from keeping domestic animals.

13) Prohibit smoking in your environment. If you're a smoker, stop.

14) Swear off alcohol during the pollen season. Such beverages contribute to swelling in the nasal passages.

15) Plan vacations away from your home-pollinated area to pollen-free locations.

While I realize that some of these suggestions are more than extreme, they are valid nonetheless. My advice to patients troubled by allergies is to make appropriate changes that are feasible, take one of the prescription antihistamines I mentioned and see an allergist if symptoms persist or are intolerable.

Three options for cat allergy

Q. I am terribly allergic to cats. However, I have a beautiful cat to whom I am very attached.

Because of a prostate problem, I cannot take over-the-counter decongestant medications. My doctor has given me shots, which are ineffective. I don't want to get rid of my cat. What can I do to relieve my allergic reaction?

A. Many antihistamines, especially those to which decongestants have been added, may slow urination in men with enlarged prostate glands. Furthermore, most nonprescription antihistamines have the additional disadvantage of sedation, which can make daytime use troublesome.

Some patients in your situation would bite the bullet and hustle their felines off to another home.

Other patients might consider desensitization injections administered by a trained allergist.

As a third option, I suggest the prescription antihistamine Allegra, which is safe, non-sedating and has not been reported to affect the urinary tract. Ask your doctor about this.

Hives result from allergies

Q. What are urticaria?

A. Urticaria are simply hives—allergic reactions in the skin caused by a wide variety of agents, ranging from stress to pollen or drug sensitivity. The hives itch, appear as slightly raised irregular patches, and can disappear rapidly only to form on another portion of skin. Treatment includes cold compression, antihistamine drugs, and steroids (for severe cases). Urticaria are not by themselves harmful, but they can be maddening and may reflect a serious allergy that should be addressed. Therefore, a person with repeated or extensive attacks of hives should consult an allergist and have special testing to identify the cause of the urticaria.

Nose & Throat

Treat strep throat to avoid more serious problems

Q. What is the significance of a strep throat? What makes strepto-cocci so special?

A. Streptococci are merely yet another group of bacteria that cause human disease. They commonly infect the throat, to cause marked pain and fever.

Unlike other bacteria, strep have an unusual feature: untreated infection may lead to additional, more serious disorders, such as rheumatic fever and kidney disease (nephritis).

Therefore, the significance of a strep throat is that it can, if untreated, result in adverse consequences elsewhere in the body.

A simple throat culture will diagnose strep infection, which can easily and inexpensively be cured with several days of penicillin or a similar antibiotic.

Sinus problem may be allergies

Q. Why is it so difficult to get relief from a sinus problem? I've suffered for 35 years, have been to ear-nose-and-throat specialists and continue to be miserable all the time.

A. I wish I could help you. Have you considered seeing an allergist? Perhaps your "sinus" problem isn't sinus at all. Allergic reactions, such as rhinitis, can cause sinus congestion and are easily treated with antihistamines and steroid nose sprays.

Sinus surgery should be last resort

Q. After a prolonged episode of explosive coughing, fever, malaise and headache, I was referred to an ear-nose-and-throat specialist, who ordered a CT scan of my sinuses. Bingo! The study confirmed significant infection in four of my sinuses.

Nonprescription Drugs Have Side Effects

Q. Can over-the-counter drugs be harmful?

A. In certain circumstances, yes.

Nonprescription drugs provide substantial profits for the pharmaceutical industry, as well as a genuine concern among health professionals. OTC medications are increasingly in demand. It's not that these drugs cost less than their prescribed counterparts. Quite the reverse. Gram for gram, they cost about the same. Moreover, patients' health insurance may cover prescription medicines—but not the same drug in OTC form. Thus, the main advantage of these compounds is, for people eager to take more control over their health, convenience.

OTC products can pose some dangers. For example, patients taking prescribed antidepressants may become confused and delirious from timed-release cold capsules. Many OTC cough-and-cold medications can raise blood pressure, worsen glaucoma, cause drowsiness, affect coordination and lead to urinary retention, especially in the elderly. Aspirin and similar OTC analgesics frequently cause stomach upset, gastric problems and delayed blood coagulation. Acetaminophen, when consumed with alcohol, can irritate the liver.

In particular, patients can inadvertently overdose on such drugs when, for instance, they supplement prescription medications, such as high-dose Motrin, with OTC Advil or Medipren, both of which contain the same active ingredient (ibuprofen) as does Motrin.

To complicate matters further, many people don't consider OTC's to be drugs at all. Therefore, when asked by a doctor what medicines they are taking, they mistakenly fail to inform the physician of the OTC medication. This can set the stage for diagnostic dilemmas, such as indigestion and bleeding from unreported analgesics, or unpredictable and dangerous drug interactions, such as that between antihistamines and sedatives. As Americans gravitate toward OTC remedies, the phenomenon of polypharmacy emerges. Patients may self-medicate with one drug to overcome the side effects of another.

Regulations regarding OTC medicines remain relatively stringent in the United States, unlike other countries where drugs—such as antibiotics and codeine—are readily available without prescriptions. This easy access can lead to severe allergic reactions, addiction and inappropriate self-medication. However, even with strict regulations about OTC, Americans must be cautiously parsimonious in choosing to take these medications. Any substance, prescription or not, has potential side effects, can cause illness and may react unfavorably with other OTC preparations, herbal remedies and compounds.

Consumers should heed these suggestions:
• Avoid self-medicating for trivial and temporary ailments.
• Read labels carefully.
• Check with a doctor about possible drug interactions.
• Be honest with your physician about which OTC products you are taking.
• Consider OTC remedies to be as potentially hazardous as prescription drugs.
• Seek medical attention for symptoms that persist for more than a few days or recur.
• Avoid OTC drugs if you take prescription medicine, unless your doctor approves.

While OTC drugs may be convenient and easy to obtain, most are surprisingly potent and may lead to serious consequences.

The specialist prescribed an extended course of antibiotics, which I finished three weeks ago. But I am still hounded by "tight" sinuses, cough and fever. The otolaryngologist assures me that the situation will resolve, but he also says that sinus surgery might be necessary. What can I do to resolve the situation?

A. Far be it for me to diagnose your malady or suggest treatment. I can say, however, that your otolaryngologist appears to be on the mark. Like most responsible physicians, he will consider surgery only as a last resort.

In my experience, sinus infections can be very difficult to treat, in part because they are cavities in the bone and antibiotics don't easily penetrate them. Thus, you may require antibiotic therapy for several weeks, far longer than the treatment for ordinary infections.

I suggest that you follow the otolaryngologist's advice that I assume will be another four to six weeks of antibiotic coverage. Then the issue of surgery can be reconsidered.

Husky voice needs investigation

Q. When my voice became husky, I was diagnosed with a paralyzed vocal cord. How did I get this condition?

A. Each of the two vocal cords is activated by a nerve. When this nerve malfunctions, the cord becomes paralyzed. Therefore, your doctor—with the help of an ear-nose-and-throat specialist—must investigate the cause of the paralysis, which could be due to trauma (especially after neck surgery), a tumor (pressing on the nerve) or a neurological disorder (such as multiple sclerosis or stroke). Additional mechanical causes of vocal cord paralysis include aortic aneurysm (ballooning out of the upper aorta), lead poisoning and viral infection of the nerve.

I don't know how or why you developed this affliction, but I believe that your physician should do more than merely note the paralysis on examination. Additional tests to consider include CT or MRI scans to search for a growth or other correctable lesion. The vocal cord paralysis is simply a symptom; now you need a diagnosis.

Dry mouth may be due to nasal blockage

Q. I am plagued by dry mouth while sleeping. This results in frequent awakening with trips to the bathroom to use a mouthwash and brush my teeth. What can I do to overcome this?

A. If, because of nasal blockage or allergies, we breathe through our mouths (instead of our noses) at night, the constant drying action of room air may evaporate saliva and lead to "cottonmouth." By adding additional moisture to the inhaled air—by means of a humidifier—you may be able to overcome your problem with minimal inconvenience.

In addition, stop using mouthwash; many brands actually irritate the lining of the mouth, aggravating the sensation of dryness. Also, don't brush your teeth during the night because this activity will fully awaken you and disrupt your sleep. Finally, consider placing a glass of water on the bedside table so that you can take a sip, if needed, without having to get out of bed.

I should add that dry mouth is a consequence of the immune disease called Sjogren's syndrome—as well as disorders of the salivary glands—so you might consider bringing your dry mouth to your doctor's attention, just to make sure that the problem shouldn't be more aggressively addressed.

Don't support your local hanky industry

Q. What would you recommend as therapy for a lifelong postnasal drip that causes me to carry a dozen Kleenex tissues in my pocket wherever I go? My doctor has prescribed Clarinex, Allegra and Zyrtec, but the medicines give only a few hours of relief.

A. This can be a tough problem to solve, especially if you have allergies (to pollen or dust, for example), work in a dusty environment or smoke cigarettes (or live with someone who does).

Obviously, you are fed up with supporting the hanky industry and have not responded to a battery of antihistamines. Therefore, I urge you to see an allergist. After performing skin and/or blood tests, the specialist should be able to pinpoint the substance(s) to which you are reacting. Then, armed with this information, you can either attempt to avoid the irritant or undergo desensitization shots against it.

Eyes & Things Ophthalmic

Brief review of glaucoma and cataracts

Q. What are the symptoms of glaucoma and cataracts? I'm sure there are elderly people, like myself, who want to know more about these serious eye diseases.

A. Glaucoma, a pressure increase of the fluid within the eyeball, is a major cause of blindness. Its cause is unknown, and it is common in elderly patients. Symptoms include headache, halos around lights, impaired dark adaptation, blurred vision and frequent change of glasses. Treatment with drops, pills or surgery is almost always successful.

Cataracts, the progressive clouding of the clear lenses in front of the eyes, also affect vision. They are painless. Cataracts are often part of the aging process but can also be caused by diabetes, exposure to X-rays or sunlight, inflammation and certain drugs (notably cortisone).

Symptoms include progressive diminution of vision. Treatment, with lens extraction and other surgery, is curative.

Both glaucoma and cataracts should be diagnosed by professional eye specialists (either ophthalmologists or optometrists). Screening for these two diseases should be an integral part of any routine eye examination.

Hole in retina may not be repairable

Q. My wife has been diagnosed with a hole in the retina of her right eye. The optometrist states that nothing can be done to restore the vision in that eye. She is desperate, and we would value your opinion.

A. The retina is a thin coating inside the back portion of the eyeball. It is rich in nerves and enables us to see objects when light, focused by the lens, strikes the retina.

There are a variety of diseases, including detached retina and retinal degeneration, that can damage this sensitive tissue. From your brief description, I cannot diagnose your wife's affliction with certainty. Therefore, I'll give a general answer.

Retinal disorders often result from injury and, unfortunately, from the aging process. Many patients suffer from visual difficulties as they age. By and large, retinal diseases are challenging to treat; unequivocal improvement is usually more the exception than the rule.

For example, retinal degeneration, a poorly understood disease, leads to patchy areas of thinned, non-functioning retina, causing what appear on examination to be retinal "holes." This produces a spotty loss of vision because the diseased tissue does not register images. Patents ordinarily complain of visual loss, flashing lights or spots floating in the visual field. Some instances of retinal degeneration respond to special laser surgery.

So do many cases of retinal detachment, which produces similar symptoms and is associated with a painless wrinkling or pulling away of the retina from the underlying tissue.

As you can appreciate, retinal disorders require meticulous examination by eye specialists to determine whether the causes are treatable or not. Since your wife has valid concerns about her vision, I urge her to seek a second opinion from an ophthalmologist who specializes in retinal disorders. Although the optometrist may be correct, a second opinion won't hurt and might help your wife avoid progressive deterioration of her sight.

Macular degeneration relatively common in the elderly

Q. My mother visited her eye doctor recently and was told she has macular degeneration. Please discuss this devastating condition.

A. Of the plethora of eye diseases that affect vision, few are as serious as age-related macular degeneration (AMD). This disorder, of unknown causes, attacks part of the retina called the macula, the nerve cells that are responsible for central vision. Degeneration of the macula results in an inability to focus on objects. Although peripheral vision is usually spared, preventing total blindness, the loss of central vision results in a significant handicap because this vision is critical for reading, driving, recognizing people's faces, and doing detail work. Thus, AMD is the leading cause of severe loss of vision in adults over 50 years of age.

Although the exact basis of AMD remains a mystery, the condition may be hereditary. In other instances, smoking, chronic exposure to direct sunlight, a lack of vitamin A, and some medical conditions appear to play a role.

Librarian's Lament

Q. I'm a librarian. It's a rare day that someone doesn't ask me for reference material about a disease or a treatment. These people seem to come directly to the library from the doctor's office, complaining that the physician hasn't taken the time to explain a disease or the potential effects of the drugs used to treat it. It seems to me that practitioners are abrogating their responsibility, when they simply diagnose, write prescriptions and ship patients off without a word of explanation. Is my experience unusual?

A. Unfortunately not.

While most practicing doctors attempt to meet their patients' needs, not all can do so. Knowledge—as you point out—is precisely where many patients get shortchanged.

Yes, explanations take time. Yes, it's frustrating to review the same material repeatedly. Yes, some patients don't get it the first or second time.

However, I agree with you: The benefits of knowledge are enormous. And physicians ought to take this aspect of the doctor/patient relationship more seriously. Thanks for writing.

There are two types of AMD: the dry (atrophic) form and the wet (exudative) form. About 90 percent of patients have the dry type, which usually begins with the development of tiny yellow deposits (drusen) in the macula that can cause visual distortions, such as wavy lines, dark spots in the visual field and difficulty seeing fine details.

The wet form of AMD affects about 10 percent of patients, is progressive and, therefore, more serious than the dry type. It is related to the formation of abnormal blood vessels that can leak fluid and blood beneath the macula, causing more profound loss of sight.

In most cases, early AMD affects one eye only, but both eyes may eventually become impaired. This damage is permanent. As a result, most medical attention has been directed toward early therapy that may arrest the degeneration.

Those people who notice even slight visual disturbances should be examined by a doctor as soon as possible. Frequent eye examinations are crucial for patients with AMD because, although the disease may not change for months at a time, it will never improve on its own. It is also crucial to have regular exams because if dry AMD changes into the wet form, more aggressive therapy becomes mandatory.

Eye surgeons have several techniques to treat wet AMD. These include laser photocoagulation (during which the laser beam burns the abnormal blood vessels to stop their growth), photodynamic therapy (during which a special dye is injected into the bloodstream and activated by a laser beam to shrivel the blood vessels) and macular surgery (to repair the macula itself).

While none of these treatments will cure AMD or reverse the damage already present, the therapy will often retard the loss of vision.

With respect to the dry form, there is no consistently effective treatment or cure. However, because of deficiencies in antioxidants in some patients with AMD, many ophthalmologists are actively prescribing a "cocktail" of vitamins, zinc and antioxidants in hopes that the combination will prevent retinal damage or at least arrest the progression of AMD.

In summary, age-related macular degeneration is a serious and relatively common disorder. Again, it appears in two forms. The "wet" type is less prevalent, more serious, and can be treated—but not cured—by various laser/surgical techniques. The "dry" type is more common, progresses more slowly, may transform into the "wet" variety, is untreatable and incurable. There is hope, however, that a vitamin/antioxidant supplement may slow down the progression of the disorder.

Appropriate eye specialists should examine patients with AMD at regular intervals.

Blepharitis = inflammation of eyelid margins

Q. I suffer from blepharitis. Four ophthalmologists have not been able to help me. Should I see a dermatologist?

A. Blepharitis is an inflammation of the eyelid margins, usually caused by bacterial infection (such as staph) but sometimes due to allergies or skin conditions, such as eczema or seborrhea.

Antibiotic creams or drops usually clear up bacterial blepharitis. However, noninfectious cases are much more difficult to eradicate.

If your ophthalmologists have been unable to solve your problem, I agree that a dermatologist is the next logical step. The skin specialist may be able to help you—or refer you to an allergist if necessary.

Dry eyes may be related to autoimmune disease

Q. After having suffered from dry eyes and mouth., my daughter was diagnosed with Sjogren's syndrome. She was told that the disease is incurable, yet I have read that it is treatable. Please explain.

A. Sjogren's syndrome, a chronic inflammatory disorder of many bodily organs, is believed to be an autoimmune disease—one of several disorders, such as lupus and rheumatoid arthritis, marked by the body's allergic reaction to its own normal tissues. No one knows why the immune system overreacts and tries to destroy healthy cells as though they were foreign invaders. Autoimmune diseases are quite common.

Sjogren's syndrome affects primarily the eyes and mouth (which become extremely dry) and the joints (stiffness and pain). In addition, about one-third of patients develop enlarged parotid glands, the salivary glands in the cheeks.

Severe Sjogren's syndrome causes dryness in other tissues as well, including the skin, nose, respiratory tract and vagina. The intestinal tract and liver may be affected (shrinkage and malfunction), as can the heart, lymph nodes and kidneys. Although the syndrome usually exists in a mild, chronic form and treatment will slow progression of the disease, the affliction may, in rare instances, be complicated by lymphoma, a type of lymph gland cancer.

Like many medical conditions, Sjogren's syndrome is treatable—but not curable. It's important to make this distinction. Most diseases are treatable (insulin for diabetes, drugs for hypertension and so forth), but surprisingly few disorders are curable, antibiotic treatment for infections and chemotherapy for cancer notwithstanding.

Therapy for Sjogren's includes eye drops (to keep the corneas moist), mouthwashes and sugarless gum (to wet the mouth) and steroid drugs (to reduce inflammation).

In my opinion, your daughter should be seen by a rheumatologist, who can offer a program of treatment and supervision, in conjunction with her primary care physician.

Ears & Things Auditory

Second opinion in order for long-term ear infection

Q. For years I have had an ear infection treated with antibiotics and cortisone. My new doctor has prescribed prednisone. The druggist was hesitant to fill this prescription for internal use. Please advise if it is safe for an otitis media problem.

A. Some patients with repeated middle ear infections (otitis media) suffer from allergies that cause the normal tubes, which vent the middle ear chambers, to close. This can set the stage for bacteria to grow and cause pain, as well as the possibility for permanent damage. Cortisone (and similar drugs, such as prednisone) may help counteract such an allergy.

While the usual treatment for otitis media is antibiotics, I can understand why your previous physician prescribed cortisone, as well— and why your present doctor has chosen to give you prednisone.

Because this is not standard practice, however, and prednisone can cause side effects (such as diabetes and osteoporosis), I can also understand the pharmacist's reluctance to dispense such a powerful drug.

I do not know whether you need such "double therapy." Ask your new doctor about this and request that he speak to the pharmacist. You need to have the situation resolved. Another suggestion: Make an appointment with an ear-nose-and-throat specialist. I believe that a second opinion is in order.

Simple aging may be part of tinnitus

Q. My tinnitus is driving me nuts. Do you know anything about treating it with Valium, Elavil or B12 shots? I'm ready to try anything.

A. A constant noise in the ear (tinnitus) can be very annoying. It is sometimes caused by ear infections or wax accumulation, both of which can be treated.

Tinnitus is also part of the aging process and is a common consequence of ear damage from environmental noise. Obviously, aging is untreatable; however, prudent protection of the ears in noisy environments will prevent damage.

The methods of treatment you mention, including tranquilizers, antidepressants and vitamin shots, don't work and are really not worth trying. You should be examined by an otolaryngologist to see if there is any therapy for your condition. If not, you'll have to learn to live with it.

The cause of a perforated eardrum

Q. Please explain the term "perforated eardrum." Can the word "perforated" refer to any other part of the hearing mechanism?

A. The eardrum is a tough but thin membrane that separates the middle ear chamber (containing the tiny bones that help us to hear) from the outer ear (the external ear canal).

The eardrum may rupture from an injury (such as pushing a cotton swab too deeply into the ear) or from a middle ear infection that increases the pressure in the ear and causes the drum to burst.

In either event, a perforation (hole) is formed. Ordinarily, the perforation itself causes no symptoms and will heal, over time, without therapy. However, if the perforation is large—or if the trauma or infection is recurrent—the drum may not mend.

Such a chronic perforation is often associated with persisting inflammation of the middle ear, leading to a watery drainage, tinnitus (ringing in the ear) and loss of hearing. In these instances, antibiotic therapy is recommended, and otolaryngologists must operate to place a patch over the hole or otherwise repair the drum.

The word "perforation" is not customarily used to describe any other component of the hearing mechanism, although the word is a perfectly valid expression that describes a hole or defect in any organ, structure or tissue.

The cause of nerve deafness

Q. My elderly aunt has been diagnosed with nerve deafness. Is this caused by sinus infections?

A. No, it isn't. Nerve deafness is due to a disorder of the nerves of hearing, deep within the skull, that transmit auditory impulses to the brain.

Aside from the nerve deafness of old age, the most prevalent type is the result of chronic exposure to loud sounds.

Although the discharge of firearms, the sound of jet engines and the

Hearing Aids

Hearing aids can help those with certain types of sensorineural hearing loss. These battery-powered devices increase sound volume by means of a small microphone to pick up sound, an amplifier to magnify sound signals and an earphone to increase volume.

There are several different types of hearing aids. Some conduct sound by means of the mastoid bone, rather than an earphone; some are contained entirely in and behind the ear, while others have a body-worn battery and amplifier; and some hearing aids magnify high frequency sound only.

To ensure that the appropriate hearing aid is chosen, testing and fitting must be done by an audiologist—a professional who specializes in evaluating hearing and fitting hearing aids.

noise of certain occupations have traditionally been recognized as causes of deafness, ear specialists have become increasingly concerned about other components of modern life.

For instance, jackhammers, subway trains, rotary lawn mowers, unmuffled gasoline engines, and a host of other noisy activities will, over time, cause loss of hearing. In addition, electronically amplified music, so much the rage among the young, is clearly producing an entire generation of hard-of-hearing people.

If a noise is loud enough to be uncomfortable or if it causes tinnitus (ringing in the ears), it will produce nerve deafness. In the ear, such noise makes the hearing mechanism vibrate too violently, literally shaking cells off the organ that transforms soundwaves into electrical impulses that the brain interprets as sound. Once the cells have been lost, they are gone forever; they do not regenerate. Repeated exposure to loud sounds dislodges more and more cells, until permanent loss of hearing appears.

Such deafness occurs in the sound frequency called the "middle" or "conversational" range. Consequently, victims typically have difficulty hearing what is being said to them in a crowded room; they cannot discriminate speech when there is background noise. Also, they are forced to turn up the volume on radios and TV sets.

Ear Infections and Disorders

Ear infections and disorders are common, but distressing. Even minor infections can cause major hearing and balance impairment. The ear contains a number of parts and is relatively complex for its size, and a problem affecting just one part can greatly impair functioning.

Most ear problems can be treated easily. If treatment is delayed, however, the infection may cause permanent hearing loss or bone infection. Many ear problems have similar symptoms (such as ear pain, pressure and impaired balance or hearing), and a serious infection can be mistaken for a minor problem. Therefore, it's wise to seek medical treatment for any ear problem that last for more than a few days.

The ear's structure

The ear has three general divisions: the outer ear, the middle ear and the inner ear.

The outer ear consists of the external ear structure and the inside passage that leads to the eardrum.

The eardrum, which is stretched over the ear canal, separates the outer ear from the middle ear.

The middle ear contains three connected bones: the hammer (malleus), anvil (incus) and stirrup (stapes). It also contains several openings, including the Eustachian tubes, which equalize air pressure between the eardrum and the outside.

The inner ear contains the labyrinth and the cochlea. The labyrinth, which helps maintain balance, consists of three semicircular canals. The fluid-filled, snail shell-shaped cochlea plays a major role in hearing. The auditory nerve is attached to the cochlea and labyrinth, and transmits hearing and balance messages to the brain.

Soundwaves flow through the outer ear to the eardrum, causing it to vibrate. The middle ear bones magnify these vibrations, which are transferred to the fluid in the cochlea. This fluid stimulates the tiny hair cells lining the cochlea. The auditory nerve then transmits this stimulation to the brain, where the stimulus is "translated" as sound.

Hearing loss

There are two types of hearing loss: conductive and sensorineural.

Conductive hearing loss: This type of hearing loss occurs when ear wax, fluid, otosclerosis or a mechanical defect in the middle ear keeps soundwaves from reaching the inner ear. Hearing generally returns when the cause is corrected.

In otosclerosis, abnormal bone growth within the inner ear immobilizes the stapes (or stirrup) bone, through which soundwaves must pass. The result is a type of conductive hearing loss that can be corrected by stapedectomy (surgery to replace the stapes).

Stapedectomies are successful in the vast majority of cases, but about 5 percent of patients will become totally deaf in the ear that was operated on. However, otosclerosis itself can progress rapidly; if left untreated, it can lead to complete deafness in both ears.

Sensorineural hearing loss: In this type of hearing loss, sounds reach the ear, but nerve failure keeps them from being passed on to the brain. This may be caused by damage to the auditory nerve, the cochlea or the brain, and may occur with aging, as a side effect of some medications or after exposure to loud noise.

Sensorineural hearing loss caused by damage to the cochlea cannot be reversed by surgery or other medical treatment.

Acoustic trauma is a type of sensorineural hearing loss that follows a blow to the ear or exposure to excessive noise. Loud and/or high-pitched noise damages the hair cells within the cochlea, which play an important role in conducting sound.

Presbycusis is severe sensorineural hearing loss that occurs gradually with age. It's caused by damage to the ear's neuroreceptor cells and affects men more often than women.

In most instances, this kind of nerve deafness is preventable. I implore teenagers to turn down the volume and protect their ears in noisy environments. Individuals in high-noise occupations must wear ear protection. There is nothing "macho" about putting up with loud sounds that are bound to cause irreparable ear damage.

Hearing aids and ear wax

Q. I've worn hearing aids for years and attempt to remove the excess wax every month or so. Why do I find about three times as much wax in one ear as in the other?

A. I don't know, but it's true. People tend to develop ear wax accumulations selectively, in one ear or the other. Of course, the situation is aggravated by hearing aids that push the wax further down into the ear canals, making removal more difficult.

You can obtain advice about ear cleaning from your family physician, who will call upon an otolaryngologist if you need a specialist.

'I don't know' means I don't know

Q. In a recent column, a reader asked: "I've worn hearing aids for years and attempt to remove the excess wax every month or so. Why do I find about three times as much wax in one ear as in the other?"

You responded: "I don't know. People tend to develop ear wax accumulations selectively, in one ear or the other. You can obtain advice about ear cleaning from your family physician."

Perhaps the reader's letter was edited, but it appeared that his inquiry, which concerned differences in ear wax accumulation, only required an explanation. Instead, you referred him back to his family physician, without answering his question.

A. What is it about the phrase "I don't know" that confuses you? I made some comments about ear wax, but I was honest in stating that I couldn't answer the reader's question. Would you prefer that I give him a long, confusing, drawn-out and complicated opinion?

My experience is that my readers expect me to be forthright and succinct. This is how I chose to answer a question to which I didn't have an answer.

"I don't know" is an answer.

Incidentally, I also stick to this pattern with the patients in my practice. If I don't know the answers, I'll admit that and refer such patients to specialists. For example, last week in the office, as an emergency, I saw a 55-year-old architect who had chest pain of two hours' duration, associated with some difficulty breathing, cough and weakness. He was otherwise healthy. His exam was normal. I said: "Ted, I don't know the cause of your symptoms, but I am very concerned." I had his wife drive him to the hospital emergency room for appropriate testing. He was found to have pericarditis (an inflammation of the heart covering), was admitted to the hospital, discharged three days later, and is now happily back to normal, playing squash.

Most good physician I know are willing to say "I don't know" and ask for help in selective instances. I view this as a positive attribute.

Where was I? Oh, ear wax. Did I get off the subject? Sorry.

Half-capful of alcohol for water in the ear

Q. I went swimming a few days ago and, after coming out of a deep dive, I realized that water had entered my right ear. I've tried all kinds of tricks, including a headstand, to get it out. The water remains and is affected my hearing. Can you recommend something that would help?

A. Before answering your question, I need to know why you didn't go to your primary care physician to obtain assistance. Your letter is dated mid-June and here I am, answering it five months later. This problem could probably have been solved in five minutes in the doctor's office.

Now to your question.

Although a water-plugged ear can result from serious barotrauma (for example, a ruptured eardrum at significant depths), most people suffer hearing loss after swimming because water enters the ear and, because of wax, cannot escape.

Therefore, your first step is to pour a half-capful of rubbing alcohol into the ear. The alcohol may loosen and dislodge the wax (if wax is present), as well as combining with the water and evaporating it away.

If this simple strategy is ineffective, see your doctor for an ear lavage to remove what I suspect to be a wax accumulation. The next step after that is to see an otolaryngologist, if necessary.

Cancer

Different types of tumors grow at different rates

Q. How long does it take for a tumor the size of an apple to form in the colon? Would heavy drinking contribute to the growth?

A. Some tumors, such as prostate and bowel cancer, usually grow slowly over years; other malignancies can reach the size of an apple in weeks. Therefore, the answer to your question depends on the type of tumor.

For example, some cancers contain cells that appear so abnormal that a pathologist cannot identify the source of the growths. Such lesions are so malignant that they spread rapidly and kill early.

On the other hand, other lesions show fairly organized cellular structures and are considered to be less aggressively malignant than the types I mentioned above. Such characteristics can be determined by biopsy, and are of crucial importance because effective therapy depends on whether the type and source of the cancer can be determined. For instance, the presence of cancerous lung cells in a lymph node has more far-reaching consequences than the appearance of abnormal lymph gland cells in that organ. In the first instance, the finding confirms the spread of cancer (metastases), whereas the second situation suggests lymphoma, a relatively easy malignancy to treat.

Excessive alcohol consumption is statistically associated with certain malignancies in the gastrointestinal tract.

Cancer-talk, in plain language

Q. Please explain what a doctor means, when stating cancer is differentiated or undifferentiated. Last month, I underwent a hysterectomy because of uterine and ovarian cancer. My doctor's comments went about a mile over my head when he said it was undifferentiated.

A. All cancer arises from normal tissue. In other words, cancer cells are normal cells that have gone awry. Thus, malignancies often retain many of the characteristics of the "parent" cells. For example, lung tumors that spread to the liver may continue to exhibit lung-like qualities.

To the extent that cancer cells retain some normal appearance, they are called "differentiated." When malignant cells lose their markings and the pathologist cannot determine their tissue of origin, they are termed "undifferentiated."

This distinction is important. Let's say, for instance, that a woman has an enlarged lymph gland under the arm. Lymph node swelling is common in many nonmalignant conditions, such as bacterial and virus infections.

This gland, however, continues to grow and the physician appropriately orders a biopsy. The lymph node is removed and examined in the lab. The pathologist notes that under the microscope, the cells look malignant but they have a peculiar glandular appearance resembling breast tissue. The pathologist will then report to the physician that the lymph node contained "malignant cells, consistent with well-differentiated carcinoma of the breast."

At this point, the doctor must search for a "primary" lesion in the breast. Once found, this small nest of cells, the original cancer, will be removed and the patient will require follow-up radiation and/or chemotherapy.

On the other hand, the malignant lymph node may contain only cancerous lymph-gland cells, a "well-differentiated" lymphoma (lymph gland cancer), for which treatment, including chemotherapy, is entirely different.

Finally, the biopsied gland may be invaded by highly malignant cells so abnormal that the pathologist cannot recognize an organ of origin: undifferentiated cancer.

As a general rule, the more differentiated the malignant cells, the closer they correspond to normal tissue and the easier they are to treat. Undifferentiated cancer is, in the main, so aggressive that it carries a poor prognosis.

In your case, the surgeon evidently removed a highly malignant cancer that—presumably—arose from your uterus or ovaries. I say "presumably" because in the presence of undifferentiated cells, no one can be absolutely sure, without chemical analysis of the cells themselves. Despite this unsettling news, there are several treatment programs—involving various combinations of chemotherapy—that may be used to treat your condition. Ask your gynecologist about this.

I might add that not all practitioners feel comfortable talking to patients about cancer. Such doctors may cover up their discomfort by using excessively technical terms, which—unintelligible to the average patient—discharge the physician's responsibility to provide "necessary" information.

In my opinion, no patient should leave a doctor's office without first having had a comprehensive explanation about what is wrong. This explanation should be given in understandable language and the patient should persist in questioning the doctor until the situation is absolutely clear.

I urge you to return to your physician or surgeon for an in-depth discussion of what was found at surgery, what should be done about it and what to expect in the future. I'd also want to make sure that your doctor plans to refer you to an oncologist, a cancer specialist, for a second opinion and a treatment program. This step seems to me to be a vital one, inasmuch as you were given bad news without much advice about prognosis and follow-up.

Remember, the practitioner is there to serve you. Your understanding of your affliction is not a privilege—it's a right.

Cancer may have a genetic basis

Q. Is the tendency to cancer inherited? Are some people genetically susceptible to lung cancer, regardless of their smoking habits? How fast does lung cancer spread?

A. You raise a question that has fascinated doctors for years: Is a predisposition to cancer inherited? Experts await the definitive answer.

Yet, there are unmistakable clues. Cancers of the ovaries and breasts, for example, seem to show a genetic pattern. Moreover, epidemiological studies certainly suggest that a tendency to cancer runs in families. That is, if most of your immediate family died of malignancies, you are at a greater risk of developing a malignancy than, say, a person whose family members lived to ripe old ages.

No one can yet say that lung cancer is inherited, but authorities continue aggressively to search out inheritance patterns and, perhaps, a marker in the blood stream, much like those that are present for many cancers in females. Therefore, the answer to your question is a qualified "yes"; the tendency to cancer is probably genetically determined, but is by no means a certainty.

Heart disease also seems to have a genetic predisposition, but remember that if we live long enough, we're bound to get cancer or heart disease, the two most common diseases of old age. In adopting a personal lifestyle, the prudent individual would be wise to take into account his or her family history. This is why good doctors try to obtain as much information about a patient's family history; the pattern may provide presumptive evidence of present or future health problems, such as diabetes, hypertension and many other medical conditions, including cancer.

Let me illustrate this with a personal anecdote. My great-grandfathers and grandfathers died of heart attacks (known in the old days as "acute indigestion"); my own father had arteriosclerotic heart disease for which he had successful bypass surgery. My great-grandmothers and grandmothers died of cancer; my mother succumbed to a lung tumor. Thus, I infer, heart disease seems to run in the male lineage of my family, cancer in the female line. If you were to ask me what I will probably die from, I'd say heart disease.

However, because of my mother's affliction, I stopped smoking cigarettes years ago and attempt to avoid exposure to known carcinogens. This approach seems sensible to me, even though I doubt I will get cancer as a result of my mother's genes. Nonetheless, I would be foolish to tempt fate by smoking two packs a day and working in a coal mine. Thus, I take my family history into account, but am not governed by it.

The speed with which lung cancer grows and spreads is largely a function of the type of malignancy. Some malignancies are highly aggressive, resist treatment and quickly spread to cause death. Others grow more slowly and are amenable to therapy. I am not aware of any genetic variation in this pattern.

Early detection aids cancer recovery

Q. A friend had a pain in his right ribs for three months that was ultimately diagnosed as cancer of the liver. Is there a test that people with a high risk of cancer can take periodically to catch the trouble as soon as possible?

A. Pain is often the first sign of cancer; this symptom deserves a thorough medical investigation in any patient. Unfortunately, however, by the time the malignancy causes pain, the tumor may already have spread or grown to the point where treatment is not satisfactory, only palliative. Cancer of the liver is such a tumor. Difficult to treat at best, painful liver cancer is almost always a problem because the discomfort indicates the malignancy has spread to the liver covering or to the surrounding tissues.

Therefore, while I understand your frustration about your friend's ailment, I suspect that unless the cancer had been diagnosed before he had pain, little could have been done to alter the course of his illness.

> 66 The speed with which lung cancer grows and spreads is largely a function of the type of malignancy. Some malignancies are highly aggressive, resist treatment and quickly spread to cause death. Others grow more slowly and are amenable to therapy. 99

You're correct that early diagnosis of cancer greatly improves the chances for cure. This is why doctors try to identify patients with high-risk factors, such as cigarette smoking, a family history of malignancy and exposure to industrial pollutants (such as asbestos). Also, this is the reason physicians encourage women to have Pap smears and mammograms. Further, men and women over the age of 50 are urged to have periodic screening for hidden blood in the stool, frequently an indicator of early cancer or premalignant lesions of the bowel.

At present, there is no test that will effectively identify early cancer in healthy people. Rather, doctors focus their attention on high-risk patients with symptoms, such as fatigue, weight loss and change in normal body functioning. True, there are blood tests that indicate the possibility of malignancies of the reproductive tract and the liver, but these tests are not sensitive enough to discover small cancers as part of a general screening procedure.

Perhaps your friend's cancer could have been diagnosed earlier by a CT scan (special X-rays) of the liver. However, as I stated, our methods of detection do not, in general, yield results that lead to a cure, once pain has developed.

Cancer is not considered contagious

Q. Is cancer either contagious or infectious? Most of us retired men in our community know we may develop prostate cancer, thus the question.

A. The cause of cancer is unknown. However, most authorities agree that malignancies are not contagious or infectious in the traditional sense of a strep throat or pneumonia.

In particular, breast and prostate cancer, which are common in women and men, do not appear to be spread from one person to another. Such growths are more likely to be related to factors within the body, such as hormone imbalances.

Many cancers appear to be related to genetic tendencies; the disease runs in families, for example.

Whether some malignancies have a viral origin is unclear. Obviously, in such cases, an element of contagion would be possible, but no experts have defined the potential risks. I'll keep my readers informed.

Accepting or rejecting treatment personal decision

Q. I had a gallon of fluid removed from my right chest cavity. A lung specialist said it contained cancer cells, but it's treatable! Can I avoid chemo and radiation? I'm 82 and don't want to go through this.

A. As a general rule, cancer is treated with surgery, radiation and/or chemotherapy. Which method or combination treatment depends on many factors: the type of cancer, the aggressiveness of the malignancy, potential spread of the tumor, the patient's age and general state of health, and—very important—the person's preference about how to be treated (or not treated).

Without knowing your type of cancer and whether it has spread, I cannot comment on the best path for you to follow; that decision I'll leave to you and your oncologist, working as a team.

I will make a brief comment, however. Cancer cells in the fluid from your chest (malignant pleural effusion) is an extremely serious condition that, in most cases, is the result of a highly malignant lung cancer that has spread into the chest cavity—and very likely, even beyond that. Therefore, while "treatable," it is probably not curable. In all likelihood, we're talking about prolonging your life for a few months at most. And what about the quality of that life?

Your age makes surgery very risky; chemotherapy may make you sick. Radiation may be your best bet. This is a topic that your should review with your oncologist.

When my mother was diagnosed with lung cancer several years ago, the doctors found that it had spread to her liver. They offered her a combination of radiation and chemotherapy. "How much time have I got without it?" she asked. "About six months." "How long if I take treatment?" "A year."

She chose therapy, in part because she wanted time with her infant grandson. Exactly a year after treatment, she died.

These situations and decisions are very difficult—and very personalized. For example, I've had many cancer patients who refused treatment, were kept comfortable and died quickly.

Please have a frank and in-depth consultation with a cancer specialist. At this point, you need information and support for any decision you have to make.

Inflammation may signal breast cancer

Q. What can you tell me about inflammatory breast cancer? I'm a 74-year-old female, post mastectomy for this condition. Now my other breast has gotten progressively more sensitive and sore, yet, because there is no lump, my doctor is content with a mammogram every six months. He's actually angry that I got information from the National Cancer Institute. Is his approach a good one?

A. Some (but not all) breast cancers are associated with inflammation that can be identified in a biopsy specimen. The reason for this inflammation is unknown, but the condition is associated with a virulent type of malignancy leading to a swollen, tender breast that may not be lumpy. A mammogram may not necessarily reveal this type of cancer.

I don't want to second-guess your doctor, who is more familiar with your condition. However, given your previous inflammatory cancer, I'd be suspicious that your remaining breast might be similarly affected. If you were my patient, I'd probably push for a biopsy, all things being equal.

I'm sorry to hear that your physician was upset that you did your homework. Your actions seem reasonable to me, inasmuch as it's your life and future that are on the line.

I believe that you could be best served by obtaining a second opinion from another qualified surgeon. If the consultant agrees with your doctor, all well and good.

On the other hand, if he is suspicious—as I am—he may recommend biopsy. In either case, you will at least be able to resolve this difficult problem.

Breast cancer can run in families

Q. My sister has been diagnosed with breast cancer. Are the rest of us in the family more likely to have this problem? I had a mammogram two years ago and perform regular self-examination. Is the testing properly done standing or while lying down?

A. There is a statistical tendency for breast cancer to occur in certain families; in many cases, this is due to a genetic abnormality that is inherited. If, for example, your mother, maternal aunt and sister had breast cancer, you would be considered to be in an extremely high-risk category. In contrast, were only your sister to have breast cancer, your risk is also increased, but to much less a degree. I do not believe that you need to worry unnecessarily about an isolated case of breast cancer (your sister's) in the absence of a more compelling family history.

Nonetheless, you should continue to have mammograms, preferably annually. In addition, you should perform self breast examinations every month or so. Such an examination is done in both the standing (or sitting) and lying positions. In the first instance, you should inspect your breasts in a mirror to discover any asymmetry, dimpling or other irregularity. Then, while supine, you must carefully palpate each breast in an organized manner, section by section.

Follow your doctor's recommendations about appropriate breast examinations and suitable monitoring.

How breast cancer progresses

Q. With all the publicity about breast cancer, I'm still not sure how this malignancy kills. What is the sequence of events from a lump to death?

A. Cancer cells are marked by two important characteristics: uncontrolled growth and loss of normal function. Each healthy cell in the body is under the control of chemical factors that either stimulate it to grow or to cease dividing, depending on the body's needs. In order to maintain health, cell growth must be turned on or shut off when appropriate. In addition, each cell has a built-in genetic program that causes it to die when its time has come. This process is called apoptosis (pronounced apo-tosis).

Malignant cells don't behave this way. They grow and divide rapidly and uncontrollably; they are immune to the body's growth-governing factors. In addition, cancer cells don't do what they're supposed to do. They stop cooperating with other cells. It's as though all their energy is directed toward one goal: growth.

Because of these characteristics, cancer cells usually kill patients by interfering with normal cells. They push them, squeeze them, steal their blood supply and—eventually—replace them; normal cell growth is no match for malignant growth.

Here is a simplified sequence of events in a case of untreated breast cancer:

The cancer begins as a single, mutant cell deep in the breast. For reasons nobody yet understands, the body's immune system fails to recognize this cell as "foreign" and imperfect. (Early malignant cells are ordinarily immediately destroyed by "killer cells" that are an integral part of the immune system.) The cancer cell divides again and again in a rush of uncontrolled activity.

Most new cancer cells remain in the breast, eventually forming a lump or nodule that appears, in many cases, to be fueled by the female hormone estrogen. However, other malignant cells escape into the blood stream and the lymphatic system, where they travel to the nearest lymph nodes (in the armpit and along the ribs). In the lymph nodes, they continue to divide and conquer, forming new nodules.

As the lymph glands become saturated with cancer cells, more malignant cells spread beyond the nodes via the lymph circulation. This hop-and-skip process is repeated until the cancer cells are carried to vital organs, such as the lungs or liver, where they displace healthy cells and interfere with normal cellular functions. Eventually, the lungs and liver become studded with masses of malignant tissue. After several months, the patient's organs fail, infection may set in and death ensues.

Thus, the treatment of breast cancer, as for other malignancies, requires therapy to remove or deactivate as much diseased tissue as early as possible. This is followed by radiation or medicine to slow the growth of abnormal cells that are left. Using modern techniques, such as anti-hormone therapy, specialists are often successful in killing cancer cells or retarding their growth, thereby enabling patients to live longer, more independent lives.

Therefore, it is vitally important to identify breast cancer early—by examination and mammography—so that treatment can begin before malignant cells have spread (metastasized) to lymph nodes or remote locations. Once such spread has occurred, most cancers are more difficult to treat.

In the past decade, the therapy for breast cancer (and other malignancies) has improved dramatically; cures are now the rule, thanks to early detection and aggressive medical/surgical management. Also, on the horizon, is the possibility of an anticancer vaccine that would permit killer cells in the immune system to recognize and destroy malignant cells before they have had a chance to multiply. Thus, in essence, such a vaccine would enhance our defenses, perhaps to all types of cancer cells. Such a breakthrough, although years away, would completely alter our concept of malignant disease, which would be relegated to the has-been status of smallpox and plague. Here is truly an example of the wonder of scientific achievement. We all need to support the researchers who are working on this challenge.

Is biopsy needed for breast lump?

Q. Seven years ago I had a mastectomy because of a lump in my left breast that was found to be malignant. This week my doctor found a lump in my right breast that did not show up on a mammogram. He suggested I do nothing for six months since he believes it is nonmalignant and is a fibrocystic growth. Could a fibroid be felt on physical examination and not seen on mammogram?

A. A benign fibrocystic growth is more dense than the surrounding normal breast tissue. This is the reason it can be felt as a lump.

Ordinarily, such growths are visible on a mammogram. However, they usually can be distinguished from malignancies; for one thing, they ordinarily do not contain flecks of calcium, as do many breast cancers.

I do not know why the fibrocystic area was not visible on the mammogram. Perhaps you have so-called "cystic" breasts, so that several areas of hyper-dense tissue were evident, obscuring the area in question. Thus, the X-rays were inconclusive. Ultrasound would probably have solved the problem, but, apparently, was not used.

In any case, you should definitely continue to be monitored. As you know, breast cancer on one side enormously increases a woman's risk of having a malignancy in the opposite breast.

Consequently, if the fibrocystic area grows—or even if it remains stationary for several months—you may want to consider biopsy, just to be on the safe side. One last option: Seek a second opinion from a surgeon who is well-versed in breast diseases.

Breast cancer not related to lifestyle

Q. I don't smoke, drink or do drugs. I am slim and physically active. I eat prudently. I've just been diagnosed with breast cancer. There is no family history, but my father died of prostate cancer at 71. What improvements can I make in my life to mitigate the condition?

A. Regrettably, bad things happen. Ill health can befall even the most prudent person. A corollary: Behaving yourself does not insulate you from diseases most of which appear to be carried in the genes. Nonetheless, folks who don't take care of themselves get sicker sooner and die earlier as a consequence of unhealthful lifestyles. And that's just the point.

You have evidently not abused your health in the past. As a result, you're probably in exceptionally good shape, a characteristic that could have an enormous impact on overcoming your genetically-defined breast cancer. For instance, were you an obese smoker and heavy drinker, you probably wouldn't respond as well to therapy for your breast cancer, which may include surgery, chemotherapy and/or radiation.

Thus, your many years of sensible living may now pay off dividends. You can approach your unanticipated breast problem with a healthy body and mind. Follow your physician's specific advice about what actions you can take to beat your breast cancer. At the same time, relish the knowledge that by showing wisdom in your lifestyle, you may have made possible the likelihood of cure.

Breast densities are not necessarily ominous

Q. Please explain what "increased densities" on a mammogram are all about.

A. When X-rayed, all tissues give characteristic patterns on X-ray film. The pattern depends on the density of the tissue being examined. Bone, for example, is extremely dense and will, therefore, absorb more X-rays, leading to a white image on the film. In contrast, fat is much less dense; more X-rays pass through it to expose the film and cause a darker image.

The breast is composed of tissues of varying densities: fat, glandular elements, cysts, scar tissue, and—in some cases—calcifications. Thus, the X-ray pattern in a mammogram reflects a variety of tissues within the breast.

It's the radiologist's duty to interpret the shadows on the X-ray films and tell the patient's physician whether the images are normal or suspicious. In general, breast cancer is denser than normal breast tissue—and may contain tiny flecks of calcium that tip off the radiologist to a potential problem.

The fact that you had "increased densities" on your mammogram is not necessarily worrisome; it simply means that you have some dense tissue in the breast that is probably normal—but should be followed up with either a repeat mammogram in six months or a biopsy now. The fact that your densities did not contain calcium is a very encouraging finding and probably means that you don't have a serious breast problem. Nonetheless, you should ask your doctor about this.

Fibrocystic disease and breast cancer

Q. I've had fibrocystic breast disease for years. When a recent biopsy was done, it showed atypical ductal hyperplasia. What does this mean? Also, I am awaiting the results of a lymph node biopsy and would like information about therapy should the tissue be malignant.

A. Fibrocystic disease of the breast (squishy cysts interspersed with scar tissue) is benign, although women with this condition show a slight increase in the risk of developing breast cancer at a later date. However, once the fibrocystic tissue shows atypical ductal hyperplasia (abnormal changes)—as it may in about 5 percent of cases—the risk of cancer increases dramatically, especially if there is a family history of breast malignancy.

You are being evaluated appropriately with biopsies to determine if cancer exists in your breast. If it is present, it should be removed and suitable additional therapy, such as radiation or antihormone pills, given. If the biopsies are negative, you will need to have close follow-up: for example, mammograms every six months and re-biopsy of any suspicious lesions.

In my opinion, you are jumping the gun by asking about further therapy for a breast malignancy you may not have. Take the problem a step at a time and follow your doctor's advice. If and when you might develop a serious problem is still unknown, but should there be cancer, it would certainly be treatable—even curable—under the supervision of an oncologist, a cancer specialist.

Tamoxifen therapy is worth the discomfort

Q. I was diagnosed with breast cancer and had part of my breast removed, followed by six weeks of radiation therapy. Fortunately, none of the lymph nodes under my arm contained cancer cells. Now, my oncologist wants to prescribe tamoxifen. However, I am reluctant to take it because of the risk of other cancer or blood clots. Your opinion, please.

A. Depending on whether a breast cancer is sensitive to estrogen as determined by special tests on the biopsied specimen, most specialists urge women with this disease to take tamoxifen, an anti-estrogen drug. This is standard procedure, and I encourage you to heed your oncologist's recommendation.

You had a serious disease that, happily, did not spread to the lymph glands. You should be cured, after surgery and radiation. Nonetheless, you are at increased risk for another breast cancer. The purpose of tamoxifen is to prevent this by blocking the effects of estrogen. (As you know, many breast cancers are worsened by estrogen stimulation.)

True, tamoxifen is associated with a wide variety of side effects—including hot flashes, vomiting, liver inflammation, blood clots, and others, which are diagnosed by examination and blood tests.

However, such reactions are not common, and I believe that the benefits of tamoxifen far outweigh the disadvantages. Uterine cancer has been reported in women on tamoxifen but, if you're willing to undergo periodic gynecological examinations, this should not be a contraindication.

In short, follow your oncologist's advice.

Benign mass probably benign, but play it safe

Q. My last three annual mammograms showed what appeared to be a benign mass. Should I have the lump biopsied?

A. Probably not. If you have a breast lesion that has not changed, by mammography, in three years, and if the radiologist is convinced that it has no X-ray features (such as sprinkled calcifications) to suggest malignancy, you needn't have a biopsy.

On the other hand, if the X-ray interpretation is equivocal or if your primary care physician has doubts about the benignity of the mass, you should proceed with biopsy—whether or not the lump has changed in size.

Let me add a cautionary note. If you have a family history of breast cancer, display no other evidence of benign fibrocystic disease and are worried about the possibility (however remote) of breast cancer, I'd urge you to have a biopsy. The procedure (needle biopsy under ultrasound guidance) is safe, takes only a few minutes, and—if normal—will remove lots of stress from you and your doctor. Frankly, I'd rather recommend a biopsy that proves negative than to advise no biopsy and then, years later, kick myself in the butt because you had breast cancer. Please follow your physician's/gynecologist's suggestions in this matter.

Most ovarian cysts are innocuous

Q. I've had several ultrasound examinations that revealed ovarian cysts. My gynecologist is not concerned, and I wonder at what point I should become worried.

A. Ovarian cysts are common. They are small collections of fluid that form on the surface of an ovary after ovulation and disappear with time. They are harmless and, by and large, do not require treatment unless they bleed or cause severe discomfort.

In general, such cysts have a characteristic appearance on ultrasound testing: They look like fluid filled bubbles. If, after examining you and reviewing the imaging pictures, your gynecologist is satisfied that the cysts are benign, I believe that you can trust his judgment and ignore them.

Should there be a question, however, the doctor can confirm the diagnosis by laparoscopy, during which he looks at the cysts (and, if necessary, biopsies them) through a lighted tube introduced through the abdominal wall.

Fortunately, in most cases, this procedure is not necessary to diagnose simple ovarian cysts.

Abnormal cervical cells must be investigated

Q. What is cervical dysplasia? My daughter has it and we are at our wits' end. What's the treatment?

A. Dysplasia means cells that are abnormal in size, shape and appearance. Apparently, your daughter had a Pap test that showed dysplasia of the cells of the cervix, the opening of the uterus.

Such cells could well indicate chronic irritation or infection. These conditions are easily treated.

On the other hand, cervical dysplasia may be a forerunner of cancer, and, I suspect, this is what concerns you.

When faced with this problem, most gynecologists recommend further testing, such as a cone biopsy. During this office procedure, part of the cervix is trimmed away and examined under a microscope in an attempt to identify cancer cells that could be the cause of the dysplasia. Fortunately, the presence of dysplasia does not automatically indicate a serious disorder; nonetheless, the association does exist and must be investigated.

Once a cancerous growth has been excluded by biopsy, gynecologists ordinarily urge treatment of the dysplasia. This includes antimicrobial drugs, safe sex for women with multiple partners and frequent follow-up visits.

Hodgkin's disease is often curable

Q. I've recently been diagnosed with Hodgkin's disease. If the lymph nodes in my armpits are swollen, would it help if they were surgically removed?

A. Hodgkin's disease is a type of lymphoma, cancer affecting the lymph glands.

The disorder usually begins with swollen lymph nodes, commonly in the neck and upper body, that may be associated with fever, night sweats, weight loss and malaise. As the disease progresses, anemia, jaundice, swelling of the ankles, and difficulty breathing appear.

Hodgkin's disease is diagnosed by lymph-node biopsy, which shows a typical cancerous pattern. Once the diagnosis is established, the disease must be staged; that is, its extent must be verified because the type of treatment depends on the location of the involved glands—and whether other organs, such as liver and bone, are also affected. This is accomplished by X-ray tests and surgical exploration.

Stage I is disease in a specific, localized area, such as the neck.

Stage II reflects involvement of "skip" areas either above or below the diaphragm.

Stage III indicates tumor on both sides of the diaphragm, including the spleen.

Stage IV is extensive involvement outside the lymph system.

In the past few years, treatment for Hodgkin's disease has been remarkably improved. The affliction is now curable in most cases. Patients with Stage I and II disease are treated with radiation therapy; those with Stage III and IV disease must undergo extensive irradiation, with or without combination chemotherapy (anticancer drugs).

I cannot tell from your question what the stage of your disease is; it could be Stage II or, if lymph glands in your pelvis are affected, Stage III or IV. You will probably benefit from radiation alone, although some oncologists (cancer specialists) follow this with chemotherapy as well. Having the lymph nodes under your arms removed will make little difference in the prognosis.

Myeloma not related to lung cancer

Q. I'm a 74-year-old ex-smoker who had 40 percent of my right lung removed two years ago because of cancer. Now, without any warning or reason, I have been diagnosed with multiple myeloma. The doctor told me that the two cancers are unrelated. I've always lived life carefully. How, therefore, could I have developed myeloma?

A. No one knows the cause of multiple myeloma, a form of cancer that affects plasma cells, a type of blood corpuscle. Presumably, nothing you did (or didn't do) caused this malignancy, which alters blood proteins and leads to anemia and kidney failure, among other consequences.

The good news: Chemotherapy is ordinarily effective, enabling patients to live many years in remission.

The fact that you have had two apparently unrelated cancers suggests an underlying abnormality in your immune system. Some experts believe that cancer cells grow when the body fails to identify such abnormal tissue and, therefore, cannot destroy it.

You must closely follow your physician's instructions about how to monitor your myeloma (with blood tests) and what treatment is appropriate.

Esophageal cancer is challenging to treat

Q. My husband was recently diagnosed with cancer of the esophagus. Is radiation therapy the best approach? I'm afraid that his lungs could be damaged by this treatment. What about chemotherapy?

A. Esophageal cancer is notoriously difficult to treat because any therapy is bound to interfere with normal eating and swallowing. Further, this malignancy is ordinarily not discovered until it has grown quite large and may have metastasized (spread) to surrounding tissues.

Modern radiation therapy, during which treatment can be accurately focused on the affected area, is certainly a possibility. While it may not cure the disease—in the strictest sense—it will surely shrink the tumor and permit your husband to eat relatively normally.

Depending on the size and type of esophageal cancer, chemotherapy (with drugs) may also be considered. However, this usually causes side effects (such as hair loss, malaise, poor appetite and pain), which patients may find unacceptable.

Some experts advise radiation treatments (to shrink the tumor) followed by surgery (to remove it).

While it's true that radiation could cause lung damage by burning normal tissue, I believe that the potential benefits outweigh the unpleasant consequences. What you and your husband need most is professional guidance about which treatment will accomplish the greatest benefit. A cancer specialist (oncologist) can supply the information. Therefore, I recommend that your husband's therapy be planned and supervised by such a specialist.

No matter which option your husband chooses, he is—I'm afraid—in for an unpleasant experience and an uncertain prognosis. Nonetheless, an oncologist would be your best resource. Don't make up your mind about therapy until you can obtain more information on which to make a rational judgment.

Is follow-up necessary for bladder cancer?

Q. I'm an 80-year-old male who had a cancer removed from my bladder. My urologist wants to perform a cystoscopy every three months for the first year, every six months for the second, and once in the third. Is this necessary? Since my only symptom was the passing of blood in my urine, can't I just wait to see if it recurs and do something then?

A. Look at bladder cancer as a form of skin cancer—with the exception that it grows on an internal skin surface and is, therefore, harder to see. Like a skin malignancy, bladder tumors can easily be removed if they are small and haven't spread.

Also, like skin cancers, they tend to bleed readily.

Your urologist is correct in demanding close follow-up. If your bladder cancer recurs, he can easily remove it during cystoscopy, a technique of examining the bladder lining. As each month progresses and you remain cancer-free, the risk of a recurrence is lessened.

Thus, the doctor quite properly wants to perform cystoscopy at periodic intervals; more frequently at first, then less often. True, you could probably monitor the situation by checking your urine for blood, but the tumor may not bleed until it is quite large, making the job of removing it harder and increasing the risk that it will spread.

No sane human being looks forward to having someone shove a tube into his or her bladder. However, in this instance, such a procedure may actually save you from more extensive and expensive surgery. Especially with bladder (and skin) cancer, an ounce of prevention is, truly, worth a pound of cure. Follow your urologist's recommendations.

Skin malignancy needs follow-up

Q. My husband had a mole under his arm that was diagnosed as a basal cell carcinoma and removed. Since he had done nothing about the mole for two years, could it have metastasized to other organs?

A. Basal cell carcinoma, a common skin malignancy, often resembles an enlarging mole or a sore that doesn't heal. Like any cancer, it has the potential to spread. Therefore, if your husband disregarded the cancer for two years, it could have metastasized.

However, this type of cancer if more likely to spread into the tissues beneath the skin; therefore, if the doctor included wide borders of normal tissue when he excised the lesion, there is probably less risk of metastasis.

Your husband should follow the doctor's advice with respect to appropriate follow-up examinations and, if necessary, additional surgery.

Understanding leukemia prognosis

Q. I have a coworker who has chronic leukemia. Would you comment on the different types and expected life span?

A. For practical purposes, leukemia—cancer of the white blood cells—is divided into acute and chronic forms; either type of blood cell (lymphocytes or myelocytes) can be affected. Thus, a patient can have either acute or chronic lymphocytic leukemia or acute or chronic myelocytic leukemia.

In general, the acute forms are much more dangerously aggressive, causing rapidly progressing illness and death, unless treated.

On the other hand, chronic leukemia is less serious. For example, the affliction may be discovered by accident during a blood test in a person who is free of symptoms.

Nonetheless, chronic leukemia must be treated or it—like acute leukemia—will progress to death, albeit at a somewhat slower rate than its acute counterpart.

Symptoms of leukemia include fatigue, weakness, weight loss, pallor, fever, easy bruising, and swollen glands.

The diagnosis is made by blood tests and examination of the bone marrow.

Most cases of chronic leukemia can be successfully treated with drugs, such as hydroxyurea; radiation therapy and steroids may be required.

Although some types of chronic myelocytic leukemia may be fatal within three or four years, some patients live much longer. Chronic lymphocytic leukemia has a more favorable prognosis, with some patients living as long as 20 years.

The cause of acute and chronic leukemia is unknown. Some studies have suggested a genetic disposition. Massive exposure to radiation (such as occurred during the Chernobyl incident) usually leads to a particularly vicious type of leukemia. A few authorities suspect that strange virus infections may produce the disorder.

During the past decades, the most striking benefits in cancer therapy have been in the treatment of leukemia, especially in children. While therapy for most cancers has not affected the death rate—or changed it only slightly—treatment for leukemia has been revolutionary.

Therefore, the diagnosis of leukemia no longer carries with it the horrendous stigma of an early and uncomfortable death. Rather, the affliction is treatable—even curable—in the majority of cases.

Blood counts are key with leukemia

Q. About five years ago my doctor told me I had chronic lymphatic leukemia, for which my blood is checked every three months. So far, I haven't had any problem but if I should in the future, what can I expect?

A. Chronic lymphatic leukemia is a type of blood cell cancer involving the infection-fighting white blood cells called lymphocytes. The cause is unknown. The disease is marked by swollen lymph glands, fatigue, fever, loss of appetite, breathlessness, anemia and malfunction of the immune system. Symptoms may take years to appear.

The diagnosis is made by blood tests and bone marrow examination.

In general, the prognosis is favorable: Survivals of up to 20 years are common, which isn't bad considering that most patients are diagnosed at or above the age of 60.

Therapy with anticancer drugs, radiation and cortisone is usually effective but need not be used unless patients develop progressive symptoms or until the lymphocyte count exceeds 75,000 per microliter (normal is 4,000-10,000).

You seem to be following a relatively typical pattern. You should continue to be monitored at the discretion of your physician. When you develop symptoms or if your lymphocyte count rises, he can refer you to a hematologist for treatment.

Oral cancer: What's the treatment?

Q. I've been diagnosed with oral cancer and have undergone surgery eight times on my tongue. What information can you share on squamous cell carcinoma?

A. Squamous cell carcinoma is a type of malignancy arising from the cells of the skin and the lining of body cavities. Like any cancer, it will spread uncontrollably unless treated. Symptoms depend on the site of the tumor, as well as the extent of the metastases (spread) at the time of the diagnosis.

For example, squamous cell carcinoma of the oral cavity is usually diagnosed earlier (because it can be seen and felt) that a similar tumor in the lung, which may not be recognized until it has grown large enough (or spread) to cause cough, blood-tinged sputum, weight loss, and a shadow on the chest X-ray.

The treatment for a malignancy depends largely on its size and location. Surgery, radiation, chemotherapy, or a combination of these methods are usually employed, with varying results.

With respect to your specific case, I suggest that you discuss your condition and prognosis with your oral surgeon (or an oncologist), who is the person most familiar with your particular tumor.

How to treat cancer of the mouth

Q. Is lichen planus a precursor to cancer? I first experienced this after a reaction to iodine following hysterectomy. It cleared up and didn't appear again until after gum surgery. I never smoked or drank and have no diseases that would cause leukoplakia, which later developed. I've now had a tongue operation after a cancerous tumor was found on the floor of my mouth. Would you recommend radiation therapy? What is happening to me?

A. Lichen planus, a recurring inflammatory eruption that often affects the oral cavity, is not itself precancerous. However, any kind of chronic ulcer in the mouth may lead to cancer. Moreover, early cancers in this area can resemble lichen planus.

As in your case, lichen planus frequently occurs after exposure to certain drugs, such as those containing bismuth or iodine.

Leukoplakia, whitish inflammations in the mouth, were once believed to be premalignant. The current theory is that they are not. Further, they are unrelated to lichen planus.

You have had a serious form of cancer that affected the floor of your mouth and required partial removal of your tongue. At this point, the less important question is how the cancer developed. The more important issue is what you're going to do about it.

Radiation may be appropriate, as may chemotherapy. In making your decision, you'll have to be guided by an oncologist. Follow the specialist's advice.

Early signs of colon cancer

Q. What are the signs of colon cancer?

A. Most colon cancers grow slowly; consequently, early malignancies usually produce no symptoms whatsoever. As the tumor enlarges, it may leak blood into the intestine. This may be the first sign of a problem. However, the blood in the stool may be invisible to the naked eye and can only be diagnosed with a chemical test (Hemoccult and others) that identifies the presence of blood.

Eventually, the cancer grows large enough to cause signs and symptoms, including changes in the pattern of evacuation, abdominal pain, weight loss, malaise, weakness and obvious blood in the stool.

Colon cancer is, for the most part, curable if it is discovered in its early stages. This is the reason adults with a family history of malignancy—and any person over the age of 50—should undergo periodic colonoscopies.

Celiac disease—lymphoma connection?

Q. You once stated that celiac disease is associated with a risk of lymph node cancer. Since I suffer from celiac disease, I would appreciate a clarification and/or expansion of this statement since it was rather startling and totally unexpected news to me.

A. Lymphoma (lymph node cancer) can be a complication of celiac disease, a form of malabsorption caused by a sensitivity to the cereal protein gluten. The tendency to lymphoma is not known to be affected by a strict adherence to a gluten-free diet. Therefore, patients with celiac disease should be monitored by gastroenterologists with X-ray tests and biopsies.

Ask your doctor about this. Although the risk of lymphoma is small, it is real.

Is a second colon operation necessary?

Q. About a year ago I had a colonoscopy. A polyp was discovered and I underwent a right hemicolectomy. It was benign; however, my doctor insists that I need to have another colonoscopy now to determine if any precancerous polyps were missed. Do you think I need another one so soon?

A. Yours is an unusual story, because surgeons usually do not remove part of the colon (hemicolectomy) for benign polyps.

As a general rule, any polyps are removed at the time of the colonoscopy, the intestine is left intact and the situation is monitored with repeat colonoscopies every four or five years. Therefore, I cannot comment on your doctor's strategy, because I'm not sure of his rationale.

If you had a benign polyp, the physician should have been able to detect other polyps (if any were present) during the first colonoscopy. Hence, a second procedure should not be necessary for several years. On the other hand, a malignant polyp would require more aggressive therapy, such as you described, again with colonoscopic surveillance every few years.

It sounds to me as though your doctor believes he missed something and now wants to cover his buttocks by repeating the colonoscopy. Or perhaps the polyp he removed was, in fact, premalignant and he is being overly cautious.

I'm as confused as you are. Consequently, I suggest that you insist on a second opinion from a gastroenterologist, who—after reviewing the records of your previous procedures—can advise you when (and if) another colonoscopy would be appropriate. In addition, the consultant should be able to tell you if you were subjected to unnecessary surgery.

From the limited information you supplied in your question, I'd have

What Is a "False Positive" Test?

A negative test is considered to be normal. A positive test is one that is outside the normal range. This doesn't necessarily mean that something is seriously wrong, however. A chest X-ray, for instance, may show small areas of inconsequential scarring that make the film "positive," but nothing needs to be done about it.

Because no test is 100 percent perfect, negative tests may not reveal an abnormality that is truly present. For example, a mammogram may not show a tiny early cancer.

Therefore, the issue of positive vs. negative has to be taken in a clinical setting, using other criteria to refine and define the diagnosis.

to conclude that someone fouled up. I think that your best bet is to place yourself under the care of a specialist who can fully explain this complex situation and carry out the required follow-up examinations.

Wife of smoker not to blame

Q. My husband just died from lung cancer at age 63. A committed smoker, he was diagnosed with pneumonia five years ago and two years ago had an abnormal chest X-ray. Despite radiation therapy, antibiotics and chemotherapy, he passed. I have an unsettling question about how this could have gotten so bad without us knowing. I blame myself for not responding to his cough and weight loss.

A. Spouses of smokers often blame themselves for deaths from lung cancer that are unquestionably the responsibility of the patient. In most instances, a spouse cannot cause a partner to stop engaging in self-destructive behavior. This is a personal decision that a person makes when he or she is ready.

Your husband died of complications from a habit that is well known to cause lung cancer. Nothing you or anyone else could do would have affected the outcome. This was his decision—and his alone.

While I am sorry for your loss, I prevail upon you to absolve yourself of responsibility. You are not to blame.

Living with effects of chemotherapy

Q. My wife recently underwent a series of chemotherapy treatments for lung cancer. Although the cancer is now in remission, she is experiencing persistent tingling in her feet and hands. Is this from the medicine?

A. Probably. Chemotherapy refers to treatment of malignancies using powerful antimetabolite drugs. In essence, these compounds are extremely poisonous and affect cells' ability to reproduce and grow.

Because cancer cells divide and grow uncontrollably and much faster than normal cells, the theory is that chemotherapy selectively alters and kills cancer cells. However, healthy cells are unavoidably poisoned as well. This leads to malaise, nausea, hair loss, anemia, and a host of other expected complications, including neuropathy (nerve damage).

Your wife, who has completed a course of chemotherapy over what I assume to be several weeks, may well be suffering from drug-induced neuropathy. In general, it's the nerves of sensation, not muscular movement, that are affected; thus, she is experiencing numbness, tingling and pain, without weakness or loss of coordination.

You should ask her doctor about this, but in my experience, the neuropathy of chemotherapy usually disappears in a matter of weeks after the cancer treatment has been stopped.

The side effects of chemotherapy are very unpleasant—so unpleasant, in fact, that some patients may refuse treatment rather than risk weeks of feeling sicker than they would from the cancer itself. However, these side effects are inevitable: the price one has to pay for drug therapy.

To my knowledge, there is no standard treatment for the neurotoxicity of chemotherapy. If your wife is patient, her symptoms should diminish with time.

Is there hope for a cancer cure?

Q. After an eight-year battle with breast cancer, my wife died two years ago. The people at the hospital and hospice were wonderful to me, and they ultimately suggested grief bereavement sessions. I attended several, yet the anguish is still present. The attendance at these sessions waxed and waned. At every session, someone would voice an opinion that pharmaceutical companies, the doctors, and/or big business were holding back the research or marketing of a cancer cure for a more auspicious moment. This was like rubbing salt in my wounds. If answering this will embarrass you, I understand. Otherwise, please respond.

A. Breast cancer is one of the chief causes of death in women. It is inconceivable, as well as unconscionable, that any responsible authority or corporation would deprive such women of a cure because of financial or other nonmedical considerations.

There is, as you know, available treatment for breast cancer, ranging from hormones to radiation. True, these therapies are imperfect, but they are the best we've got. Many research scientists are working feverishly to discover a cure for cancer. You can be sure that a breakthrough would be widely reported and used, when it occurs. Such a moment would, indeed, be auspicious.

Based on studies—including the recent work implicating a genetic factor as a cause of certain breast and bowel malignancies—more and more specialists are beginning to believe that the next exciting medical marvel will be cancer prevention by genetic manipulation. Unfortunately, such progressive therapy is still decades away.

I can well understand the anger, frustration and sense of loss that you and the members of your bereavement sessions continue to face. But rather than blaming the "system" for not having developed a satisfactory cure for cancer, I think that you can work through your grief more effectively by putting the past behind you, getting on with your life, and using the support of the bereavement group to make new choices and accept new challenges. Granted this is not easy, but it certainly beats focusing on past losses.

Rare mushroom may someday yield anticancer agent

Q. Have you heard of the rare maitake mushroom of northeastern Japan that is reported to be an anticancer agent? A report that appeared in the Cancer Chronicle sounds pretty impressive.

A. Powder made from the rare Japanese maitake mushroom is the latest cancer-cure fad. Whether this material will prove effective as a cancer treatment depends on the results of studies now under way in Europe.

Information is hard to come by because maitake mushrooms are very rare, even in Japan, and must be grown in carefully controlled environments. If there is some useful substance in the mushrooms, it will eventually be identified, synthesized and made available to the public. But that's a long way off. Don't hold your breath.

What You Should Know about Skin Cancer

You probably know someone who has or has had skin cancer. Skin cancer is the most common of all cancers, and more than 500,000 new cases are diagnosed each year in the United States. One-third of all cancers are skin cancers, and one in every seven Americans is affected. When all age groups are taken into account, more men than women get skin cancer, but among younger age groups, almost as many women as men develop the disease.

The sun is the cause of at least 90 percent of all skin cancers, and almost all skin cancers are preventable. Skin cancer is completely curable when treated in its earliest stages.

Skin cancers are more common among people who have lightly pigmented skin or who live at latitudes near the equator. Among blacks, because of heavy skin pigmentation, skin cancer rates are negligible.

Rates of skin cancer are rising, according to Dr. Stephen Katz, chief of dermatology at the National Cancer Institute, and this trend has made dermatologists very concerned. Factors in the increase include the popularity of sunbathing, more leisure time for outdoor activities and the fashion of wearing skimpier clothing that allows more skin to be exposed.

Basal cell carcinoma

Basal cell carcinoma is the most common form of skin cancer, affecting more than 400,000 Americans each year. In fact, it is the most common of all cancers, accounting for one-quarter of all new cancers.

What to look for:

Because chronic overexposure to the sun is the cause of almost all basal cell carcinomas, they occur most frequently on the exposed parts of the body—face, ears, neck, scalp, shoulders and back. They may, however, develop on non-exposed areas.

Basal cell carcinoma can sometimes resemble noncancerous conditions, such as psoriasis or eczema.

The Skin Cancer Foundation recommends looking for the following signs:

—An open sore that bleeds, oozes or crusts and remains open for three or more weeks. A persistent non-healing sore is a very common early sign.

—A reddish patch or irritated area, frequently occurring on the chest, shoulders, arms or legs. Sometimes the patch crusts or may itch or hurt. At other times, it may cause no discomfort.

—A smooth growth with an elevated, rolled border and an indentation in the center. As the growth slowly enlarges, tiny blood vessels may develop on the surface.

—A shiny bump or nodule that is pearly or translucent and is often pink, red or white. The bump can also be tan, brown or black, especially in dark-haired people, and can be confused with a mole.

—A scar-like area, white, yellow or waxy, that often has poorly defined borders. The skin itself appears shiny and taut. Although a less frequent sign, it can indicate the presence of an aggressive tumor.

Types of treatment:

The diagnosis of basal cell carcinoma is confirmed with a biopsy in which a small piece of tissue is examined for malignant cells under a microscope. There are several ways to treat this cancer, most of them surgical, and all can be performed on an outpatient basis under local anesthesia. The choice of treatment will depend on the size and location of the tumor and the patient's age and general health.

Basal cell carcinoma almost never spreads to vital organs, but it can destroy surrounding tissue, especially around the eye, ear or nose.

Malignant melanoma

Malignant melanoma is the most serious form of skin cancer. Fortunately, the death rate for melanoma has begun to level off for the first time in decades, suggesting that educational measures for physicians and the general public about early detection may be having an effect.

Causes of melanoma:

Sunlight exposure appears to play a major role in melanoma, although the relationship is less well documented than that for basal cell carcinoma. Other factors involved are genetic elements, immunologic factors, and possibly viral and chemical carcinogens.

About 1 to 2 percent of infants are born with moles on their skin, called congenital nevi. In those that are very large, more than 10 inches in length, melanomas develop in 5 to 10 percent. Some melanomas seem to arise from acquired moles that develop in almost everyone during early life. In other cases, melanomas seem to run in families.

Melanomas may also develop in the eye or in hidden areas such as the genitals, and predisposing causes for these lesions are unknown.

Dr. Arthur Sober and his associates at Harvard Medical School have reported that individuals who have had blistering or painful sunburns as children or adolescents have a two to three times greater risk of developing melanoma. Dr. Sober suggests that individual traumatic sun exposures may be more important than chronic levels of exposure.

What to look for:

The trunk is the predominant site for malignant melanoma in males (42 percent) and the legs in women (34 percent). There are several types of melanoma, and not all are dark-colored. According to the Skin Cancer Foundation, the following warning signs in a new or existing pigmented area of the skin or a mole may indicate melanoma:

—Change in size, especially sudden or continuous enlargement.

—Change in color, especially multiple shades of brown or black, mixing of red, white and blue or spreading of color into surrounding skin.

—Change in shape, especially development of irregular or notched borders.

—Change in elevation, especially raising of part of a pigmented area that used to be flat.

—Change in surface, especially scaliness, erosion, oozing, crusting, ulceration or bleeding.

—Change in surrounding skin, especially redness, swelling or development of colored blemishes next to the pigmented area.

—Change in sensation, especially itchiness, tenderness or pain.

—Change in consistency, especially softening or hardening.

How is melanoma treated?

Treatment for melanoma is always surgical excision. The extent of the surgery will depend on the extent the lesion has penetrated the deeper tissues. Nearby lymph nodes may also be excised if the tumor has metastasized to them or if the severity of the lesion indicates a high probability of metastasis.

It is now possible to predict with considerable accuracy which malignant melanomas are curable and which are not. Thickness of the tumor is a key indicator. Malignant melanomas that are removed when they are less than 3/4 of a millimeter (about 1/32 of an inch) in thickness are cured in virtually all cases. Progressively thicker melanomas have correspondingly poorer prognoses.

Protection against skin cancer

The most important thing you can do to prevent skin cancer is to avoid excessive sun exposure. Minimize exposure during the hours of 10 a.m. to 2 p.m., when the sun's rays are the most damaging. Wear protective clothing, and by all means use a sunscreen.

Some of the most effective sunscreens contain PABA compounds. If you find you are allergic to PABA-containing sunscreens or they irritate your skin, sunscreens containing cinnamates, benzophenones or anthranilates are also effective.

Sunscreens are classified by Sun Protection Factor (SPF) ratings, according to the degree of sunblocking effect. Most dermatologists recommend using a product that has an SPF of 15. Sunscreens should be applied 15 to 30 minutes prior to exposure to allow the product to penetrate the skin, and reapplied frequently, especially while swimming or perspiring heavily.

Sunscreens should be used when outdoors at high altitudes where there is less atmosphere to absorb the sun's rays, on overcast days, during outdoor winter activities, and even in the shade, if you're near reflective surfaces. Sand, snow, concrete and water can reflect more than half the sun's rays onto your skin.

Keep young infants out of the sun. Begin to use sunscreens on children at six months of age and then allow only moderate sun exposure. In view of the recent evidence on the relationship between childhood sunburns and later skin cancer, teach children sun protection early. Sun damage occurs with each unprotected exposure and accumulates over a lifetime.

Be aware of all the warning signs, and perform regular self-examination of your skin. The Skin Cancer Foundation suggests "EYBSOYB"—examine your birthday suit on your birthday":

Undress completely in a well-lighted room with a full-length mirror. Examine your hands, including spaces between fingers and fingernails. In the mirror, look at the backs of your forearms and elbows. Observe the entire front and both sides of your body in the mirror. With your back to the mirror, look at buttocks and backs of thighs and legs. With your back to the mirror, use a hand mirror to examine back of neck, back, buttocks and back of arms. Examine your scalp in the same way, using both mirrors. Sit down and prop one leg up on a chair, and use the hand mirror to examine the inside of the leg, including the groin and genital area. Repeat on the other side. Last, examine both feet, including the spaces between the toes, and the soles.

Concerns about cancer follow-up

Q. In the past three years, I've had both breasts removed because of cancer and, last year, had an excision of a melanoma on my back. My previous oncologist insisted on annual checkups to detect and treat any remaining (or new) cancerous tissue.

However, my employer has changed insurance companies, and my new HMO doctor says that such follow-up is unnecessary. She insists that I check myself for lumps and skin lesions. I don't feel comfortable with this advice. Should I follow it or go out of plan and pay out of pocket?

A. Although you are probably cancer-free at this time, you are undoubtedly at risk for trouble in the future. Thus, I share your concern. In my opinion, your HMO is more focused on the bottom line than on the health of its participants.

The first step I would take is to scream bloody murder. The HMO needs a lesson in ethics and appropriate medical care. Return to your original oncologist for a planning session. If he still believes that annual follow-up is prudent, he can write to the HMO appeals board and request that the company pay for you to go out of plan and/or provide you with yet another opinion from a qualified cancer specialist. You are not helpless in this situation. If the consensus is to examine you at regular intervals, the HMO will probably back down and acquiesce—especially if there is even a hint of legal action. But, at this point, your priority is to obtain objective and sound opinions about your best option.

Is routine CT scan a good idea?

Q. A close friend of mine just died of cancer of the pancreas. Her doctor told me that there is really no way to diagnose this condition until it reaches an advanced state. Her cancer was eventually discovered with a CT scan.

It occurred to me that a good preventive health measure might be to obtain periodic CT scans in, say, all people over 65. What do you think of this proposal?

A. I used to think that it was an unnecessary waste of money and resources. But, I must admit, I've had second thoughts, since several of my patients have asked me the same thing. One even went so far as to undergo the procedure and was quite relieved at the favorable, normal results. (He paid for it himself.)

You're correct that many cancers (especially of the ovary and pancreas) are difficult to diagnose in their early stages. Doesn't it then make sense to perform routine CT scans on healthy older adults every year or so? Maybe.

CT scans ordinarily cost between $800 and $1,500. I'm told by my radiologist colleagues that the radiation exposure is acceptable. Given the potential benefits, why wouldn't a well-heeled—and perhaps well-healed—consumer spend this amount for the purpose of detecting a curable cancer or other affliction (such as an abdominal aortic aneurysm) as part of a routine examination?

I don't have the answer.

However, I'd be willing to bet that more and more people are going to consider this option seriously. Medicare and health insurance won't pay for routine CT scans, but I think that this issue is worthy of public debate. It's something we all—doctors and patients—ought to think about.

To my knowledge, there have been no definitive reports or studies in the medical literature that address this proposal. We probably need some research on the topic.

I'm sure that scientists in a large teaching hospital will eventually conclude that the enormous cost outweighs the meager benefits. But if your life is saved, the cost to you is trivial.

Therefore, I'm keeping an open mind about this revolutionary concept. For my patients who want a routine CT scan and are willing to pay for it out of pocket, I'll probably acquiesce and order it.

Shark cartilage worth a try?

Q. My husband suffers from untreatable kidney cancer. He had one removed already because of this, is a diabetic, and needs some direction. A friend suggested shark cartilage as a possible cure. Is this a logical move on top of the eight medications he's already taking?

A. The therapy for untreatable cancer of any type depends on the roll of the dice. Because the condition is, by definition, untreatable (usually because it is too far advanced), any experimental therapy—no matter how outlandish—may provide last-ditch hope for cancer patients who cling to life. And, in fact, an occasional, terminally ill patient will seem to respond to unconventional treatment.

I watched the "60 Minutes" segment on the use of shark cartilage in cancer patients and was impressed that the substance seemed to show promise. However, there are—as yet—no studies convincing enough to sway most cancer specialists.

Because your husband is already taking so much chemotherapy, I'd be reluctant to add another drug—especially an unproved substance. Nonetheless, it probably wouldn't hurt; ask his oncologist about this. It seems to me that your husband has nothing to lose—and, perhaps, much to gain—from shark cartilage therapy.

Cancer does have spontaneous cures

Q. I don't understand why you pan Mexican clinics that treat cancer with alternatives to traditional therapy. Chemotherapy and radiation further weaken the immune system—just what a cancer patient does not need.

Speaking personally, 13 years ago I was diagnosed with untreatable small cell carcinoma of the lung that had spread to my heart and esophagus. I was given three months to live. In desperation, I went to the Bio-

Medical Center in Tijuana, Mexico, for immune-booster shots. I am now cancer-free: living proof that this therapy is effective, and has been in over 80 percent of patients during the last 50 years. The program costs only $3,500 and appears to be superior to U.S. cancer treatments. Wake up and help cancer victims!

A. Your personal experience is certainly stunning. However, if the Mexican injections are so effective, why haven't they been widely publicized in the world's medical literature? In our epoch of instant information, millions of patients could be helped if the Mexican findings were valid and could be disseminated. But that hasn't, to my knowledge, happened so far.

Also, as I'm sure you know, cancers can undergo spontaneous cure for reasons that no one understands.

I agree with you that methods to improve our immune responses to malignant cells makes far more sense than our current, primitive approach which is centered around killing both healthy and cancerous cells with poisons in hopes that somehow the malignant cells will die faster. This is why, as I have repeatedly speculated, the future cure for cancer will probably lie in a series of vaccines given early in childhood, much as standard immunizations are given today. In my world of optimism, I see my granddaughter's great grandchildren getting their cancer shots along with measles and mumps vaccines. But that day isn't here yet.

Today, we are clearly stuck with cancer therapy that is far from being universally effective, the one exception being therapy for certain forms of childhood leukemia. But this deficiency doesn't mean that medical science should descend to alchemy. We need studies that show which cancer treatments are promising and which are not. Given your enthusiastic endorsement of alternative therapy south-of-the-border, why have the Mexican doctors failed to publicize their astounding successes? Perhaps because such successes are no greater than those derived from traditional treatments.

The subject of cancer prevention and therapy is vitally interesting to most people for obvious reasons. Therefore, research scientists have an obligation to test any possible cure, no matter how outrageous, in hopes that it may provide the basis for a sound anticancer program that will benefit many generations of human beings.

15

Sex

—

Alcohol can affect potency

Q. I always enjoy your column and hope you will do one on impotence.

A. I receive a constant stream of letters inquiring about impotence (now known as erectile dysfunction, or E.D.), one of mankind's most ubiquitous ailments—the inability to achieve (or sustain) an erection. The causes of E.D. are legion and range from circulatory deficiencies (common) to psychological factors (rare).

In my practice of general internal medicine, the most frequent cause of E.D. is prescription medication. Almost any drug used for hypertension, heart ailments or depression can affect sexual functioning, often with disastrous consequences to an intimate relationship. Consequently, my standard approach for such patients is to alter, stop or change the drugs. In many cases, potency returns in a matter of days.

Another surprising cause of E.D. is alcohol abuse. I'm not referring to the skid row bum. In contrast, I see perfectly normal, successful men who are "social drinkers"—with sexual problems. Many of these men are retired, and it is in this group that the effects of moderate alcohol can be most damaging, because, as we age, we become less tolerant of the substance. In a male of 70, a couple of stiff drinks before dinner followed by a nightcap at bedtime can have a disastrous effect on potency. Therefore, in such situations, I urge them to cut down on alcohol (or, better yet, eliminate it) for a few days. This can produce astonishing results.

Of course, many cases of E.D. are due to severe circulatory problems, such as the premature arteriosclerosis seen in male diabetics. In these instances, referral to a urologist is prudent because special therapy—such as vascular surgery or penile implants—may be necessary.

Finally, there is no doubt that Viagra has revolutionized the treatment of E.D. The prescription drug is safe and effective, but should be avoided by men who take nitrate drugs for cardiac conditions.

Sexual Dysfunction

Sexual dysfunction is a widespread phenomenon. Studies have shown that 43 percent of women and 31 percent of men have had some sort of sexual difficulty. Fortunately, the majority of these instances can be treated and overcome.

The sexual response in both men and women consists of four distinct but related phases: desire, arousal, orgasm, and resolution, a cycle that is highly variable and depends on a complex interaction of both physical and emotional factors.

A lack of desire (libido) is the most common problem in women and may affect as much as 22 percent of females.

On the other hand, men have more difficulty with the latter part of the cycle. While 5 percent of men experience a loss of libido, and another 5 percent suffer from erectile dysfunction (E.D.), almost 30 percent of men have a problem reaching orgasm.

In large part, sexual problems worsen with age. Postmenopausal women note vaginal dryness, a loss of arousal and/or discomfort during intercourse. Treatment with an estrogen-based cream or an estrogen-filled ring (EstraRing) is often effective, as are lubricants, such as Vagasil, Replens and Lubrin.

Likewise, as men age, they find that it takes longer to achieve an erection and the erection may be short-lived. A healthy 40-year-old has a 5 percent chance of developing E.D.; by age 65, that figure jumps to 25 percent.

In both sexes, sexual dysfunction has many causes, including diabetes, arteriosclerosis, multiple sclerosis, prostate cancer, spinal cord injuries, cigarette smoking, overindulgence in alcohol, low levels of the male hormone testosterone, stress, depression, fatigue, arthritis, certain medications (such as beta blockers for cardiovascular disease), recent surgery, and problems with interpersonal relationships (familiarity, anger, resentment, and dissatisfaction with a partner).

Treatment of sexual dysfunction often includes counseling. Women should discuss their concerns with their gynecologists; men need to address their issues with a urologist.

A man can achieve an erection in a three-step process. The

first is arousal, when he has mental images or physical sensations that make him want to engage in sexual activity. During the second step, the nerves in his brain communicate this desire to the nerves in the penis, which increases blood flow to the organ. In the third stage, the penile veins constrict, trapping the blood in the penis, which then becomes erect.

Erectile dysfunction has traditionally been treated with penile implants, vacuum constriction device, MUSE (a disposable application inserts a tiny pill into the penis), and injections of compounds into the penis itself.

However, at present, the newer drugs for E.D. are vastly superior and have literally revolutionized the therapy for this common affliction. Called phosphodiesterase inhibitors, the drugs enhance the effects of nitrous oxide, a chemical that relaxes the smooth muscles of the penis, leading to an increase in the volume of blood reaching the penis.

Viagra (sildenafil) was the first drug in this class that was approved by the Food and Drug Administration in 1998. Since then, the FDA has approved Levitra (vardenafil) and Cialis (tadenafil). Although the drugs are usually taken about an hour before anticipated sexual activity, Cialis has a longer period of activity—up to 36 hours—thus it has been termed "the weekend pill" in Europe.

Phosphodiesterase inhibitors must be avoided by patients who take nitrates for cardiovascular conditions, because the combination can lead to a dangerous reduction in blood pressure, causing faintness. For other men, however, side effects (such as headache, skin flushing and indigestion) are relatively rare. In the unlikely situation that an erection may last for more than three or four hours, emergency medical attention is mandatory.

I am frequently asked how often normal couple have sex. The intervals between encounters varies widely depending on age and many other factors. I suppose three to four times a month would be average. Conventional wisdom is that if someone desires sexual relations once a month or less—and if either partner considers this to be a problem—then there is cause for concern and professional help should be considered.

The good news: Most cases of E.D. are treatable, even curable; which therapy depends on the cause.

New drugs improve libido, ability

Q. Please settle an argument. I say that herbal aphrodisiacs are useless, but my friend swears by them.

A. Sexual dysfunction is an age-old complaint, primarily among men, that has provided the basis for an astounding and ancient tradition of medication called aphrodisiacs.

Of course, the ancients' view of pharmacology was as primitive and incorrect as their understanding of impotence and other sexual problems. Almost any substance was, at one time or another, touted as a love potion. For example, centuries ago, chicken eggs were believed to improve sexual interest (libido). Unicorn's horn, a nonexistent remedy, once enjoyed wide popularity as an aphrodisiac, which makes me marvel at the skills of medieval con artists.

When first introduced into Europe, chocolate, potatoes and tomatoes were hailed as sex enhancers. This undeserved reputation didn't last, however, and the products became what they are today: prosaic edibles.

Suggestion has always played a crucial role in identifying an aphrodisiac. For instance, rhinoceros horn is shaped like a phallus, as are certain roots. Rhubarb and octopus are fleshy and firm. Garlic and pepper are "strong." Other substances, such as bull or goat testicles, have an obvious association with sexuality. Ginseng root, a staple of Chinese folklore, possesses antiinflammatory characteristics resembling those of aspirin; therefore, it's supposed aphrodisiac quality may actually be the result of its pain-relieving effects.

Belief is another important factor in aphrodisia. Basically, if a person believes that a compound will benefit him, it will in a high percentage of cases. This is called the "placebo effect" and, in some studies of sex enhancers, it can approach 50 percent.

The Food and Drug Administration has concluded that no safe, over-the-counter aphrodisiac is worth the money to pay for it. Most are harmless, but at least one, cantharidin, also called cantharis, can be lethal. Known under the sobriquet of "Spanish Fly," this powder is prepared by crushing and drying the "blister beetle," which is found in Near East and Mediterranean countries. Even tiny amounts of this powder, when ingested, may cause intense inflammation of the urinary tract, a situation that can lead to genital stimulation. In order to relieve the discomfort (by "scratching the itch"), some unfortunate victims engage in extended sex. This doesn't work. Toxicity, seen as kidney failure and shock, usually appears within 24 hours.

Take heart. Modern medicine has come up with at least four drugs that improve sexual interest and/or ability.

1) Levodopa. Used in treating Parkinson's disease, this medication often improves sexual functioning in the elderly.

2) Selegiline. Useful in slowing the development of Parkinson's disease, this medication enhances sexual ability without side effects or harm. Studies are being performed to test whether the drug may someday be used to counteract the waning sexual interest and ability so prevalent in the elderly.

3) Testosterone. Helpful only for men who have documented hormone deficiency, the drug has not been widely accepted because of the possibility that it may increase the risk of prostate cancer.

4) Viagra. This prescription medication has achieved worldwide recognition as the superior treatment for erectile dysfunction. The medicine stimulates certain muscles to trap blood in the penis, leading to more satisfactory erections. Although ordinarily safe, it should not be used by men who are taking nitroglycerine compounds for heart disorders.

In conclusion, reader, you are correct; your friend's generalization isn't. Fortunately, modern medicine is moving beyond the fly-by-night, street-corner world of traditional and ineffective aphrodisiacs. We are entering a new era of drugs that may actually cure one of mankind's oldest and most persistent complaints.

Even doctors sometimes make bad puns

Q. What is the difference between Cialis and Viagra? Is one better than the other?

A. To my knowledge, the only difference between the two products is that Cialis has a larger "window of opportunity"; hence, it has been termed the "weekend pill" by Europeans.

Let me share with you a personal experience that you may find amusing. Several months ago, I was visited ("detailed") by a representative of the Lilly company, which markets Cialis. She asked me if I had any questions about the product. I said no, except that I was curious about how the drug was named. She could not answer. So I did.

Alice was a very skillful and experienced "lady of the night" in Detroit. When male patients complained to their doctors of waning sex performance or interest, the physicians advised them to go "see Alice." This referral usually cured the problem; hence the name Cialis as a drug therapy for erectile dysfunction.

Of course, my supposition is simply an attempt at humor. Or is it real?

Topical estrogen may help vaginal dryness

Q. My 70-year-old wife experiences painful intercourse because of vaginal dryness. All her doctor can suggest is a simple lubricant. We would be open to holistic remedies or lifestyle changes—such as additional rest. Or should she see a gynecologist?

A. By all means, she should see a gynecologist. Vaginal dryness that leads to painful intercourse is a common symptom that many postmenopausal women experience. Although various lubricants are often helpful, your wife might be able to overcome her problem were she prescribed topical estrogen cream on a regular basis. The gynecologist can advise her.

Sex drive still strong in woman with one ovary

Q. I am a 66-year-old woman who had an ovary removed in 1973. I still want sex. Is there something wrong with me?

A. Not on your life. The loss of one ovary (or both) should not necessarily affect your libido (sex drive). After hysterectomy, some women say that they experience a decrease in libido, but this is far from a consistent perception. Women do not need more than one ovary, any more than men need more than one testicle. Enjoy the gift of sexual awareness.

Bypass surgery may affect sexual arousal

Q. Ten years ago, my wife was discovered to have a 90 percent blockage of her aorta. This was followed by surgery during which the doctor performed a bypass procedure and a sympathectomy. Since then, she has had no sexual desire of any kind. Just what was done to her?

A. During the operation your wife required (to bypass the blocked portions of her aorta and to sever certain nerves causing arterial constriction), the surgeon probably damaged some of the nerves necessary for sexual arousal. If I'm correct in this assessment, the situation is permanent. In my opinion, she should have been informed of this potential consequence before surgery. I suggest that you ask your family physician to find out (from the operative report and hospital record) what, exactly, the surgery entailed. He can then discuss this with you and explain the specifics about which you are concerned.

Masturbation safe and sane

Q. I'm a 64-year-old Catholic widower. After my wife died three years ago, I began indulging in regular masturbation. I know that the Church disapproves of this practice, but will it harm me physically?

A. Not in the slightest. Masturbation is a safe and harmless way to resolve your sexual tension until you feel comfortable enough to reach out to a prospective partner.

Cancer not passed on via sex

Q. Is the spouse of a man with prostate cancer (and an elevated PSA) at risk for cancer if she has relations with him?

A. There is no medical evidence suggesting that prostate cancer is spread through intimacy, nor is cervical cancer in women spread to men. In fact, I cannot think of a single malignancy that can be spread from one person to another by ordinary human contact.

Wife blames husband's roaming on Viagra

Q. I compliment you on your statement that wives should be consulted before doctors prescribe Viagra. If my husband's physician had performed pre-Viagra counseling, my marriage might not be in shambles.

My husband and I never had a particularly exciting sex life, in part because he couldn't maintain an erection. So he decided that the problem was that, after 32 years of marriage, he was no longer sexually attracted to me. He refused counseling. Instead, he talked his doctor into giving him Viagra. The doctor assured him that he could have great sex, so my husband had an affair with a bimbo. Obviously, the sex was wonderful. However, I found out about this escapade, my marriage went down the tube, my life has been ruined, and I am in the process of a divorce, feeling unloved and betrayed.

A. Your situation is, unfortunately, all too common. New, younger sexual partners can have an enormous impact on men with erectile dysfunction—and, for obvious reasons, Viagra can play a huge role in the scenario. I understand why your natural response is to blame the drug for your husband's infidelity, but I do not believe that this indictment is necessarily justified. The most important consideration is, in my opinion, that your husband refused to address his problem with the help of professional resources—in particular, a marriage counselor. His reluctance to examine the root of his difficulty suggests to me that his concerns about sexual performance probably preceded his use of Viagra—perhaps by months or even years. So, as I

> **Masturbation is a safe and harmless way to resolve your sexual tension until you feel comfortable enough to reach out to a prospective partner.**

states above, this situation is very complex. Perhaps you could be helped by some counseling yourself; at the very least, such an option might enable you to place the unhappiness and betrayal behind you, while you put your life in order.

Father children at any age?

Q. Can a man father a child at any age? When does he become infertile?

A. As men age, their sperm become less vigorous and numerous, but conception can occur as long as one sperm meets a receptive female ovum. The problem, as you know, is getting the sperm to the right place at the right time. If an older man is unable to achieve an erection or orgasm, the motility of his sperm becomes a moot point.

There are numerous medical reports of elderly men fathering children in their 80s and 90s. I suppose the most famous example is Charlie Chaplin who, as I recall, became a father in his 80s.

Therefore, the answer to your question is straightforward: Regardless of age, if an elderly man is able to have intercourse, he can impregnate a partner. As a sidelight, he could probably also provide viable sperm for artificial insemination.

Seventy-two-year-old patient can't get Viagra samples from his doctor

Q. I'm 72 and have erectile dysfunction. I take 13 pills a day for hypertension and a heart problem. No nitroglycerine, however.

I asked my female internist for some free samples of Viagra. She refused and said I should act my age. She concluded (incorrectly) that I would tell the other old war veterans if she gave me samples and that would "break the government."

I'm even willing to purchase the Viagra if she would agree to prescribe it.

Is this what happens to men as we get old? Do we have to ignore our sex drives? We don't want nay more babies, just a little sex now and then.

Do you think sex will make a person feel younger or act older? Will it keep the heart from pumping? Will a man die with a smile on his face?

A. May older men continue to have sexual urges. However, for a variety of reasons, they may not be able to perform.

This often is a side effect of prescription drugs. Therefore, I believe that your first step is to review, in detail, your medications with a sympathetic physician. Your present female doctor does not appear to fit this bill.

Consequently, I recommend that you search for a second opinion from another practitioner who can modify or change your prescriptions, refer you to a urologist or provide you with samples of Viagra or other similar medicines to counteract your erectile dysfunction.

This may enable you to die with a grin or, at least, feel a little younger and have a strong, pumping heart. (I hope your wife agrees, but don't count on it!)

16

Osteoporosis

Osteoporosis is treatable

Q. Please discuss osteoporosis. How can the disease be stopped from progressing?

A. Osteoporosis is a disease primarily affecting the elderly. It is marked by a progressive loss of calcium from the bones, making them brittle and susceptible to fractures. While the tendency to osteoporosis appears to be inherited, the affliction is worsened by inactivity, smoking, low levels of estrogen (occurring during and after menopause) and other hormonal factors that are, as yet, incompletely understood.

We all lose calcium from our bones during middle and old age. However, many experts believe that those of us with low bone-calcium to begin with will develop more severe osteoporosis at earlier ages. Thus, the stage may be set during adolescence and the 20s for bone problems in old age. Individuals who consume large amounts of calcium and have rugged bones in their youth may not suffer significant osteoporosis later. This is especially important for women during the reproductive years because pregnancy causes an enormous drain of calcium from an expectant mother, whose bones may weaken if she doesn't use calcium supplements during her confinement—and later, too, if she nurses.

Osteoporosis itself is painless. However, once bones become "washed-out" and demineralized, they crack more easily. In general, this takes two forms: frank fractures (such as a broken hip) and compression fractures of the spine. This latter entity is extremely uncomfortable because of the pain caused by progressive crushing of the vertebral bones. Compression fractures are a major cause of disability and handicap in the elderly.

Briefly, the treatment of osteoporosis includes exercise, calcium supplements with vitamin D, hormone therapy (for women) and drugs, the newest being Actonel and Fosamax. Although mild/moderate osteoporosis can be treated by family physicians, severe and advanced cases should, in my opinion, be under the care of endocrinologists or metabolic specialists.

Osteoporotic fractures are treated as ordinary fractures: casting (when appropriate), surgical fixation and braces/analgesics for spinal compression fractures.

Osteoporosis probably is genetic

Q. All my life I was assured that I could avoid osteoporosis if I took hormone replacement therapy and calcium supplements.

That was a lie. I feel cheated.

Now, at 62, I have been diagnosed with severe osteoporosis, even though I religiously followed my gynecologist's advice (hormone replacement therapy) and my family physician's urging that I take calcium supplements, exercise regularly and stop smoking.

How much exercise is "plenty," how much calcium is "appropriate" and what can I do now?

A. Although I acknowledge and accept your concerns, I do not believe that your physicians were

> 66 We all lose calcium from our bones during middle and old age. However, many experts believe that those of us with low bone-calcium to begin with will develop more severe osteoporosis at earlier ages. 99

incorrect in their analysis. For most women, the development of osteoporosis can be limited or reversed by HRT and other treatment, coupled with calcium and vitamin D supplements.

I suspect that you are the product of your genetic heritage: You inherited a tendency for osteoporosis. In such instances, HRT and calcium therapy are not sufficient; your need Fosamax or Actonel and more aggressive treatment.

I recommend that you exercise five or six times a week for 30 minutes a day, continue your calcium supplements (1000-2000 milligrams of the mineral plus 500 units of vitamin D) daily, discuss HRT with your gynecologist, and consider additional therapy with Fosamax.

I do not believe that you have been "cheated." Rather, your body is responding to the unavoidable consequences of aging. Acceptance of this inevitability will help you to adjust to the reality of the situation. But, for now, you need to address the osteoporosis problem with your family physician.

How much calcium for osteoporosis therapy?

Q. I am a woman, 70, with osteoporosis. What is the customary dosage of calcium supplements and vitamin D? How often should I see my doctor for my condition, and how long should I continue therapy?

A. Before answering your questions, let me give you a short primer on vitamin D. This vitamin is essential for normal bone growth and integrity. The Recommended Dietary Allowance is 400 International Units a day for the average young adult, an amount that is easily obtained in a well-balanced diet.

Supplemental vitamin D is recommended for postmenopausal women. However, excess consumption of D can be harmful, leading to weakness, fatigue, anemia, depression, kidney damage, high blood pressure, and elevated blood cholesterol levels. Therefore, people who take such supplements must be careful not to overdose; an amount exceeding 2000 IU is sure to cause toxicity.

The current recommendation for calcium intake depends on a person's age. Usually, about 1000 milligrams a day is appropriate for most of us. Pregnant women require slightly more and postmenopausal females (and those with osteoporosis) need significantly more, about 1500 mg a day.

Most calcium/vitamin D pills, such as Os-Cal+D, contain 500 mg of calcium and 125 IU of the vitamin. I suggest that you take 1500 mg of calcium plus 375 IU of D. This is supplied by three Os-Cal 500+D tablets, or the equivalent in similar products, per day.

If you have significant osteoporosis, however, you need more than just calcium and vitamin D. You ought to consider prescription options, such as once-a-week Fosamax, that will not only arrest the bone disorder but will also drive more calcium into your bones, thereby improving the osteoporosis profile.

In order for the mineral/vitamin supplement to be effective, it must be continued indefinitely.

I don't know how often you should visit your doctor. This depends on your general health and the severity of your osteoporosis. Ask your physician to advise you. Most authorities believe that a bone density test,

Tough-to-Diagnose Problems May Require Referral to Superspecialists

Q. I am a previously active man who has pain and stiffness. The condition began about a year ago, and now I have severe pain, even on stair climbing. I have not been a runner and am in good health. X-rays, MRI scanning and blood analyses (including a Lyme test) were normal. I've seen two orthopedic surgeons. No help or diagnosis. I've taken many anti-inflammatory drugs. No help. I am depressed and frustrated. Any advice? My doctor is at his wit's end.

A. Challenging diagnoses are a frustrating experience for patient and doctor alike—obviously, more for the patient. From your brief note, I assume that the common causes of knee pain have been ruled out by rather extensive testing. Therefore, you are in a special category. In a word, you are unique.

It also appears that you have exhausted the medical resources in your community.

In situations such as this, I have learned over the years to request help from superspecialists. As a result, I have forged valuable bonds with the staff members at the two medical schools in my state. And I have rarely been disappointed with the help they have provided for patients with obscure diagnoses.

Therefore, I believe that your best bet would be to make an appointment in a diagnostic clinic at a teaching hospital in your

repeated at regular intervals every year or two, is a satisfactory way of monitoring the situation—particularly in women with severe disease who are taking Fosamax or other drugs, such as Actonel.

Remember that along with mineral/vitamin supplements and prescription medicine, there are additional strategies you can use—such as regular exercise and discontinuation of smoking—that will have beneficial effects on bone health.

Does osteoporosis therapy have to be continued?

Q. Five years ago, at age 67, I was diagnosed with moderate osteoporosis and was placed on weekly Fosamax therapy. A recent bone area. I did not suggest an arthritis clinic or an orthopedic clinic because I'm not at all sure that your pain symptom stems from arthritis. I'd rather make sure that your discomfort is not muscular or vascular. But I get ahead of myself.

The diagnostic clinic is, in my view, the place to start. Before your appointment, make sure that you have with you all the pertinent records from your own physician. A complete background, hand-delivered, will be of inestimable value to the examining physician, and will certainly save you much inconvenience and expense. (For example, you won't necessarily need to be retested with MRI and blood analyses if you have the films and lab reports with you.) Don't—I repeat, don't—fax or mail this information in advance. Although I love tertiary medical centers, all too often incoming records get mislaid, misfiled or simply discarded. Guard your records carefully and turn them over only to a doctor.

I believe you will be best served by this approach. I know that it has worked for me. For those physicians who may read this and object, I say: Hey, I don't know everything. I often need help (even with inconsequential issues!). So it's nothing personal when I refer patients to specialists. What is important is that the patients get help; my ego doesn't suffer. And I am providing the kind of service that my patients expect and need. I'm just doing my job for the folks I care about.

density test showed that my osteoporosis has regressed; my bones are now normal.

My primary care physician wants me to continue the medicine, but my orthopedist said I could stop it. Which doctor should I listen to?

A. There is an old story about Paul Dudley White, a brilliant and legendary Boston cardiologist. Many years ago, at the peak of his career, he was asked to make a house call on a very rich socialite in New York City. Her physicians were at their wit's ends because, although the woman needed digitalis therapy for her heart disease, the drug—in a dose of one pill per day—made her very ill. The doctors needed to know if some alternative would be appropriate. The patient begged Dr. White to visit her and gladly offered to pay him for his time, travel expenses and consulting fee.

The cardiologist arrived at her townhouse, questioned her, performed an appropriate examination and noted that the digitalis did truly make her ill; yet he agreed that not taking it would be dangerous.

At that point, Dr. White proved his clinical superiority and did something the socialite's doctors hadn't even considered. He advised the patient to cut the digitalis pills in half! Problem solved. The woman ended up receiving the lesser dosage and lived to a ripe old age. Sometimes, particularly in medical practice, common sense does make sense.

Back to the osteoporosis issue.

At your age, your bones will lose a significant amount of calcium and without therapy, your osteoporosis could well reemerge. On the other hand, I agree with your orthopedic specialist that weekly Fosamax is probably more than you require. Therefore, I suggest a compromise a la Dr. White. Cut back your Fosamax to one pill every three or four weeks. This should stabilize your bone calcium concentration. You must be monitored with a bone density exam every year. If your density falls, you can increase your Fosamax. If your bones remain strong, a further reduction in the drug's dosage might be in order. Ask your primary care physician if he would endorse this approach.

17

Diabetes

What's new in diabetes research?

Q. I'm an insulin-dependent diabetic with a family history of the disease. I have four children and figure that at least one will develop diabetes in the future. Is there any current research underway that might make diabetes a thing of the past?

A. Researchers in many medical centers are actively working to discover the exact cause of diabetes, an inherited inability of the body to metabolize sugar efficiently because not enough insulin—or the wrong kind—is produced in the pancreas. As far as definitive therapy is concerned, there have been no outstanding breakthroughs, although transplant of pancreatic tissue and/or cells does show promise.

To date, most diabetics must rely on traditional treatment: a low-sugar diet, weight loss (if the patient is obese), pills to stimulate the pancreas to produce more insulin, or insulin injections to overcome the deficient production by the pancreas.

Many authorities consider diabetes to be an autoimmune disorder, which causes people to become allergic to their own normal pancreatic cells. This is probably accentuated by a genetic predisposition.

Therefore, any revolutionary advance in curing diabetes may well depend on new knowledge related to the diagnosis and prevention of autoimmunity. For example, new evidence implicating a viral infection in children who develop diabetes is being aggressively studied.

Insulin doesn't damage arteries

Q. I'm a diabetic and have taken insulin injections for more than 25 years. Could the insulin be damaging my arteries?

A. Insulin itself does not adversely affect circulation or damage arteries. The diabetes is the culprit, by accelerating arteriosclerotic blockages, leading to premature heart and kidney disease.

Living with Diabetes Mellitus

Most of us know that there is virtually an epidemic of obesity among adults and children in the United States and many of the industrialized countries of the world. What we may not realize is that obesity is helping to fuel an epidemic of diabetes as well, because obesity is one of the major risk factors in developing this disease.

Diabetes Mellitus is the term doctors often use to describe diabetes (differentiating it from a rare disorder called diabetes insipidus). Diabetes is a disease in which blood glucose levels are above normal because people with diabetes have trouble turning food into energy. The basic chemistry is that, after a meal, food is broken down into a sugar (glucose), which the blood then carries to cells throughout the body. Using the chemical insulin, made in the pancreas, cells process blood glucose into energy.

People develop diabetes for one of two reasons: Either the pancreas doesn't produce enough insulin, or cells in the muscles, liver and fat don't use the insulin properly. The end result is that the glucose stays in the blood, elevating blood sugar levels, while the cells are starved for the very energy they need.

Blood sugar levels fluctuate throughout the day, rising after a meal and returning to normal within a couple of hours. Normal levels tend to increase slightly but progressively after age 50, especially for those who don't exercise or move around much. Nationwide, about 6 percent of the population has some form of diabetes. People who have diabetes need to control the disorder through a combination of proper nutrition, exercise and medications (insulin or oral diabetes pills).

There are two types of diabetes mellitus, Type 1 and Type 2. It is the more common Type 2 that is on the rise, with 17 million cases in the United States, according to the latest report from the Department of Health and Human Services. That's an increase of 8 percent from the most commonly used previous estimate. Untreated, this is a disease that can lead to many short-term and long-term complications, so diagnosis and treatment are important. Prevention is even more important. The good news is that there are things people can do to bring those numbers down and to avoid some of the risks.

Symptoms of diabetes

According to the National Diabetes Information Clearinghouse, many people have no signs; symptoms can be so mild they're unnoticeable. However, here are some signs to look for:

- Increased thirst
- Increased hunger
- Fatigue
- Increased urination, especially at night
- Weight loss
- Blurred vision
- Sores that don't heal

Should I be tested for diabetes?

All people 45 and older should be tested for diabetes. If you're younger, but have risk factors such as being overweight and inactive, or have high blood pressure or high cholesterol—or if diabetes runs in your family—you should be tested. All at-risk groups, such as blacks, Native Americans, Asian Americans, Hispanics and Pacific Islanders should be tested.

Steps you can take to prevent diabetes

If you're overweight, lose weight and make maintaining a reasonable body weight a lifelong goal. If you're not sure what your proper weight should be, check a Body Mass Index (BMI) chart or ask your doctor. Being overweight can keep your body from making and using insulin properly. Make wise food choices most of the time, and be physically active every day. If your blood pressure is 140/90 or higher, in addition to losing weight and making wise food choices, reduce your intake of salt and alcohol, and see your doctor about whether you need to be taking medication to lower your blood pressure. If your cholesterol is high, watch your diet and ask your doctor whether you need medicine to reduce your cholesterol.

Moreover, the degree of arterial damage is directly related to how well the diabetes is controlled; that is, whether the blood sugar level can be brought under strict control and maintained in a normal range.

Your doctor can recommend the ideal doses of insulin for your needs, in conjunction with a suitable diet and a program of regular exercise. You should adhere to his suggestions.

The only real drawback to insulin therapy is the risk that, on occasion, you may self-administer too much of the drug, with resulting hypoglycemia (weakness, faintness, hunger, sweating and rapid pulse). As you know, such episodes are treated with orange juice or other sugary drinks.

Recently, authorities have developed a new device to help combat the problem of over- or under-administration of insulin. The device, called the Paradigm system, has just recently been approved by the Food and Drug Administration. Made by Medtronic MiniMed Inc. and Becton, Dickinson and Co., this new device automatically calculates and administers the insulin dose after each meal. Patients must still, however, check their blood sugar levels and program in how many carbohydrates they plan to eat at that meal. Because the device does the math for the patient, the likelihood of administering too much or too little insulin is greatly reduced or eliminated. Therefore, specialists hope this will result in better management of diabetes.

A pager-sized glucose monitor beams the input information directly into an implanted insulin pump using wireless technology. Simply put in meal plans and the internal calculator does the math, taking into account insulin sensitivity and insulin already in the blood. Patients using this new device still have the final say. A button on the device allows that dose to be accepted or overridden if for some reason more or less insulin is needed.

The product is available by prescription. It costs approximately $6,000. While that may seem like a hefty price, I believe it may be well worth it. It will provide better control and quality of life.

Arteriosclerosis and diabetes

Q. Five years ago, I was diagnosed as being diabetic. I take 250 milligrams of Diabinese daily. Since then, all my teeth became loose and were pulled, my nails split easily, I'm losing my hair and I've found it increasingly difficult to become sexually aroused. I'm 50 and female. I hope you can shed some light on this.

A. Circulatory insufficiency is one consequence of long-term diabetes. Diabetics tend to develop arteriosclerosis at a faster rate than do normal people. This blood vessel narrowing deprives tissues of oxygen and nutrients. Therefore, diabetics are more prone to develop infections, skin ailments, dental abscesses, heart disease and vascular problems, and sexual dysfunction. Check with your doctor to make sure that your diabetes is under control and that you do not have an internal imbalance of hormones or a low-grade infection.

Visual problems in diabetics common

Q. I am an 85-year-old diabetic. Recently, my sight has been hazy. Is there any exercise or food to strengthen my eyes?

A. Visual problems in elderly diabetics can reflect retinopathy, a complication of the diabetes itself, especially if it is not well controlled. Cataracts are also common in diabetes. I am not aware of any exercises or foods that could improve your vision. Rather, I urge you to undergo a thorough eye examination by a licensed professional. Once the precise cause of your "hazy" vision is diagnosed, you can obtain treatment. If the problem is as simple as presbyopia (loss of close-up focus due to age), reading glasses will correct this deficiency. On the other hand, diabetic retinopathy may require laser surgery, and cataracts may need a lens implant. Clearly, you must have an ophthalmic exam and, in my opinion, such an examination should be repeated at least annually. Remember, too, that you have to keep your blood sugar levels in the normal range to reduce your risk of heart and kidney disease as well. Therefore, you should also keep in close contact with your primary care physician or diabetes specialist.

Medicine won't make up for unhealthful lifestyle

Q. I am alarmed at the number of pills my husband has been prescribed: seven a day, including Glucophage and lisinopril.

Unfortunately, he won't watch his diet. After a month on the Atkins diet, he lost 30 pounds and was able to reduce the amount of his antidiabetes medication. But he cannot resist sweets, breads and pasta. I'm in a quandary.

A. Seven pills a day is not excessive for a diabetic hypertensive who is overweight. Therefore, in my view, the number isn't crucial. Your husband's denial is, however.

Diabetics must eliminate concentrated sweets (sugar and sugar-containing products) from their diets, and lose weight if they are obese. From your brief description, I gather that your spouse has trouble addressing this issue. The fact that he lost a phenomenal amount of weight in a relatively short time on the Atkins diet confirms my suspicion that he must begin to take more responsibility for his health.

For example, were he to take the situation seriously, he could diet until his weight becomes acceptable, and then determine if he needs medication (or how much). Weight reduction might not only enable him to cut down on his Glucophage; it might also reduce his blood pressure, thereby enabling him to modify his dose of lisinopril. In the most favorable circumstance, he might be able to take one Glucophage (or none) and one lisinopril (or none). But the decision to take full responsibility for health issues is the important consideration. I recommend that you discuss this with him and his physician, who, I am sure, would endorse such a plan.

Your husband's attitude is, unfortunately, a national concern. People often search for the easy answers to self-induced disorders. Obesity has become a serious problem among both children and adults in our society. The easy and common solution is to ignore the situation and rely on medication to help overcome the consequences of being overweight. The preferred and cheaper solution is to diet, exercise regularly and avoid medication when appropriate.

I urge you to share your insights and concerns with your husband's physician Working as a team with a positive goal in mind, you may be able to modify your husband's attitudes, habits and behavior—all to his enormous advantage.

A balance program may fit the bill

Q. My husband, 70, has Type 2 diabetes. He is starting to lose his balance when he walks. Are there any exercises that might help him?

A. Diabetes, in conjunction with the normal aging process, often leads to balance problems. This is a complex issue relating to vision, muscular reflexes, proprioception (the perception of body positioning) and neuropathy (nerve damage).

In my experience, such patients can be helped by a formal balance program. These programs are frequently available in hospitals through the physical therapy departments. Ask about this at your community hospital. If such a program is not available, inquire at your nearest teaching hospital. Your—and your husband's—efforts will be well-rewarded if he can receive training by professionals.

18

Stroke

_____

Understanding stroke complications

Q. My father passed away from complications of a stroke. Please discuss this condition.

A. There are two kinds of stroke: hemorrhagic and thrombotic.

The former, which is relatively unusual, is often associated with a weakened blood vessel (aneurysm) in or near the brain, head injuries or hypertension.

In such instances, a small artery ruptures, releasing blood, under pressure, into the brain, with resulting destruction of tissue. Hemorrhagic strokes are diagnosed by CT or MRI scans and, if treatable, require surgery to stop the bleeding.

In contrast, thrombotic strokes—the most common form—are caused by blood clots that form on the linings of major arteries, for example, the carotid arteries in the neck, break off and are carried in the bloodstream to the brain, where they become wedged, depriving vital tissue of nutrients. These strokes are also diagnosed by CT or MRI scans.

Regardless of cause, strokes produce neurological symptoms that range from slight confusion and temporary difficulty speaking to major nerve damage, paralysis, and coma.

By and large, the outcome of a stroke depends on its severity and location. Extensive brain damage often results in death or, at the very least, a severe and permanent handicap. Strokes occurring in vital tissue will often be fatal.

In addition to the acute dangers of strokes, patients often experience life-threatening complications during convalescence; for example, pneumonia or new strokes. Therefore, any person with a stroke needs careful supervision in a hospital, and the caregivers must aggressively treat complications as they arise.

Strokes—The Basics

What is stroke?

Stroke, a form of cardiovascular disease, results when the blood flow to the brain is stopped, depriving the brain of the oxygen and nutrients it needs. The blood can't get through because a blood vessel bursts or becomes clogged with a blood clot. Another name for stroke is cerebrovascular accident (CVA).

Brain cells can survive only a few minutes without oxygen. When the cells die, the part of the body that the cells had controlled is no longer able to function. This may affect the senses, speech, behavior, thought, memory, walking, and balance and may cause paralysis, coma or even death.

The warning signs of stroke

Don't ignore the warning signs of stroke! Although stroke usually comes on suddenly, often completely unexpectedly, there may be warning signs. By being alert to these signals, you may be able to get help faster and save a life or minimize damage. The five main warning signs of stroke are:

• A sudden weakness or numbness of the face, arm or leg on one side of the body.

• Loss of speech, or having trouble speaking or understanding someone else who is talking.

• Sudden dimness or loss of vision, particularly in only one eye.

• Sudden unexplained headaches or a sudden change in the usual pattern of headaches.

• Unexplained dizziness, unsteadiness, or sudden falls, especially when associated with any of the symptoms listed above.

In addition, about 10 to 20 percent of strokes are preceded by another phenomenon called "transient ischemic attacks" (TIAs), temporary and intermittent "mini-strokes" that last for only a few minutes or hours. TIAs are caused by temporary interruptions in the blood supply to the brain and can occur just a few days or up to several months before a stroke, with similar symptoms.

Since the symptoms of TIAs are often vague and confusing and the body returns to normal so quickly, people tend to ignore them and never mention them to a doctor. That can be very dangerous, however, because TIAs are serious warning signs of stroke. The problem remains hidden and may get worse. About 50 percent of people who have survived a stroke report a history of TIAs. Therapy for TIAs and preventive action must be started as soon as possible to avert a full-blown stroke. Treatment options include drug therapy to delay blood clotting or to prevent clots from forming, as well as surgery to clear out clogged arteries that supply blood to the brain.

Recovering from stroke

The outlook for stroke patients today is very encouraging. With proper rehabilitation, 90 percent of patients who have suffered significant strokes can be taught to use a wheelchair. Over 70 percent can become independent in the activities of daily living, and close to 50 percent of those who had been previously employed can return to work.

Recovery will take time, effort and patience, and some adjustments may be necessary. But those who have survived a stroke have already come through the worst part. They are alive and, with proper rehabilitation therapy, can look forward to productive, happy lives.

Routine management of stroke patients requires speech and physical therapy, medication to control high blood pressure, antibiotics for infection and, in the case of thrombotic strokes, anticoagulant drugs, such as aspirin or Coumadin.

Because stroke patients may have difficulty swallowing, nutritional needs may have to be met with intravenous supplements or feeding tubes.

Strokes frequently occur suddenly and without warning. This is a concern for most people, who do not wish to have advanced life support if there is no hope for a future life of independence. Thus, a living will in which the signer requests to not be kept alive by artificial means if severely disabled is especially important under these circumstances. Modern medical technology has the power to keep most patients alive indefinitely—even those in coma from strokes—when there is no chance of reasonable recovery.

While I am sorry to learn of your father's death, perhaps he would have chosen this option in preference to living with a serious handicap, such as massive paralysis or machine-dependent life-support.

Some strokes can be prevented by stopping smoking, taking medication for diabetes and hypertension when appropriate, and paying attention to warning signs, such as "mini-strokes" for which aspirin therapy may prevent a full blown stroke.

TIA serves as serious warning

Q. My very active mother, 71, recently had what the doctor called a TIA. She has no recollection of what went on for several hours, but her mind skipped back about a year and she kept asking the same question over and over.

What is a TIA? My mother has high blood pressure and is 25 pounds overweight. Does that have any bearing on the case? Are there any preventive measures she could take?

A. A transient ischemic attack, or TIA, is fundamentally a short-lived stroke. A small blood clot momentarily blocks one of the arteries that supply oxygen to brain tissue. The event is transient (temporary), ischemic (causing lack of oxygen) and certainly an attack, as it occurs without warning. If the clot is small—and it usually is, with TIAs—the body immediately mobilizes anti-clotting factors to dissolve it. Within hours, the patient ordinarily returns to normal and suffers no adverse consequences except, perhaps, for some confusion and amnesia.

TIAs are warnings of bigger and more serious things to come. Therefore, they should not be taken lightly. In your mother's case, there are clearly two actions she could take.

First, her blood pressure must be brought under control. For a number of technical reasons, chronic hypertension is associated with a wide variety of cardiovascular diseases, stroke and TIAs included. Although weight loss may not affect her brain circulation, it will probably help to lower her blood pressure, so she should try to lose weight.

Second, patients with TIAs are often helped by medicine that reduces the blood's tendency to form small clots. One aspirin a day, two or three times a week, is probably the safest and least expensive medicine.

Some specialists would consider putting your mother through more extensive testing, which might involve X-ray studies of her carotid arteries. I do not know enough about her to form an opinion, but you can ask your own doctor if blood-pressure reduction and the use of aspirin would be sufficient.

Memory lapse linked to mini-stroke

Q. My father is 77 and very active, both physically and mentally. However, during the past year, for about 15 minutes at a time, he has become disoriented. He cannot remember what day it is or what happened the previous day. He cannot place familiar people or recent events, but he walks and talks normally. We answer his questions and assure him he will remember everything in a little while and he does! Within an hour his memory returns and he goes on with his day. He's had an MRI and other testing. There's no evidence of mini-strokes. His doctor has no explanation and only suggests one baby aspirin a day. What's happening?

A. I'll bet your father is, in fact, experiencing micro-emboli (mini-strokes) that do not show up on the MRI test because they are too small. Apparently, his doctor agrees with me, because he prescribed aspirin, which retards clotting and is the treatment of choice.

Over time, as your father experiences showers of mini-strokes, his brain will be affected. His memory may not return and he will be less able to lead an independent, normal life. Therefore, this situation should be addressed immediately, before irreparable harm occurs.

Ask your father's doctor for a referral to a neurologist. Because most micro-emboli arise from arteriosclerotic plaque within the carotid arteries in the neck, your father needs further testing, such as a Doppler ultrasound or MRA (a test resembling an MRI that checks only for circulation), to identify the source of the clots. If obstructions in the carotid arteries are to blame, your father may require an operation to remove them.

What you have described is, I suspect, the equivalent of a TIA (transient ischemic attack), during which parts of the brain are temporarily deprived of oxygen. This is a precursor to an actual stroke, which causes permanent damage. Don't delay. Get your father to a neurologist.

When stroke follows aspirin therapy

Q. My husband was taking a baby aspirin a day on the advice of his physician. A month ago, he discontinued his therapy, because he was scheduled for minor surgery. Shortly thereafter, he had a stroke. Could this have been avoided? Many of our friends say they are taking a whole regular aspirin a day. Did my husband need more?

A. Aspirin acts as an anticoagulant. It is used as a prophylactic to prevent strokes and heart attacks in people who have previously suffered these disorders. (It is not appropriate therapy for otherwise healthy people.)

The major risk of minor surgery is excessive bleeding. Therefore, it's standard practice to suspend aspirin therapy in patients who contemplate an operation.

However, the discontinuance of aspirin carries with it certain potential consequences, of which stroke is one.

Here is how I put together your husband's situation. He properly stopped aspirin in preparation for surgery. This was followed by a stroke that presumably occurred because he we no longer anticoagulated.

Could this have been avoided? Probably. We'll never know if your husband would have had a stroke anyway, aspirin or not. But the sequence of events suggests a cause-and-effect relation.

Did he need more? No. The problem was that he stopped the low dose he was taking. Had he been prescribed eight or 10 aspirin a day—and had discontinued them as ordered—the outcome might have been the same.

Thus, I conclude—as, I am sure, your doctor did—that this was an unpredictable tragedy that could possibly have been prevented if your husband hadn't needed surgery.

As a general rule, a whole baby aspirin provides satisfactory anticoagulation in people who need this therapy.

Will stroke victim recover speech?

Q. My husband had a stroke and is in a nursing home. He still can't use his right arm or leg, nor can he talk. Is there medication to help his brain? I use a hand vibrator on his neck and arm, but I'd be very pleased if he could talk again.

A. When a stroke occurs, part of the brain is deprived of oxygen and dies, causing symptoms that depend on the location of the damage.

Your husband has had a major stroke that affected his speech center, as well as one side of his body. This is, as I'm sure you've been told, extremely serious. It's unlikely that he will ever regain the functions that he has lost.

Nonetheless, the prognosis is not necessarily grim. By retraining other nerves and brain tissue to compensate for the affected portions, physical therapists and speech therapists may be able to treat your husband's weakness and speech difficulties. This is a long and arduous process, as you can imagine, and he may require extended institutionalization while he works hard to recover.

Here is the bottom line: Your husband's damage, although permanent, can be moderated by a lengthy process of rehabilitation.

Incidentally, the vibrator treatment you are giving him will not improve his condition, but it may feel good to him—and to you, because at least you are doing something. Your best hope is to rely on the expert care being rendered by the professional staff in the nursing home.

Is mini-stroke to blame?

Q. My 72-year-old sister has, on three occasions, lost vision in her left eye. After the second instance, her doctor prescribed Coumadin for a presumed "mini-stroke." Her prothrombin time is 14 seconds. An MRI was normal. A carotid Doppler failed to reveal any blockages. Is she receiving appropriate therapy?

A. Older people may experience the effects of periodic blood clots to the brain. Sudden, temporary loss of vision in one eye, brief periods of confusion and forgetfulness or short-lived weakness may indicate that a "mini-stroke" (or TIA, transient ischemic attack) has occurred.

The diagnosis may be difficult to make, because definitive tests, such as MRI or CT scans, may be normal in the presence of tiny strokes. Under such circumstances, physicians often prescribe anticoagulant drugs, such as Coumadin. Also, these patients frequently undergo carotid ultrasound/Doppler examinations to determine if blockages in the neck arteries are a source of blood clots. Even with normal test results, however, anticoagulant therapy may be advisable.

Your sister has a clinical presentation that suggests small strokes: Tiny blood clots formed in one of her arteries, broke off and were carried to the brain, where they produced temporary visual disturbances. I believe that her doctor was correct to prescribe Coumadin, because—if left untreated—the next blood clots could cause more widespread, permanent damage, perhaps death.

However, now that she is taking Coumadin, the speed with which her blood coagulates must be monitored with a blood test called the prothrombin time. In an untreated person, the prothrombin time is about 12 seconds. Patients on therapy should clot more slowly, at about 18 to 20 seconds.

Therefore, while your sister is taking treatment, it isn't enough. She needs more of the drug to raise her blood test into the therapeutic range. She should return to her doctor, who will modify the dose of Coumadin.

Although full-dose Coumadin therapy is no guarantee that your sister may avoid a future stroke, it will certainly help prevent such a consequence.

Doctor's warnings make good sense

Q. My mother is recovering from a stroke. She has been told to stop smoking and follow a low-fat diet. But she's impossible. She insists that her doctor told her to stop smoking because that's what all doctors tell their patients. Her idea of a low-fat diet is to eat bacon only three times a week. I'm a 35-year-old health-care worker, but what do I know? I'm only a kid, as far as my mother is concerned. If you will reinforce the doctors' prohibitions, maybe my mother will listen to you!

A. Then, again, if she's like MY mother, she won't. You're always a child to your parents.

Seriously, your mother's doctors are absolutely correct, as you know.

Aside from the much-publicized effects of tobacco smoke (including heart disease, lung cancer and emphysema), many folks forget that the nicotine (and other compounds) in cigarette smoke affect the vascular system by causing constriction of arteries and, probably, a tendency for blood clots to form in these arteries.

For obvious reasons, these last two effects can substantially increase the risk of stroke—a situation your mother undoubtedly wishes to avoid, despite her stubbornness. Therefore, discontinuation of smoking is of paramount importance for anyone who has suffered a stroke.

Similarly, cholesterol deposits on arterial linings predispose to stroke and heart attack. The reasons for this are complex, but certainly involve the tendency of blood clots to form on rough, irregular arterial walls. Thus, smoking and high blood cholesterol probably exert an unwanted, combined effect that could be catastrophic for someone who has already had a stroke.

There, I've said it. Will your mother heed my advice?

Loss of nerve cells should be aggressively addressed

Q. I am a 75-year-old woman who blacked out for almost an hour. Because I drive, I asked for an MRI to make sure I didn't have a stroke. The report concluded with the following sentence: "There are deep white matter changes, more than usually seen for this age, and compatible with ischemic micro-angiography." What does this mean? My doctor assures me that I am fine.

A. I take issue with your physician. In everyday English, the MRI report is saying that your brain is shrinking, because of loss of nerve cells probably caused by mini-strokes. If, indeed, this is the case, I believe that the issue should be aggressively addressed—at minimum by a neurological consultation, a carotid artery ultrasound test and the daily use of 81 milligrams of aspirin. Also, in my opinion. The prudent practitioner should order a brain wave test (EEG) and a Holter monitor (a 24-hour cardiogram to check for abnormal heart rhythms).

If you were to faint again while driving, the consequences could be disastrous. Therefore, I favor an active effort to diagnose the cause of your blackout so that you can be prescribed treatment to prevent a future occurrence. Ask your doctor to reconsider his position.

Is a mini-stroke treatable?

Q. You recently wrote that "mini-strokes" are treatable. However, my mother's doctor says that her dementia, which is caused by such strokes, is untreatable. Was she diagnosed too late?

A. Some people, as they age, suffer tiny strokes caused by blood clots that travel to the brain and become wedged, depriving the tissue of oxygen and leading to very slight nerve malfunction.

A patient may be totally unaware of these painless episodes or may—at most—experience a momentary "lapse," with loss of memory and slightly slurred speech.

Although each "attack" may be trivial, year after year these tiny strokes continue to occur; eventually when there is enough cumulative nerve damage, symptoms—such as forgetfulness and impaired judgment—will appear. Thus, mini-strokes are a common cause of dementia, the end result of tens—possibly hundreds—of isolated instances of blood clots in the brain.

In the early stages, this situation is treatable, using anticoagulant drugs, such as plain aspirin. But there is a hitch: Doctors have great difficulty diagnosing mini-strokes before symptoms develop. The problem is that our testing is just not sensitive enough to do the job.

Obviously, the later stages, when permanent impairment is evident, tests—such as CT or MRI scanning—will show the damaged areas in the brain. Unfortunately, at this point, therapy is largely un-successful, as in your mother's case. Therefore, most doctors do not rely on laboratory tests when deciding whether to treat temporary brain malfunction. Instead, we prescribe aspirin to prevent further damage.

This is a long-winded way of saying, "Yes, your mother's diagnosis was delayed.

Here is how I resolve the situation in my own practice. If an elderly patient comes to me with a history of transient, inconsequential nervous system complaints (suggesting mini-strokes), I'll order blood tests, a CT scan, a carotid Doppler (ultrasound examination of the carotid arteries in the neck), and an EEG (brain wave test).

This will tell me if the patient has had bleeding into the brain, a seizure disorder or some other identifiable cause for the symptoms. If the tests are negative (normal), I assume that a mini-stroke was to blame, and begin therapy with one adult aspirin a day. In many cases, this ap-proach seems to prevent further damage from occurring.

However, once the neurological deficits are obvious, aspirin treat-ment is usually insufficient; I have to be content with treatment of the symptoms, as they progress. This may mean ultimate nursing home placement.

When stroke damage does not improve

Q. I had a stroke a year ago and still don't have the use of my left hand. Is there any way to reverse the nerve damage? I'd gladly permit a surgeon to make a hole in my skull and allow a brain mechanic to make repairs.

A. I have often, in fits of whimsy, likened doctors to automobile mechanics. When you think about it, our jobs are surprisingly similar and range from routine maintenance to the installation of new parts.

Unfortunately, when it comes to the brain, the simile unravels: Brain tissue cannot be "fixed" or replaced.

When a stroke occurs—either from hemorrhage or a blood clot—sensitive nerve cells are deprived of oxygen and die. This means that the organ supplied by those cells ceases to function normally. Weakness, dif-ficulty speaking and visual problems—to mention just a few conse-quences—appear and are permanent.

Nonetheless, variable degrees of improvement are the rule because strokes are always associated with brain swelling, which makes matters worse. Over time, as the swelling diminishes, symptoms become less noticeable: Speech and strength may return, albeit not to pre-stroke levels.

Also, with an active program of rehabilitation, most stroke patients improve, as the brain, nerves and muscles are trained to compensate for the damage.

Your stroke occurred a year ago, so I am convinced that your hand is not likely to regain strength. Rather than hoping for a surgical miracle, you would do better to continue your rehab program and follow your physiatrist's advice about physical therapy, as well as his suggestions about preventing another stroke—for example, by taking an aspirin a day.

Regaining balance after a stroke

Q. I'm 87 years old and had a stroke last year that left me weak on one side. Following this, I fell and broke my hip. Although I can get around with a cane, my balance is terrible and I am very afraid of falling again.

I am under the care of a very capable orthopedic surgeon, who confessed that he cannot help me with my poor balance. How can I regain my lost balance and confidence?

A. With hard work and patience, you may be able to gain back some of the skills you have lost. You should be enrolled in an intense rehabilitation program, under the supervision of a physiatrist (a specialist in rehab medicine). Such programs are available through most hospitals, as well as from private nonaffiliated therapy groups. You will be trained in a series of active and passive exercises to retrain your damaged muscles and nerves. In addition, the therapists will teach you techniques to help you compensate for your poor balance. There may also be many minor alterations that you can make in your home which will render your environment safer. Such alterations include better lighting, use of hand rails, avoidance of scatter rugs, relocation of your furniture, an elevator for your stairs, a change to more secure footwear, and the use of home health aides to assist you in everyday living.

As I mentioned, your recovery will take hard work and commitment under professional guidance, but the potential benefits may make all the effort worthwhile.

Heed the warnings of TIAs

Q. I'm healthy 69-year-old woman with a normal blood pressure. Last year, I had a TIA that lasted about six hours. I recovered completely.

Two months ago, while driving, I suffered a severe headache and slight confusion. This was followed by a similar episode a week later.

My doctor diagnosed migraine, which I've never had before, and put me on Elavil, an antidepressant. Should I be doing something else?

A. You bet you should.

A TIA (transient ischemic attack) is a temporary stroke, usually caused by a small blood clot that becomes wedged in brain tissue. Unlike a completed stroke, in which permanent damage occurs, a TIA resolves within 24 hours because the body dissolves the clot before it can cause damage. Nonetheless, this is a significant warning that a more disastrous neurological event is waiting in the wings—especially since you have had two further attacks. At this point, your physician should be aggressively searching out the source of the blood clots.

In my opinion, you need a CT or MRI scan of your brain (to check for bleeding), as well as a Doppler ultrasound of your carotid arteries. These tests will, among other things, show the presence of arteriosclerotic plaque, the presumed origin of the clots.

It is reprehensible that your doctor diagnosed migraine (extremely unusual to develop at your age) without obtaining the tests I mentioned. If he is disinclined to follow up with the testing, insist on a referral to a neurologist. In my view, you're sitting on a time bomb.

If you haven't had bleeding into the brain, you should be treated with anticoagulant drugs—at the very least, aspirin. If significant arterial blockage is present, you may have to consider surgery or other techniques to unblock the arteries. In any case, you can ill afford to wait— because if I'm correct, you're a candidate for preventable, serious future consequences.

Managing a post-stroke patient at home

Q. My 75-year-old brother suffered a disastrous stroke 10 years ago that left him with marked right-sided weakness and speech difficulties. At present, he lives at home and is cared for by his wife, with the help of minor assistance (housecleaning and food preparation). What is his prognosis? The doctor mentions the possibility of seizures and indicates that my brother will not appreciably improve. This is difficult to accept.

A. Following a stroke, most patients reach the peak of their recovery within six to 12 months. A stroke causes death and dysfunction of vital nerve tissue, often marked by partial (or total) paralysis and speech handicap.

Rehabilitation programs that involve speech training, occupational therapy and physical therapy are paramount in helping stroke patients recover. The goal is to increase independence by "reeducating" muscles and nerves to compensate for the damage caused by the stroke. There is, understandably, a limit to the degree of recovery. Your brother appears to have reached his limit.

Provided he doesn't have a second stroke—a definite risk for such patients—your brother will probably remain pretty much as he is now. Of course, you have to take into account the fact that he, like the rest of us, will progressively weaken with age. In elderly stroke patients, this can cause problems because they're already weaker to begin with.

Seizures can sometimes follow strokes, especially during the acute phase when brain damage is most severe and is aggravated by cerebral edema, posttraumatic swelling of brain tissue. However, if your brother has been free of seizures, he is likely to remain so.

Again, the major factor to consider is the risk of another stroke, which makes prognostication difficult. Your brother should follow his physician's advice—particularly about continuing rehab, medication to control hypertension (if it is present) and the possibility of anti-clotting therapy, such as daily aspirin. In addition, your sister-in-law must remain open to the probability that, at some time in the future, she will be unable to function as the primary caregiver. She may burn out or simply be unable to assume the responsibility of a severely handicapped spouse. At that point, a skilled nursing facility (or more hours of professional home care) may become mandatory.

Your brother's family doctor, with the help of specialists (such as neurologists and physiatrists), can offer considerable assistance in the present difficult times, as well as in the future, with more difficult times that lie ahead.

19

Bladders & Things Urinary

Bladder obstruction must be cleared

Q. What can I do to improve ailing kidneys? I have frequent urinary infections and diminished urine output. Tests show that my bladder doesn't empty completely. Would a special diet help the problem?

A. I don't agree that your primary problem is "ailing kidneys." Rather, you appear to have a bladder outlet obstruction.

When the bladder fails to empty completely, the residual, stagnant urine provides an ideal environment for bacterial growth: it is dark, moist and warm. Once the bladder is infected—a condition known as cystitis—the microorganisms may work their way up into the kidneys, leading to nephritis, an exceedingly dangerous situation. If left untreated, such a complication can eventually cause renal failure.

Consequently, I'd direct attention to the bladder outlet. Once the obstruction is treated (with medicine or surgery), the whole system will once again be free to drain completely and, after a brief course of antibiotics to eradicate any remaining infection, you should return to normal.

In my opinion, fluids and special diets will not help you. What you do need is a consultation with a urologist, who will document the presence of urinary blockage and recommend therapy.

Urinary infection not necessarily kidney infection

Q. At age 70, I developed a kidney infection, yet I have no symptoms. My doctor simply suggested that I increase my fluid intake. Can you tell me more about this?

A. First of all, I doubt you have a kidney infection. If you did, the doctor would certainly have prescribed antibiotics, rather than merely encouraging you to drink more. Untreated kidney infection is dangerous because it can lead to renal damage, hypertension and kidney failure.

True, you may have a urinary infection; however, this does not necessarily mean that your kidneys are involved.

Urinary infection may involve the bladder and other structures in the lower urinary tract. Such an infection ordinarily causes burning, frequency and blood in the urine. Some patients, especially the elderly, may experience no symptoms whatsoever. (In some older folks, the infection may be associated with a decline in cognitive function; they become confused and disoriented.)

Nonetheless, if your urinary tract is infected, you need treatment. Increased fluid intake is beneficial because it dilutes the infection—but does not eradicate the inflammation.

In order to diagnose the condition and prescribe the proper antibiotic, your doctor will need a urine culture. During this special but simple examination, bacterial growth is identified and then tested against a panel of antibiotics. In this way, the most effective antidote is determined.

I suggest that you question the doctor about your diagnosis, how he arrived at it and why he chose not to prescribe antibiotics.

Two-step prescription for kidney infection

Q. I have chronic pyelonephritis, and my doctor has stated that if I have another attack, I'll be a candidate for dialysis. What can I do to prevent this from happening? Is there any way I can keep this disease in check to avoid what appears to be the inevitable?

A. Pyelonephritis is a serious, bacterial kidney infection that, if untreated, may lead to renal failure. The two most important aspects of pyelonephritis are the infection itself and the potential for mechanical obstruction, which prevents urine from draining out of the diseased kidney. Before antibiotics can eradicate the infection, any blockages must be removed. Such blockages include kidney stones and scar tissue.

I don't see how you can modify your kidney disease, providing you follow your doctor's orders. Rather, it's up to him to assume this responsibility by 1) making sure, by X-raying your kidneys, that they are not obstructed and 2) prescribing appropriate antibiotics to rid your urinary tract of bacteria.

I believe that you should be examined by a urologist and, if you haven't already, a nephrologist. Working together, these two specialists (one surgical, the other medical) should be able to pinpoint your problem and offer treatment. In my opinion, your doctor frightened you unnecessarily.

Kidney cysts common and not alarming

Q. During a recent CT scan for abdominal pain, my doctor discovered a 2-inch cyst in my right kidney. He stated that it is "nothing" and ignored it. But I'm wondering what other people do in a situation like this.

A. During medical testing, doctors often discover incidental and harmless abnormalities. Kidney cysts are such a finding.

Before the advent of CT scanning, these cysts were generally not seen on routine X-ray tests. Now, however, physicians sometimes obtain more information from CT scans than they need.

In my experience, renal cysts are common, pose no threat to health and can be ignored. When patients are given this information, they usually gladly get on with their lives and pay no attention to the cysts, which cause no symptoms anyway.

Stand up against incontinence

Q. I'm writing in hopes that my experience may help other women who suffer from the urinary incontinence that I have had for several years. My main problem is an inability to empty my bladder completely. By accident, I discovered that if I stand up to urinate (in the shower, for example), I can empty very well. So now I stand for several seconds before relieving myself—or sit down, urinate, then stand up before sitting again to finish the process.

My urologist confirms that my bladder may be "kinked" when I sit, so there is some medical justification for my discovery. At night, I do a "double void." After my initial urination stops, I walk across the room and back. Then I can do more.

A. Several women have written me describing similar techniques to overcome incontinence. Apparently, in such women, the bladder-neck is blocked in the sitting position, which prevents complete emptying. Thanks for sharing your observations.

Cranberry juice beneficial

Q. I have been assured that cranberry juice has no effect whatsoever in preventing urinary infection. I've relied on this for years. Am I just being naive?

A. No. Recent studies have shown that the juice really does exert an antibacterial effect in the urinary tract. Your reliance was not misplaced.

Food choices affect urine odor

Q. What is the significance of urine that has the odor of disinfectant? I've noticed this for more than a year, yet I am a healthy 57-year-old woman who takes no medication.

A. Your urine probably smells peculiar because of something you're eating. For instance, I'm certain you've experienced the characteristic urinary odor of asparagus, after having eaten the vegetable.

Although I cannot give you a specific answer to your question, I encourage you to perform a little detective work to see if you can identify the source. If you're unsuccessful at this, check with your doctor for a urinalysis and further testing. Perhaps you have a low-grade bladder infection that needs treatment.

20

Gastrointestinal

Diverticulitis may reoccur

Q. I was recently hospitalized for IV antibiotic therapy because of pain and fever from diverticulitis. Now I'm concerned about a recurrence. My gastroenterologist indicated that there is no cure or method to prevent future infections. Can this be true?

A. I'm afraid so.

As we age, tiny pockets may appear in the colonic lining. Called diverticulosis, these small pouches ordinarily cause no symptoms.

However, these diverticula can become inflamed and infected, leading to abdominal pain, gas, maldigestion, intestinal abscesses, or bleeding. Thus, diverticulosis may progress into diverticulitis, the acute treatment of which includes a soft diet and antibiotics. (If the bleeding is severe or the infection is extensive, surgery may be necessary to remove the diseased tissue.)

Unfortunately, there is no generally accepted method or diet to prevent diverticulitis. Although some experts prohibit roughage and fruit with small seeds (which are sometimes associated with diverticulitis), the relation of diet to the disorder is far from clear.

Therefore, your gastroenterologist is correct. While you may choose to limit your diet (to avoid foods that you've found by experience worsen your affliction), there is no consistent cure or preventive. Your acute attacks will simply have to be treated as they occur, unless you choose to have an operation to remove the part of your colon most affected.

Abdominal pain may require a specialist

Q. At age 75, I have begun to have stomach pain: indigestion and gas at night. Upper gastrointestinal X-rays were normal. My doctor has prescribed Prilosec once a day. It helps as long as I watch my diet: no ice cream, chocolate, coffee or spicy foods. I often have a bonfire in my stomach. What's going on?

A. The fact that your primary discomfort occurs at night, intensified after eating certain foods, and is relieved by Prilosec (a drug to reduce the formation of stomach acid) suggests that your problem is, in some way, related to hyperacidity.

X-rays of your stomach should have shown an ulcer or hiatal hernia if you had these conditions, but X-ray tests are notoriously unreliable in diagnosing gastritis (an inflamed stomach lining) and other subtle abnormalities in the upper intestine, including gastroesophageal reflux disease (GERD), which I am guessing you have.

Therefore, I believe you would be best served by consulting with a gastroenterologist. Ask your family practitioner for a referral.

I am certain that the specialist will be able to diagnose your condition during endoscopy, a special test enabling him to examine your esophagus, stomach and part of the small intestine through a lighted fiber optic tube.

At this point, the ministrations of your doctor have not been totally effective. You need a specialist.

Colonoscopy called for

Q. I'm 78. Six years ago, I had three benign polyps removed from my colon. Should I have another colon exam? I'm asking because all I have is Medicare, and I'd like to avoid the procedure if possible.

A. Benign polyps (small growths) can easily be removed without surgery during a special exam called colonoscopy, during which a specialist—usually a gastroenterologist—examines the entire colon with a long, flexible fiber-optic tube.

Most gastroenterologist advise periodic colonoscopy (every five years or so) for people who have had polyps.

Thus, my answer to your question is "yes." Nonetheless, you should follow your gastroenterologist's advice in this matter. Incidentally, also review the cost with him. Because you have only Medicare to help with medical expenses, the specialist may be willing to accept assignment, meaning that he won't charge you more than Medicare will recognize as a reasonable fee.

At-home steps can cure many simple cases of diarrhea

Q. Please comment on the treatment of diarrhea. I am 86 and cannot get much help from my doctor.

A. Tomes have been written about the causes and treatment of diarrhea, a subject too broad for this short column. Suffice it to say, diarrhea can result from any inflammation of the intestine, as well as from food sensitivities, poor circulation to the colon, tumors and metabolic disturbances.

When otherwise healthy people suddenly experience diarrhea (with or without vomiting), it is most commonly the result of a temporary viral infection. Called "gastroenteritis," this condition can usually be satisfactorily treated and cured within 24 hours by following these simple rules:

Confine your diet to clear liquids—water, tea, soft drinks (especially ginger ale) and beef broth.

If you are able to tolerate this without vomiting, in 24 hours begin a bland diet—no greasy or indigestible foods.

Use over-the-counter remedies, such as Pepto-Bismol or Imodium A-D, as needed.

If, within 48 hours, your diarrhea doesn't clear up, call your physician.

How to handle problems with intestinal gas

Q. I am 72 and suffer from excessive intestinal gas that seems to worsen day by day. I get it regardless of what I eat—even a cup of coffee causes the problem. What can I do?

A. Intestinal gas is one of mankind's most prevalent problems, in part because it tends to become more noticeable as we age. As you can imagine, intestinal gas has many causes, including bowel diseases, poor circulation and irritable bowel syndrome. In a healthy 72-year-old, I would first consider three common contributions to intestinal gas.

One, air-swallowing. If you rush your meals, chew incompletely or consume carbonated beverages, you may be unknowingly adding to the problem. Pay attention to this and correct it, if necessary.

Two, lactose intolerance. As people grow older, they may have difficulty digesting lactose (milk sugar). As a trial, I suggest that you swear off all dairy products for two weeks. If your gas lessens, you may choose to use Lactaid to facilitate your digestion of milk, cheese and so forth.

Three, dietary factors. As folks age, they often experience digestive problems. As a result, when certain vegetables and legumes are consumed, they reach the large bowel before they have been broken down. Bacterial action on these foods may produce excessive gas and air pockets that can be quite troublesome.

Because of these three factors, you should analyze your eating practices to see if one or more could be an issue. The next step would be to try over-the-counter anti-gas products, such as simethicone (Gas-X and others) or Beano (a natural additive that I have found helps reduce symptoms in many of my patients).

If these simple and inexpensive options are ineffective, see your doctor for additional advice.

Mexico trip may harbor more than memories

Q. I vacationed in Mexico several weeks ago and, since my return to the States, have experienced constant abdominal discomfort and flatulence, with almost daily diarrhea. I had a barium enema and a sigmoidoscopy that my doctor claimed showed no irritable bowel. He gave me no medication other than antacids. Can you help?

A. You need a meticulous stool analysis, including fecal cultures and microscopic examination, to see if you brought home more than happy memories from Mexico. In my experience, healthy patients who develop bowel symptoms after traveling abroad almost always have picked up intestinal infections.

These infections are caused by a variety of disease-producing bacteria, such as E. coli, as well as by parasites, such as amebas. Although your distress and gas could result from a common condition, such as irritable bowel syndrome, I'd want to make sure that a treatable infection is not present. Ask your doctor to order the appropriate testing.

Peptic ulcer treatment update

Q. How has the treatment of peptic ulcers changed?

A. Dramatically. Years ago, the only therapy was diet and frequent milk and cream feedings, along with bicarb of soda.

Subsequently, antacids (such as Maalox, Gelusil and Riopan) became the rage. These agents were inexpensive, more palatable, more effective and did not provide excess cholesterol.

Later, the treatment of peptic disease was revolutionized by the introduction of drugs (such as Pepcid, Tagamet and Zantac) that reduce the production of excess gastric acid, a primary case of ulcers and reflux.

Now there is even a more effective treatment: stronger drugs (such as Prevacid and Nexium) that block stomach acid are available by prescription and may be supplemented by antacids as needed.

Finally, bacterial infection (with a germ called H. pylori) is a significant cause of peptic disease in many patients. When present, H. pylori is treated with antibiotics.

The therapy of peptic disease has evolved over the past decade to the point at which powerful (but safe) medications are almost always successful in curing not only symptoms but the disorders themselves.

Black tongue normal

Q. I frequently use Pepto-Bismol for stomach upset and diarrhea. After taking it, my mouth and tongue turn black, and I experience a metallic taste. Is this normal?

A. Bismuth compounds, such as Pepto-Bismol, often cause darkening of the tongue, a metallic taste and—as I'm sure you've noticed—black bowel movements. These reactions are predictable, harmless and do not indicate a problem, either with the medicine or with your reaction to it.

Hot prune juice cures constipation

Q. I think I have read that a certain fruit juice, when taken regularly, will lessen constipation. I sure would like to know of this.

A. Eight ounces of hot prune juice every morning may take care of your chronic constipation. Prunes, dried apricots and similar foods that are high in potassium are an effective and inexpensive laxative. Hot prune juice is especially effective. Try it.

Bacteria cause of colitis

Q. I have pseudomembranous colitis. Treatment doesn't seem to work, and I still suffer from diarrhea daily. Do you have any up-to-date information on this form of colitis?

A. This type of chronic bowel inflammation, which is associated with diarrhea and bloating, is a common consequence of antibiotic therapy. The medicine causes an overgrowth of a resistant strain of bacteria called *clostridium difficile* that produces a toxin capable of damaging the intestinal lining.

The disorder is suspected in anyone who develops diarrhea following a course of antibiotics and is confirmed by detecting the toxin in a stool sample. Treatment include combination therapy with Pepto-Bismol and Flagyl, an antimicrobial drug.

Although *C. difficile* inflammation is ordinarily just a nuisance, the degree of inflammation can sometimes be severe enough to cause bleeding into the stool, abdominal pain, fever, malnutrition, and severe dehydration.

If your stool tests fail to show the bacterial toxin, you should undergo colonoscopy (examination of the entire colon with a fiber-optic tube). This will enable your doctor to make a precise diagnosis by cultures and biopsy.

Lactose intolerance usually appears before 65

Q. I am healthy and 65. However, for the past three years, I've suffered excessive gas, indigestion and diarrhea after eating dairy products. Is it possible that I could have somehow developed a lactose intolerance at this age?

A. This is certainly possible, but not common. People often develop allergies to the milk sugar lactose; however, this ordinarily occurs at ages younger than 65. The reason for such a reaction is poorly understood.

You could have a breath test to check for this abnormality, but a simpler and cheaper option is to avoid dairy products (and milk sugar) as a trial. I'd go for four to six weeks. If your symptoms disappear, you've made the diagnosis and should use Lactaid when you eat normally. If your symptoms persist, please see a physician for further evaluation, testing and treatment.

21

Arthritis

Osteoarthritis versus rheumatoid arthritis

Q. Do osteoarthritis and rheumatoid arthritis have a genetic basis? What is the difference between the two? Are there home remedies to alleviate the pain and stiffness of the conditions?

A. As we age, we become less efficient at repairing damaged tissue. During our younger years, normal wear and tear is so quickly repaired that we easily ignore the miraculous process. The joints are a prime example.

When we engage in everyday activities, the joint linings tend to wear down. When we're young, the body's reparative processes compensate for this. In older adults, however, the joint linings remain thin and worn, leading to stiffness, pain and swelling. Called "osteoarthritis," this condition will affect every one of us, sooner or later, to one degree or another. The use of ibuprofen or prescription medications will help to relieve symptoms, but there is no antidote for the aging process.

In contrast, rheumatoid arthritis is an autoimmune disease, marked by severe inflammation of the joints that can affect children as well as adults. The cause is unknown, but experts theorize that the body's immune system inappropriately attacks the joint linings, leading to pain, swelling and eventual destruction of the joints unless treatment is given. Such therapy involves anti-inflammatory drugs, cortisone, methotrexate, Enbrel and others.

Neither form of arthritis is inherited, to my knowledge; however, you can understand from my brief description that osteoarthritis does "run" in families whose members live to ripe old ages.

There are no satisfactory home remedies for these forms of arthritis—or any form, for that matter.

As a general rule, patients with age-related osteoarthritis suffer fewer handicaps and can medicate themselves with over-the-counter medica-

Understanding Osteoarthritis

Osteoarthritis is a chronic disease of the joints resulting from breakdown of joint tissue, primarily cartilage. Its symptoms include pain, aching and stiffness in the affected joints. It is an extremely common disorder in both humans and animals and has been known since ancient times. Evidence of osteoarthritis is found in Egyptian mummies and dinosaur bones as well as in modern-day racehorses.

Other names for osteoarthritis are degenerative joint disease, osteoarthrosis, arthrosis, hypertrophic arthritis and "wear and tear" arthritis. It is sometimes called simply "arthritis," but must be differentiated from rheumatoid arthritis. Although both types of arthritis have some common features and some similar treatments, rheumatoid arthritis is usually a more damaging condition that is more difficult to control.

Osteoarthritis affects about nine times as many adults as does rheumatoid arthritis. In fact, X-rays show that most people over 60 have some degree of osteoarthritis, but the majority will never experience any symptoms. Osteoarthritis is generally associated with aging, although it can be seen at all ages.

Older people are more likely than younger ones to develop osteoarthritis, presumably because of joint damage from inju-

tions, whereas patients with inflammatory arthritis—such as the rheumatoid variety—usually require medical attention and prescription drugs.

New therapy for rheumatoid arthritis

Q. I have rheumatoid arthritis. For years, I was prescribed prednisone and methotrexate (an antimetabolite that interferes with the immune system.) These didn't work. Now I have been using Enbrel with stunning success. Is this therapy appropriate?

A. Enbrel, which binds to tumor necrosis factor and blocks its interaction with cells in the body, is now considered to be vastly superior to other drugs in treating rheumatoid arthritis. It is given as an injection every week or two. There are no side effects of note, but the medicine is frightfully ries and stress that accumulates over time. Women are affected about twice as frequently as men. The Arthritis Foundation estimates that 17 million people in the United States have osteoarthritis that is severe enough to cause pain.

Treating the osteoarthritis

Treatment of osteoarthritis is aimed at controlling the pain, maintaining movement and preventing joint deformity. The measures used in treatment include medication, rest, exercise, joint protection and sometimes surgery, depending on which joints are affected and how bad the symptoms are.

Aspirin is the most widely used drug for the pain and inflammation of arthritis. Newer types of agents, called nonsteroidal anti-inflammatory drugs, are frequently prescribed instead of aspirin. Sometimes corticosteroids are injected directly into joints that have become inflamed.

Both rest and exercise, in the right combination, are important in treating osteoarthritis. A joint with degenerative changes cannot tolerate the stresses and strains that a normal joint can. However, exercise is necessary to maintain proper mobility in the affected joint. Your physician can advise you on the right kind of rest and exercise program for your arthritis.

There is no cure for this disease, but with proper care under the guidance of a competent physician, most people can obtain relief.

expensive and may run several thousands of dollars a year. If your insurance covers the therapy (or you are willing to absorb the cost), go for it.

Lupus and rheumatoid arthritis may be related

Q. Is there any connection between rheumatoid arthritis and lupus? One doctor indicated my RA was dormant; after blood tests, he prescribed Naprosyn. Another physician said my lupus count was low, the RA higher and gave me Vioxx. My wrists and arms are tender. A nurse friend has thrown in a diagnosis of tendonitis. What do I have?

A. Rheumatoid arthritis and lupus erythematosus are autoimmune disorders, two of many afflictions marked by self-allergy, when the body mistakenly identifies normal tissue as foreign and attempts to destroy it.

There is a good deal of overlap between these conditions: Patients with RA may show weakly positive tests for lupus and vice-versa. Both disease affect the joints, leading to stiffness, swelling, pain and limited motion.

From your brief description, I suspect that your basic disorder is rheumatoid arthritis. In this instance, nonsteroidal anti-inflammatory drugs, such as ibuprofen, might relieve your discomfort. Other prescription NSAIDs—such as Arthrotec, Vioxx or Celebrex—might be worth a try. Enbrel, an expensive but effective therapy, given as an injection a week, could help you. Finally, the tried-and-true therapy for RA—steroids—may have to be considered.

Although I doubt that simple tendonitis is to blame, the medications I listed (except for Enbrel) should be appropriate therapy for this condition as well.

I am concerned that your diagnosis remains in doubt, because—as you know—lupus can cause serious kidney disease that should be addressed. Consequently, I urge you to resolve this situation by seeing a rheumatologist who can, by ordering further blood tests, clarify the issue.

Update on Vioxx and Celebrex

Q. When media reports indicated that Vioxx and Celebrex were possibly associated with heart attacks, I almost had one. I am certain that may arthritis sufferers had the same reaction. For the first time in 20 years, the pain of my rheumatoid arthritis has been controlled—with Celebrex—and I don't relish having to stop the medicine and affect the quality of my life. Nonetheless, I don't want a heart attack either. What's new on this topic?

A. I am pleased to be able to give you an answer to this important health concern.

The original study upon which the hungry news media based their reports, involved an analysis of more than 8,000 patients with rheumatoid arthritis. The purpose of the study was to determine whether Celebrex and Vioxx were superior to a standard treatment (Naproxen) for arthritis. The researchers concluded that 1) the three drugs were more or less similar in their success rates; 2) gastrointestinal upset was more common in the Naproxen group; and 3) heart attacks were statistically more prevalent in the Celebrex/Vioxx group. This latter finding was not only unexpected; it was of obvious concern to the millions of people taking the drugs, as well as to the manufacturer.

For some patients, life was put on hold. Do I put up with pain or risk a cardiovascular event? Further research was certainly needed.

This research has now been carried out in Boston, New Jersey and Montreal; the findings, which were reported in the Archives of Medicine, May 27, 2002, are fascinating because of their unpredictability.

Remember that in the original study, patients on Celebrex/Vioxx were compared to counterparts on Naproxen. No placebo was used.

In the recent three investigations, placebos were used. When compared to the placebo group, the Celebrex/Vioxx patients did not have a higher incidence of cardiovascular events. When compared to the same placebo group, the Naproxen patients had a lower incidence of heart attacks.

Therefore, the authors conclude Celebrex and Vioxx are not associated with an increase in cardiac problems. Rather, Naproxen protects its users from such problems. In a phrase, the effects (and complications) of any drug must be analyzed against placebos, as well as similar medications. Celebrex and Vioxx are safe to use; Naproxen is equally effective and seems to protect against heart attacks, as well.

I doubt that this brand new information will be widely publicized because it is not as "sexy" as news reports about tragedy and wrongdoing. But it is important because it shows the value of well-performed scientific research and how such research can have a significant impact on health issues.

As some of my more perceptive readers may be thinking, where do we go from here? Is Naproxen superior to aspirin in preventing heart attacks? Should all of us be using the drug for that purpose? I don't know, but perhaps further studies may shed light on this topic.

The other secondary issue—the gastrointestinal side effects of Naproxen—has been addressed. For patients with arthritis, Naproxen is now marketed in a form that is combined with misoprostol, to reduce stomach irritation. The product, available as Arthrotec-75 or Arthrotec-50, is a useful antidote for arthritic pain and, perhaps, it also has beneficial cardiovascular effects. Remember that you first read about this here.

Paget's disease not osteoarthritis

Q. I am 88 and have suffered from osteoarthritis for the past few years. Now my doctor tells me that I have Paget's disease of the bone. Are these two conditions one and the same? Related?

A. Osteoarthritis, the gradual wearing down of joint linings, is a treat that all seniors will experience, to one degree or another, as they age. This arthritis, like wrinkles and gray hair, comes with the territory. The pain and stiffness it produces can ordinarily be successfully controlled by anti-inflammatory medications, such as ibuprofen, Celebrex, Vioxx and others.

Paget's disease is a separate entity. The cause is unknown. The affliction is marked by increased bone metabolism in a spotty distribution: Calcium is lost from such areas, and new bone matrix quickly forms—too rapidly for calcium to enter the new bone and strengthen it. Thus, Paget's disease causes pain and brittle portions of bone that may easily fracture. Therapy with Fosamax and other prescription drugs is usually effective.

While your bone/joint abnormalities may limit your activity to some extent, both your disorders are treatable. Follow your physician's advice.

The cause of 'gouty arthritis'

Q. Is there such a thing as gouty arthritis? I developed arthritis 15 years ago at age 30 and continue to be plagued by recurring bouts of pain. Certain foods tend to aggravate the problem. I need advice.

A. I think you need to see a doctor to clarify this situation. Gout is gouty arthritis. The malady causes cyclic joint pain, particularly in the feet. Patients with gout have high levels of uric acid, a product of metabolism, in their blood and tissue fluids.

Under certain circumstances—such as injury or exposure to cold— the uric acid crystallizes (much like ice in a winter pond) in joint fluid. The crystals are needle-shaped and irritate joint linings, leading to inflammation, swelling and pain that can be excruciating—gouty arthritis.

Treatment with anti-inflammatory medicine, such as Indocin, usually relieves the pain, but strong anti-gout remedies, such as Colchicine, may be required in severe or resistant cases. Acute gout attacks can usually be prevented by drugs, such as allopurinol. This is especially important because uric acid crystals can also painlessly form in the kidneys, leading to kidney damage and/or kidney stones that can cause serious health problems.

Ask your doctor to give you further advice and treatment.

Alternative remedies for gout unlikely to help

Q. I suffer from gout. I take allopurinol, magnesium and B vitamins, yet I have numerous questions about control. Does excess niacin and vitamin A aggravate the condition? Is brewer's yeast good to take or might activated charcoal be better?

A. Gout is a form of arthritis caused by an excess of uric acid crystals in joint fluid. By reducing the body's production of uric acid (a by-product of metabolism), allopurinol helps prevent gouty arthritis.

But it is not appropriate therapy for acute gout, for which ibuprofen or colchicine are better choices.

Niacin, vitamin A, brewer's yeast, activated charcoal and other "alternative" treatments do not ordinarily affect uric acid. In fact, excess vitamin A (more than 25,000 IU a day) is downright dangerous because it causes lethargy, stomach pains, joint discomfort, insomnia and other consequences.

You probably need to have your dose of allopurinol adjusted, based on periodic tests of your uric acid blood level. Your doctor can supervise this and answer your specific questions.

Eating cherries may stop gout sufferer from obtaining necessary help

Q. It is not necessary for patients with gout to take expensive prescription medication. I simply keep a can of dark cherries or cherry pie filling on hand when my husband has painful, gouty attacks. The cherries work immediately; all he has to do is eat several portions. I realize there are always problems that cannot be cured by home remedies, but this one really works.

A. I am glad to learn that your husband's gout attacks are helped by such an inexpensive and delicious remedy as dark cherries.

However, I cannot endorse this approach because gout, the abnormal accumulation of uric acid in the body, can also affect the kidneys— painlessly and without concomitant arthritic discomfort.

In my view, your husband should follow his doctor's advice about more appropriate preventive therapy for gout, such as allopurinol or ColBenemid. These drugs reduce the production of uric acid and aid its excretion.

Copper bracelets a medical fad

Q. Do copper bracelets really prevent arthritis?

A. Several years ago, copper bracelets enjoyed widespread popularity as a supposed arthritis preventive. This was nothing more than a medical fad. Such bracelets failed the test of scientific scrutiny.

Avoiding Quackery

Chronic arthritis is a frustrating disease that is often difficult to live with. Improvement may come slowly. Because sound, scientifically proven treatments do not work in all cases, arthritis sufferers are particularly likely to try any form of treatment that promises relief of pain or cure. Some unproven remedies promoted outside medical practice can be harmful. Others are not harmful but are worthless, representing a waste of money and delaying proper medical attention. The American Rheumatism Association estimates that people with arthritis spend more than $1 billion a year on questionable treatments.

Testimonials to unproven remedies often come from people whose disease happened to go into remission at the time they tried the treatment. In addition, people who believe they will recover when they try something new often do recover temporarily. This is called the placebo effect, which explains why some people respond well to treatments that are ineffective.

Many of these questionable treatments are based on diet. However, no diet has ever been shown to prevent or cure arthritis. The fact that so many different arthritis diets are promoted in various publications is a good clue that none of them works.

Ant, bee and snake venoms have been touted as arthritis cures. These remedies are dangerous because some people are highly allergic to these venoms, or become allergic after repeated

Exercise for arthritis

Q. Are there exercises for people with arthritic knees?

A. The main goals of exercise in arthritic patients are keeping joints mobile and muscles trim. However, arthritis pain may severely hamper a person's ability and willingness to exercise.

This is the reason most physicians, when confronted with arthritis problems, prefer to prescribe anti-inflammatory medicine. Such drugs—including Celebrex, Vioxx, Bextra and others—enable arthritic patients to enjoy physical activity and retain their independence.

Therefore, I recommend medication and exercise—up to a point—for any patient. I say "up to a point" because it's not appropriate for such use. Any slight improvement is not worth the significant drawbacks of this painful, expensive and potentially dangerous form of therapy.

Many ineffective devices are sold to people with arthritis, including copper bracelets and electrical or electromagnetic instruments. All of these are useless.

Other unproven remedies include ointments, liniments and special lotions, such as DMSO (dimethyl sulfoxide). DMSO has been studied scientifically, but has no proven effect on arthritis. Other products applied to the affected joint may produce a sensation of warmth, but do not relieve pain. Other preparations may relieve pain temporarily by a counterirritant effect, but they do not penetrate into the joint in therapeutic amounts, as they are advertised to do.

There are several ways to recognize unproven remedies that may be ineffective at best, and harmful at worst: A cure is usually promised, generally described as "secret" or "exclusive." Testimonials and case histories are usually offered in support of the treatment, which is often advertised in sensational articles in tabloids or in mail promotions. Drugs and surgery are often condemned as dangerous, and the medical establishment is accused of conspiracy in attempting to suppress the remedy being offered. Legitimate scientists do not keep their discoveries secret, and legitimate advances in the understanding and treatment of arthritis quickly become available to the public.

people to exercise strenuously and have to put up with the resulting excruciating pain. Some stiffness and discomfort is, of course, acceptable, but if a joint really hurts, the patient must cut back.

For those individuals with arthritis of the knees, walking and, especially, swimming are good exercises. Sometimes, with medication, these people can run, play tennis, golf, skate, bicycle and engage in other sports. This depends on the degree of arthritis and the effectiveness of the medicine. Pain should be the limiting factor.

I usually discourage arthritic patients from engaging in physically demanding activities, such as weight training, because of the additional burdens on already painful joints. There are no exercises that will prevent or reverse arthritis.

You may wish to run this suggestion by your doctor, but I advise you to exercise moderately within the limits of pain. All exercise is beneficial; the degree of activity is something you and your doctor will have to decide as a team.

Remember, too, that arthritic joints may be quite sore AFTER exercise. This can be relieved by heat and gentle passive movements.

Does this cheap, safe remedy have merit?

Q. Because arthritis seems to be a rite of passage to old age, I would like to inform you of my battle with it—and how I succeeded. I'm 81 and have hesitated writing you because people don't take me seriously in spite of the fact that I've had arthritis for many years and am a huge success story.

Simply put, success is due to castor oil. Not taken internally but rubbed on my joints. It alleviates the pain in minutes.

I have arthritis in most of my major joints. I have been told I have rheumatoid arthritis. I can keep the pain at bay with castor oil and the product causes no side effects.

This remedy was first brought to my attention about 30 years ago, when my son's knees were severely inflamed from Osgood-Schlatter disease. I rubbed the oil on his knees twice a day. This was around Thanksgiving. By Easter, his knees were completely pain-free and he was back to running. He will be 47 next month and is in great health. He occasionally uses topical castor oil.

I hope that your readers might try this home remedy.

A. In keeping with my policy to publish information about home remedies that are safe, inexpensive and may hold promise, I am sharing your letter.

Over the years, castor oil, a traditional and unpleasant-tasting laxative, has been touted to cure myriad diseases. Most of these claims are bogus. But your experiences piqued my curiosity because 1) the product is applied topically, and 2) your successes seem stunning.

Therefore, I'm going to rely on my readers' (bless their hearts!) analyses before coming to a conclusion.

Folks, those of you who are willing to try castor oil (rubbed over an arthritic joint, twice a day) will be my experimental subjects from whom I would love to hear—both pro and con—after a period of castor oil usage. I cannot tell you how long this will take, but I'll certainly write a follow-up after I hear from you.

Follow-up on castor oil for arthritis

Q. When I read your recent column about using castor oil to treat arthritis, I immediately purchased some and applied it to my big toe, where I have had painful arthritis for year.

Wonder of wonders, within a week the pain was gone. Thank you so much for your health tip. Keep up your wonderful articles.

A. Since I published this novel remedy, I have received several letters from satisfied readers, so there appears to be some justification for using topical castor oil as a cure for the pain of arthritis.

> 66 *There appears to be some justification for using topical castor oil as a cure for the pain of arthritis.* 99

As I previously wrote, I have no idea why this home remedy is effective, and I am awaiting future correspondences from readers who have tried the product with success—or failure.

Alternative treatment for arthritis

Q. Please provide further information about the use of Certo for arthritis.

A. Several years ago, I casually mentioned in this column that I had heard from some people whose arthritis had responded to Certo and I asked readers to educate me about the use of this product.

Since then, I've received scores of letters about this subject—and I thank each reader for writing. Many of the letters were glowing testimonials, some contained interesting anecdotes and a few were intriguing. In the interest of space, here is a summary of what I have learned: Certo is liquid fruit pectin, a product easily obtained in most grocery stores. (It is also available as a powder.) Certo is used in preparing jams and jellies.

Many patients who suffered severe pain from various types of arthritis were at the end of their ropes; traditional medicine, including prescription drugs, had been ineffective in relieving their discomfort. Therefore, as a last resort, they tried Certo—and it worked.

Although some folks added a tablespoonful (or a packet) to coffee, tea or orange juice once or twice a day (with good results), most readers indicated that they achieved maximum benefit by mixing one to three tablespoons of Certo in a glass of unsweetened grape juice once or twice a day. (The amount can be varied according to the severity of symptoms.)

Within a week, most arthritis sufferers experienced significant relief of pain. They then either reduced the dose or discontinued Certo altogether until they had another flare-up of pain.

One reader mentioned constipation as a side effect, another described mild indigestion, but—by and large—Certo therapy is free of complications.

I have no direct, personal experience with this novel home remedy. Certo is inexpensive, easily obtained and harmless. And many readers have testified to its effectiveness.

No one knows how it works, although one physician suggested that Certo renders lead insoluble in the body, somehow affecting arthritis by this reaction.

Regardless of its method of action, Certo appears to be a successful alternative in the treatment of arthritis. I make no guarantee about its efficacy, but if even one reader experiences relief from Certo, this column is worthwhile.

22

Back & Leg Pain

Causes of hip and back pain

Q. My problem is a constant but varying pain in my hips and back. The discomfort is always there but, at times, can be quite severe. Routine examinations, blood tests and standard X-rays were all negative. What can I do?

A. Your question is too general to permit a specific answer. For instance, you don't mention your age and what blood tests and X-rays you had. Therefore, I would be presumptuous to list the afflictions causing the pain you described.

Nonetheless, I have a couple of thoughts. Pain in the hips and back often reflects arthritis or a herniated lumbar disc.

Osteoarthritis, the age-related gradual wearing down of joint surfaces, is a common cause of hip and back pain, due to erosion of the cartilaginous joint lining. In addition, arthritis often affects the spine. This malady is usually quite evident on standard X-rays of the back (and hips) and appears as narrowing of the joint spaces and the presence of calcium deposits ("lipping") at the ends of the bones. Such X-ray changes do not always correlate with the degree of pain, however; patents with minimal changes can experience severe pain and stiffness that is out of proportion to the X-ray changes. So, before blaming your symptoms on simple arthritis, I'd have to see the X-ray reports.

In addition, standard X-ray examinations are a poor way of diagnosing soft tissue injury: by this I mean nerves, muscles, tendons and discs (the doughnut-shaped structures that separate the spinal bones). It is possible that you could have a disc that has slipped out of place and is now pressing on the spinal nerves (to your hips and legs) or, worse yet, on the soft spinal cord itself, a condition called spinal stenosis.

Consequently, despite your "normal" X-rays, the story is not over.

In my opinion, you need an MRI scan to get a good look at the soft tissues, especially the nerves and the spinal cord.

Ask your doctor about this. If you have already had an MRI and it is normal, you should be referred to a specialist in disorders of the back. If not, the MRI should be performed. The test will give vital information and will help your physician arrive at a diagnosis and suggest appropriate therapy.

Back and hip pain is a common complaint. The cause is usually easy to identify with suitable testing.

Sciatica has various therapies

Q. What can I do about a pinched sciatic nerve? My orthopedist advises surgery, one chiropractor says it's a symptom of menopause and another says my hip is "funny." Except for the surgical option, which I'd like to avoid, no one is giving me a logical explanation.

A. The sciatic nerve is actually composed of several nerves that, after having passed from the spinal cord between the doughnut-shaped vertebrae bones in the lower back, combine to supply nerve function to each of the legs, as well as to transmit sensory impulses from them. Thus, a "pinched" sciatic nerve (sciatica) customarily causes pain and tingling in the buttock and lower extremity, eventually followed by weakness if the nerve isn't decompressed.

The most common cause of sciatica is a herniated disc: a portion of the material separating the vertebrae protrudes out of place and presses on one (or more) of the nerves that make up the sciatic bundle. With treatment, such as physical therapy, steroid injections or spinal manipulation, the "slipped" disc frequently moves back into place and symptoms disappear. However, if this conservative management fails to relieve pain or weakness, surgery—to repair the disc or remove it—must be considered in order to prevent permanent sciatic damage.

Other causes of sciatica include lone overgrowth (from arthritis), compression fractures of the spinal bones (from osteoporosis), abscesses and tumors (for which surgery is usually indicated). Your question suggests that there is some disagreement among your chiropractic practitioners as to the exact nature of your sciatica. For obvious reasons, this lack of consensus must be resolved before you can consider what to do next.

Although arthritis of the hip may sometimes masquerade as sciatic pain, I tend to side with you orthopedic specialist. For one thing, sciatica is never a symptom of menopause.

To obtain a clearer understanding of your situation, you should have an MRI scan. This test will clearly show if anything is compressing the nerves. Then you will be in a better position to make an educated choice about therapy. In addition, it would probably be prudent to obtain a second—or even third—opinion from a neurosurgeon or another orthopedist.

Your question raises another important point: whom to trust. There's no question that chiropractors can help treat chronic back pain, but you must be alert to their limitations. For example, on of our local chiropractors recently referred a patient with severe back pain to me. I respect this practitioner and we work well together. He had treated the patient for about two weeks and was getting nowhere. Fortunately, the chiropractor suspected that the patient's problem was more serous than simple sciatica.

I ordered appropriate testing that revealed a small lung cancer that had spread to a vertebral bone, causing pain that mimicked sciatica. The patient underwent surgery, chemotherapy and radiation therapy to his back, with dramatic relief of pain. Consequently, I was reminded that not all "sciatica" is caused by herniated discs.

My recommendation is this: If, after two or three weeks of treatment, a patient's back and leg pain has not substantially improved, another opinion—and further testing—are mandatory. In my experience, orthopedic specialists or neurosurgeons are the best resource for people with continuing sciatica.

MRI scans are useful for back problems

Q. I am 75 and in good health. This past winter, sciatica was a problem in my right leg. Should I consider acupuncture?

A. Before suggesting therapy, I'd have to verify that you have sciatica and why.

For readers unfamiliar with the condition, here's a little background: At the bottom of the spinal cord, the nerves fan out and enter the legs, where they supply us with sensation and motor function. When these nerves are injured, compressed, pinched or inflamed, we experience (first) tingling, numbness or pain, which may (later) progress to weakness. Called "sciatica," this nerve disorder has many causes, most often pressure on the nerves from herniated discs or bone spurs from arthritis.

Before recommending corrective surgery, most physicians prescribe medical therapy, including physical therapy, pain medication, steroid injections and so forth. Other treatments, such as acupuncture of chiropractic manipulation, may be useful. If, however, conservative therapy is ineffective, surgery may be necessary.

In my opinion, you need an MRI scan to determine the location of the problem and how extensive it is. For example, a simple herniated disc may, with time, slip back into place. In contrast, significant impingement on spinal nerves (or on the spinal cord itself) is unlikely to respond to nonsurgical treatment. Check with your doctor regarding the options I mentioned. He or she can diagnose your condition, offer therapy—or, if necessary, refer you to an orthopedist or neurosurgeon who specializes in back problems.

Is it muscle spasms or a spinal disc problem?

Q. How can I determine if my chronic back pain is caused by muscle spasms or a spinal disc problem?

A. I doubt that you can. But your doctor would be able to differentiate these two common causes of back pain. A thorough examination—plus appropriate imaging studies—should tell the tale. Back spasms ordinarily have their own pattern (localized pain worsened by movement and exercise), whereas disc problems usually cause pain that radiates into the buttocks and thighs. See your physician for assistance.

Piriformis syndrome may be cause of sciatica

Q. I've had a problem with sciatica for the past five years. A searing, debilitating pain radiates downward from my left lower buttock, into my leg, and is often accompanied by numbness and weakness. Past treatment has included bed rest, massage, ultrasound, physical therapy and analgesics—all of which have produced short-lived benefits. On the Internet, I recently discovered a condition called piriformis syndrome. Could this be my problem?

A. Most cases of sciatica are caused by pressure on the nerves that travel from the spinal cord into the lower extremities. This pressure is often the consequence of a herniated disc in the lower back, not a tense muscle. The symptoms you describe suggest that the pressure on the sciatic nerve may be extreme. In such cases, permanent damage (weakness and numbness) may result if the condition is not treated aggressively with surgery and other techniques.

Rather than relying on exercises and other methods of pain control, you need an MRI scan. This test uses electromagnetic waves to produce a picture of internal organs, including the spine, which will indicate where the pressure is exerted and how serious it is. Your doctor can order the scan.

Having said this, I must elaborate on the condition you mention that is said to cause sciatica in some patients. Called piriformis syndrome, the disorder is not universally recognized by physicians. Yet, in some people, the piriformis muscle, deep in the buttock, can trap the sciatic nerves in their course down the back of the thigh and leg.

Accentuated by prolonged sitting (such as working at a computer), by strenuous twisting of the torso (such as shoveling snow), or even by falling on one's backside, the piriformis muscle goes into spasm. This may lead to low-back ache, weakness of the hip on the affected side, difficulty walking, pain down the back

> 66 Most cases of sciatica are caused by pressure on the nerves that travel from the spinal cord into the lower extremities. 99

of the thigh and numbness of the lower leg—in short, all the classic signs of a herniated disc.

Unfortunately, piriformis syndrome will not be evident on either CT or MRI scans. Rather, the diagnosis is made clinically: by a specific examination of the piriformis muscle.

In a sitting position (or while lying flat on the back), the patient flexes the knee on the painful side, and pulls the knee across the body and slightly upward. As the hip rotates, the tight piriformis muscle is stretched, yielding increasing pain as the spastic muscle is stressed.

Most medical authorities recommend that the "piriformis test" be performed by qualified personnel (doctors, chiropractors or physical therapists). However, by attempting to test themselves, many patients can actually diagnose the cause of their own back pain.

In contrast to the finding of this test, a herniated disc usually causes pain when the patient, lying on the back, flexes one knee hard against the chest and then straightens the leg.

Orthopedic specialists, who treat piriformis syndrome, recommend two home exercises that help relieve discomfort by stretching both the piriformis muscle and the hamstring muscles (in the back of the thigh); the hamstrings can also increase pressure on the sciatic nerve.

Exercise No. 1: Lie down, face up, on a comfortable flat surface (such as a thick rug on the floor). Make certain that your shoulders, midback and legs are flat against the surface. Bring the knee up (on the affected side) to waist level and plant the foot next to, but just outside, the opposite knee. Then gently pull the bent knee down toward the floor, across the body, without moving the anchoring foot. In the presence of piriformis spasm, this maneuver will cause some pain. Carefully continue pressing the bent knee downward, releasing the pressure if the pain become too intense. Do this 8 or 10 times per session twice a day. As the piriformis spasm lessens, the exercise will hurt less and the hip will rotate more easily.

Exercise No. 2: Again, lie down face up on a flat surface. Flex the affected knee up toward the chest, keeping the "good" leg flat, thereby forming a right angle with the thighs. Gradually straighten the bent knee, while keeping the "down" leg flat. Repeat this 8 or 10 times, twice a day.

I don't know whether you have piriformis syndrome. See an orthopedic surgeon for an examination, further testing and additional advice.

Wait on knee replacement

Q. What is your opinion of avascular necrosis of the knee? Could it be caused by arthroscopy I had a year ago? I've been in pain for six months. My primary orthopedist recommended a new knee. I obtained a second opinion from another orthopedic surgeon, who advised me to wait because the damage involves only about one-fourth of the knee and might heal with time and rehab.

A. Avascular necrosis of any organ means that some tissue has died because of inadequate blood supply. This can be serious and difficult to treat when it affects bone.

I do not know why you developed this condition in your knee, unless you have had major surgery on the joint. I don't believe arthroscopy is to blame. During this procedure, an orthopedic surgeon introduces a small tube into the knee joint and removes damaged tissue.

If the second specialist advises you to hold off on knee replacement, I'd do so. He may believe that the knee will recover its proper circulation over time. If it fails to do so, you can always opt for knee replacement in the future.

Gallbladder surgery not cause of leg pain

Q. Following gallbladder surgery last year, I've had troublesome pains in my right leg. First it was the front of the leg and now it's above

Quinine Is the Tonic for Leg Cramps

Q. I have nocturnal leg cramps, for which a friend suggested quinine. It worked. I have not cramped in six months.

A. Quinine is the traditional treatment for nocturnal leg cramps. In many instances, it is effective. (If you object to the cost of quinine pills, try drinking six ounces of tonic water before bedtime.)

Should the quinine not be a solution for you, try putting a bar of soap at night under the bottom sheet next to your feet. I have received dozens of letters from readers who have been helped by this home remedy.

the knee. Is this a consequence of surgery? My doctor has concluded that it's arthritis.

A. I don't know the cause of your leg pains, but I doubt that they are the consequence of surgery. Also, from you brief description, the discomfort does not appear to emanate from your joints; therefore, arthritis seems unlikely.

I wonder if you're not suffering from myalgia, muscle pain caused by inflammation or overuse. As you know, however, thrombophlebitis (blood clots in the leg veins) is a dreaded complication following surgery and can appear without warning during periods of convalescence, such as postoperative inactivity. This disorder ordinarily affects the calf—not the thigh—and is readily diagnosed on physical examination and by ultrasound testing. To make sure that your leg is free of clots, you should have an ultrasound exam of your leg. If the test is negative, your doctor may choose to refer you to an orthopedic specialist for a second opinion.

A victim of outmoded imaging

Q. For the past six months, I've suffered from extreme shoulder pain. Three doctors have three different opinions, ranging from "I don't know" to a separated shoulder. One suggested cortisone injections, followed by physical therapy. X-rays have failed to shed light on my problem. Do you have any suggestions?

A. You bet. You may be the victim of outmoded imaging testing. Let me explain.

Most of the pain-sensitive structures in the shoulder are radiolucent soft tissues, meaning that X-rays pass through them without creating much of a shadow. Therefore, standard X-ray examinations for shoulder pain seldom give particularly helpful information—unless there is a fracture of bone cysts that are the cause of symptoms.

Pain can result from problems involving the muscles, ligaments, tendons and supporting structures of the shoulder, none of which can be seen on an X-ray. For example, you may have damaged a tendon, developed bursitis or torn the rotator cuff (the stabilizing tissue around the joint). These ailments would not show up on standard X-ray exams. What you need is an MRI (Magnetic Resonance Imaging), a non-X-ray exam that beautifully shows the shoulder's soft tissues.

This is cutting-edge technology and is not available in all health centers but, believe me, it is remarkable and does not require potentially dangerous X-ray exposure. While not appropriate for all orthopedic investigations, MRI is virtually diagnostic for traumatic or non-traumatic shoulder injuries. (You have not given me enough information to allow me to judge whether trauma caused your shoulder pain.)

I suggest that you get checked by an orthopedic surgeon. Such a specialist should be able to diagnose the cause of your pain (using an MRI) and clarify the apparent confusion exhibited by your other doctors. You may eventually need medication, physical therapy or surgery, but I hesitate to recommend treatment until the precise cause of your problem has been identified.

Shin splints may mimic stress fractures

Q. What causes "shin splints"? Is there something I can do to prevent the pain?

A. During repetitive, weight-bearing, strenuous activity—such as running—part of the muscle at the front of the calf may pull away from the leg bone, leading to significant pain. This is shin splints, an overuse syndrome that is treated by rest, ice, ultrasound and physical therapy. Ibuprofen will help control discomfort during the healing process.

Because stress fractures (tiny cracks in bones that are common in runners) can cause identical pain, you should have an X-ray or a bone scan to make sure this isn't your problem. Your family doctor can order the necessary testing and coordinate your therapy.

In the main, shin splints are preventable if you heed the following suggestions:

1. Avoid running on hard surfaces, such as pavement. Dirt and grass are preferable because these surfaces are softer and cause less shock during the heel-strike.

2. Make absolutely certain that your running shoes have superior cushioning qualities, especially if (because of locale) you must run on hard surfaces.

3. Do not run in cleats. If you are a soccer or lacrosse player, run in running shoes, then change to cleats for games or scrimmages.

Heel pain and neck pain have different origins

Q. About a year ago, I began experiencing severe pain on the undersurface of my heel. This was diagnosed as plantar fascitis and I received cortisone injections for it, with good results. I've also suffered from a stiff neck and have to wear a cervical collar. Could this be caused by stress or is it related to the heel problem?

A. I believe that your heel and neck pains have different origins.

Plantar fascitis is a chronic inflammation of the fibrous sheet covering the tissues of the heel. It is common in runners and is thought to be related to injury. Treatment consists of rest, foam rubber insoles, cortisone injections and drugs to combat inflammation.

On the other hand, the type of neck pain you mention is probably due to muscle cramping and contraction. Although stress may play a central role in such a symptom, arthritis of the neck bones can also cause pain. Therefore, you should have X-rays of your neck to diagnose the condition. Thereafter, you might be helped by heat, massage, gentle exercises, myotherapy (deep massage), ultrasound treatment or chiropractic manipulation.

Battling Chronic Pain

Strong pain medication may be warranted

Q. I'm a retired nurse, 67, with severe osteoarthritis affecting all my major joints. The pain cannot be controlled with ibuprofen or over-the-counter drugs. I have not responded to nonnarcotic medication. Because of a gastric ulcer, I am forbidden to take Vioxx, Celebrex and similar medicines. I can no loner lead an active life and am virtually house-bound, sentenced to an existence that I never could have imagined when I was younger and vigorous. My 32-year-old doctor refuses to consider the judicious use of narcotic pain relievers, even though I have no history of drug dependence, depression or psychological problems. I'm not interested in mood-altering drugs; I simply want pain relief. Any suggestions?

A. Young doctors, despite their enthusiasm and up-to-date training, often have difficulty putting themselves into the shoes of the elderly or patients with chronic medical problems. Pain control can be an especially difficult issue, particularly now when various federal and state governments are seriously cracking down on physicians who prescribe narcotics too freely.

However, as you have discovered, chronic pain can affect one's life in innumerable ways. I believe that in situations such as this, doctors owe their allegiances to their patients. We're not doing our jobs if we irresolutely refuse to prescribe pain relievers to patients who truly need them. Do I prescribe a handful of narcotic pills to a new patient who makes a 5 P.M. Friday appointment? Not on your life. I will usually exhaust every other alternative while I'm getting to know that patient. If, after satisfying myself that all other resources have been exhausted, narcotics are needed, I'll prescribe them—and refer the patient to a pain clinic.

From the description in your brief note, I conclude that you seem to be a responsible person who would prudently use potentially addictive pain medication. (As you know, the risk of addiction is quite low in people who take narcotics for pain relief.) Therefore, my suggestion is that you find another doctor—perhaps a more experienced practitioner—who would be more sympathetic to your plight. Such a physician would work with you, prescribe what you need and monitor your progress.

What is RSD?

Q. Please discuss reflex sympathetic dystrophy. People think I'm crazy when I tell them what the syndrome does to me.

A. This syndrome, which is an unusual consequence of injury to bone and soft tissue, consists of shooting pain associated with shriveling of bone and other tissues, abnormal sweating and flushing of the affected area. The disorder is believed due to damage to nerves that are not under conscious control; that is, the nerves that mediate pain, sweating, blood flow and other vital functions.

Although various drug therapies have been used for decades, none has been consistently effective—including Neurontin, which was thought to hold promise. Therefore, in conjunction with intensive physical therapy, a technique called "sympathetic nerve block" is considered to be the treatment of choice. During this procedure, a local anesthetic is injected around the affected nerves. If the anesthetic provides relief, permanent (surgical) block will likely be curative.

In essence, RSD is a chronic pain syndrome that usually requires aggressive therapy. Ask your doctor about a nerve block or request a referral to a chronic pain clinic. Such resources can be found in most large hospitals.

Pain unusual consequence of stroke

Q. I suffered a thalamic stroke two years ago that left me with what my doctor calls "thalamic pain syndrome." What is this? Is it treatable?

A. The thalamus is a structure deep within the brain that, among other functions, mediates the perception of pain. Injuries, such as strokes, to this area are often associated with a type of chronic discomfort called "neuropathic central pain," which can affect any part of the body. This pain is often described as "burning or lancinating."

Treatment consists of three major components: mobilization of the affected part (to prevent "frozen" joints and muscle wasting), consideration of psychological factors (such as therapy for anxiety and depression), and the use of appropriate pain control. This include analgesics (such as Neurontin and others), hypnosis, trigger-point injections, acupuncture and other methods.

Although you are likely to have pain for a long time, much can be done to lessen it. In particular, you might be helped by attending a pain clinic; such resources are available in most teaching hospitals.

Treatment of PMR

Q. I have suffered from polymyalgia rheumatica for four years and have been taking prednisone to control my symptoms. Now I have developed congestive heart failure, which is, I've been told, unusual for a man of 60. My attempts to get off prednisone have been unsuccessful. My doctors have told me that little is known about the disease and that steroids are the only treatment. Your comments about substitutes, please.

A. Polymyalgia rheumatica is a surprisingly common disorder, marked by severe muscle pain and stiffness, malaise and fever. It is sometimes associated with a condition called temporal arteritis, an inflammation of arteries in the head that can lead to visual disturbances and blindness. There is no specific test for confirmation, but the clinical presentation (how the patient looks and feels) is usually striking and blood tests (called erythrocyte sedimentation rate and C reactive protein) are ordinarily markedly abnormal. The cause of PMR is a mystery, although many authorities believe that it is yet another autoimmune disorder, such as rheumatoid arthritis and lupus, when patients become allergic to their own normal tissues. Unfortunately, steroids (such as prednisone) are the most effective therapy and will produce complete pain relief in a matter of hours. Such a rapid response helps diagnose the condition.

I say that steroids are "unfortunately" the treatment of choice because, as you know, the side effects of prednisone (and other steroids) are substantial and invariably lead to poor immunity, diabetes, osteoporosis, cataracts and other complications when used for lengthy periods.

Thus, a trade-off must be accepted by doctors and their patients in this situation. On the positive side, long-term therapy is rarely required; most patients can slowly taper their dosages of steroids, thereby avoiding any consequences of the drugs. Yet, I have in my practice an elderly doctor's widow who cannot, absolutely cannot, stop her prednisone therapy; whenever she does reduce the dose, her pain becomes unmanageable. She has been on prednisone for four years, and will probably remain on it, despite the side effects, indefinitely. Even more important, PMR patients with temporal arteritis may require long term steroid therapy in order to prevent blindness.

To my knowledge, heart failure is not correlated with either PMR or the steroids used to treat it. Therefore, I think this issue must be addressed as a separate problem. I am not aware of an appropriate substitute therapy.

However, I do have a suggestion: the Thorne regimen. Years ago, a doctor at the Harvard Medical School discovered that the steroid therapy complications could be lessened or eliminated by taking prednisone on alternate days. If, for example, a patient required 10 milligrams of prednisone (and would experience predictable consequences), Dr. Thorne discovered that giving 20 milligrams on alternate days would be equally effective without the high incidence of side effects. So, with this in mind, you might consider such a program.

Don't remove rib to solve arm pain

Q. After 17 months of misdiagnosis for arm pain, at last a diagnosis: thoracic outlet syndrome. Surgery, to remove the first rib, has been advised. Can I avoid this?

A. Without a doubt.

I'm surprised that your diagnosis was delayed for almost 18 months, because the diagnosis of thoracic outlet syndrome is disarmingly simple (no pun intended).

The arteries to your arms exit from the aorta and travel through beds of muscle. On occasion, these muscles may enlarge (usually from increased activity) and press on one or the other artery, causing temporary reduction in blood flow. Thus, thoracic outlet syndrome is basically a case of one arm "falling asleep." Symptoms are more frequent at night; this may actually awaken patients.

The diagnostic test, which I routinely obtain, is called the Addson's maneuver. The patient holds up an arm in the lateral (away from the body) position, supinates it (rotates clockwise) and forcefully turns the head in the opposite direction. I feel the pulse in the wrist when the maneuver is performed. If the pulse disappears and the person experiences numbness or tingling, the diagnosis is established. This technique puts stress on the artery and shows that circulation is reduced when the blood vessel is stretched.

In the many patients I have seen with a positive Addson's maneuver, I have never had to refer one to an orthopedic surgeon for removal of a first rib. In contrast, a simple series of arm movements—called thoracic outlet exercises—will usually solve the problem without the need for an operation. The exercises relax the muscular bed surrounding the artery and permit adequate blood flow. Ask your physician to refer you to a physical therapist, who may be able inexpensively and successfully to solve your problem.

Ten years of elbow pain may be relieved in two office visits

Q. Ten years ago, I fell and bruised a bone in my elbow. I now have constant pain. I've taken prescription pain pills, used a brace and have followed my doctor's advice about activity. However, I don't have medical insurance and cannot afford to continue seeing a doctor, mush less undergo physical therapy. What can I do to speed healing?

A. Ten years is long time to suffer the consequences of a bone bruise. I'm more concerned that a tendon in the affected area may have become irritated and frayed. For example, "tennis elbow," which is actually more common in carpenters and others whose occupations demand repetitive movements, may require cortisone injections or surgical repair.

In view of your continuing symptom, I urge you to be examined by an orthopedic surgeon. Once the specialist diagnoses your condition, you'll be in a better position to decide what to do about it. I do not believe that more than one or two visits will be necessary to relieve your pain, and your money will be well spent.

Persisting headaches need professional attention

Q. My daughter has suffered from headaches for more than 30 years. I'm from the old school and prefer home remedies, such as two aspirin and one teaspoon of baking soda, but I welcome your input.

A. For mild headaches, such as those associated with fatigue or eyestrain, home remedies are appropriate. The baking soda/aspirin combination is often effective; really, it's just over-the-counter buffered aspirin.

Severe, persisting or cyclic headaches may reflect migraine, muscle contraction, hypertension or similar medical problems that should be brought to a physician's attention and treated with more effective drugs and stronger analgesics.

Antidepressant nortriptyline sometimes helps chronic pain

Q. For the past 12 years, I've experienced muscle tightness and spasms of my neck and back. I've seen a chiropractor and had physical therapy and acupuncture with temporary relief. Finally, a neurologist put me on nortriptyline at bedtime. Is this appropriate therapy?

A. If it works, yes. For unknown reasons, this antidepressant medication often helps people with chronic pain. Stick with your neurologist's suggestion and see if your spasms improve. If not, the doctor may choose to give you specific muscle-relaxing medicine, such as Flexeril, Robaxin and others.

Treatment of arthritis and back pain

Q. I'm 80 years old and have osteoarthritis of my major joints. For several months, I've also suffered chronic back pain. An MRI scan showed five herniated discs in my lower spine. Is there a remedy that could help me?

A. The combination of arthritis and disc disease can be an enormous challenge to treat, because the conditions may cause severe chronic pain that does not respond to the usual, nonnarcotic analgesics. In addition, at your age, you're probably not thrilled by the possibility of back surgery, because this is a major procedure with substantial risks. So let's review the medical treatment.

First, you should be under the care of a back specialist, such as orthopedic surgeon. He or she can coordinate your care.

Nonsteroidal anti-inflammatory medication, such a ibuprofen or Arthrotec, may help to relieve your arthritic pain. However, is your herniated discs are pressing on sensitive nerves, you probably will need narcotics for pain control.

Third, I urge you to receive regular physiotherapy. Using rehab techniques, such therapists may be able to reduce your level of pain.

Fourth, consider alternative methods of pain control, such as massage, acupuncture, chiropractic manipulation and transcutaneous electrical stimulation (TENS). I've had patients who responded to hypnosis and steroid injections into the inflamed spinal nerves.

Last, surgery. Except for hip and knee replacement operations, there are really no procedures to relieve the joint pain of osteoarthritis. However, if a follow-up MRI shows progression of the disc herniations (with resulting increased pressure on nerves), corrective surgery may have to be considered. Before investigating this possibility, however, I'd want first to exhaust the other (medical) options.

I'm sure that your doctor will be able to help you by using one (or all) of the modalities I listed.

Prednisone therapy for polymyalgia

Q. Two months ago I injured my back at work and developed polymyalgia rheumatica. My doctor wants to put me on prednisone but, because of the side effects, I am reluctant to take it. Would the medication bring about a cure or just help the pain of inflammation?

A. Polymyalgia, an autoimmune disease marked by chronic inflammation of muscles (and, sometimes, arterial linings), is probably unrelated to your back injury, which should be treated independently. The cause of polymyalgia is unknown, but the pain and stiffness associated with it can be quite severe, even disabling. Therefore, your physician has made an appropriate recommendation. Therapy with prednisone, a type of steroid that combats inflammation, should result in prompt relief of symptoms.

However, as you pointed out, the use of the drug carries risks, including cataracts, osteoporosis, diabetes and deficient immunity. To a large degree, these side effects are dose-related.

You will need to decide whether to proceed with the prednisone. To help you, your doctor should provide an in-depth analysis of the risks of not taking the medicine, as well as the risks of taking it. For example, side effects are uncommon until prednisone has been administered continuously for several weeks; therefore one of your options is to use it intermittently, as needed for pain. Consider using the lowest possible dose that is effective. Or perhaps try taking it on alternate days (or less frequently), which will further reduce the risks.

Prednisone will reduce inflammation and pain. Although it need not be taken indefinitely once the initial bout of polymyalgia has ended, some patients require periodic cycles of therapy, and still fewer need to take prednisone for months or years.

"Tincture of time" effective remedy

Q. Can you explain costochondritis? Why do I have it?

A. Costochondritis is inflammation of the cartilage connecting the ribs to the breastbone (sternum). The cause of the affliction is unknown but may but may be related to minor trauma or a viral infection.

The pain of costochondritis is often described as a "gnawing ache" that is worse at night and bears no relation to respiratory movement of the ribs. The cartilage itself is always tender. This fact serves to differentiate costochondritis from more serious causes of chest pain, such as angina or neuralgia.

Treatment consists of ibuprofen and "tincture of time"; the discomfort usually subsides in a matter of weeks.

Hip and heel pain not related

Q. I'm a grandmother, age 70, with chronic left hip pain that now extends to my knee. Further, I have heel pain that my doctor believes is caused by bursitis. Could this be due to a calcium deficiency?

A. I believe that you have two different conditions, neither of which indicates a calcium deficiency, a diagnosis that could easily be made by a bone density examination.

Hip pain in the elderly has several possible causes, including arthritis, tendonitis and bursitis (inflammation of the joint covering).

> 66 *[We doctors] are not doing our jobs if we irresolutely refuse to prescribe pain relievers to patients who truly need them.* 99

Arthritis leads to pain because, as we age, our joint linings become thin and worn down. This phenomenon disrupts the mechanics of weight bearing, with resulting discomfort, stiffness and limitation of motion. X-rays usually show the characteristic signs: narrowing of the joint space, a "moth-eaten" appearance of the bones making up the joint and osteophytes (calcium deposits) along the sides of the joint.

Tendon irritation, which affects the muscles that control the joint, can also cause pain and limited motion. This common affliction is often associated with calcium deposits within the tendon (calcific tendonitis) that are easily detected by X-ray tests and can be differentiated from osteophytes.

Bursitis causes discomfort, which is often severe, and stiffness. There are no characteristic X-ray findings, unless calcium deposits build up in the tissues over time.

The initial therapy for these conditions is anti-inflammatory medication, such as ibuprofen, Voltaren, Arthrotec, Celebrex, Vioxx and others. In selected cases, injections of cortisone into the arthritic or inflamed areas may reverse symptoms. Finally, severe arthritis unresponsive to these treatments may require hip replacement.

I doubt that your hip problem and your heel pain are directly related. Heel discomfort may be caused by bursitis but, more commonly, it is associated with tendonitis of the Achilles' tendon or plantar fascitis (irritation of the tissues deep in the heel). Anti-inflammatory medicines and cortisone injections usually cure the ailment.

Inasmuch as your diagnosis seems in doubt, I suggest that you be examined by an orthopedic specialist who can advise you and offer further treatment.

I might add that pain anywhere in the lower extremity can ultimately involve the thigh muscles and the knee because the pain alters your gait, may cause a limp and leads to sore muscles. In addition, low back disorders, such as sciatica and herniated discs, often play a role in hip and leg pain, so this possibility must also be investigated with appropriate tests.

Nitroglycerine spray helps diabetes-related leg pain

Q. In a column, you mentioned that nitroglycerine spray was of remarkable benefit in relieving neuropathy of diabetes, an affliction that plagues me. Neither my doctor nor pharmacist was aware of this. Could you please reprint the source you quoted?

A. My reference was an article in the journal Diabetes Care (2002).

Nerve malfunction causing leg pain commonly affects patients with diabetes; the nitroglycerine spray was discovered to have beneficial effects in such patients.

Exclude serious causes before treating chest wall pain

Q. Please comment on chest wall pain, its etiology and its treatment.

A. Chest wall pain is discomfort arising from structures surrounding the heart and lungs: ribs, muscles, cartilage, tendons and other tissues in the area. The cause of chest wall pain is poorly understood. Sometimes it results from injury or strain, often from low-grade inflammation; frequently, no obvious cause can be identified.

Treatment consists of heat, pain medication, rest and anti-inflammatory drugs (such as ibuprofen). The main consideration is to differentiate chest wall pain from the discomfort caused by heart or lung disease. For example, angina, heart attack and pneumonia can occasionally present as chest wall pain. Therefore, the diagnosis is usually made by excluding other more serious afflictions.

Ask your surgeon about 'shocky' feet

Q. I have nerve compression in my lower back, following a lumbar laminectomy. Both feet still get very hot and "shocky," and my legs throb. Will these unpleasant aftereffects ever disappear?

A. I don't know.

If you had spinal surgery within the past few weeks, you may be experiencing symptoms caused by the healing process; over time, the situation will probably improve.

On the other hand, if your surgery took place months or years ago, I'd be concerned that you might be experiencing the consequences of nerve damage that could be permanent. Lumbar laminectomy is surgery to relieve the pain and other symptoms of a herniated disc.

My standard reply to questions such as yours is "ask your surgeon," who may have a perfectly logical explanation for your continuing difficulty. If, on the other hand, your surgeon cannot answer your question, request a referral to a colleague for a second opinion.

Make informed decision before using drug

Q. My doctor has prescribed Tegretol, an anticonvulsant, for my burning feet. He claims that nobody knows why it works, but it does. Please explain this.

A. Tegretol (carbamazepine) is a prescription drug ordinarily used to control seizures in patients with epilepsy. In addition, it has been found useful in (and has government approval for) reducing the pain of trigeminal neuralgia, chronic pain involving the nerves to the face. The mechanism of action is unknown.

Some neurologists have discovered that Tegretol lessens the pain of neuropathy, pain in the legs and feet that usually accompanies diabetes. Again, the reasons for this remain a mystery, nor do the experts understand why some people are helped and others are not. Tegretol has not received government approval for this purpose.

Unfortunately, Tegretol can cause serious side effects, ranging from somnolence and dizziness to double vision and life-threatening suppression of the bone marrow where new blood cells are made. Therefore, patients taking the drug need close supervision, including periodic blood tests to measure Tegretol levels in order to avoid toxicity.

If Tegretol works for you, fine. However, I do urge you to discuss

Managing Chronic Pain

Chronic pain is a problem for millions of people. Unlike acute pain (sudden and brief—as from infection, injury or surgery), chronic pain can last for months or years. It may or may not be caused by a medical condition, and it doesn't go away when an underlying condition is treated. Instead, chronic pain becomes the focus of the patient's entire life, taking a toll on personal relationships, self-esteem, work and outside interests.

Many specialists view chronic pain as a disease in itself, rather than as a symptom of an underlying disorder. Within the past 15 years there have been numerous discoveries about the body's reaction to pain and its natural pain-control mechanisms. There have been many breakthroughs in pain control, providing management of pain that was once thought untreatable. These breakthroughs include alternatives to painkilling medications, which can interfere with daily functioning or lead to drug dependence.

Pain may be caused by illness, stress or emotional problems, or even by surgery or treatment for an illness. In some cases, a patient develops a "pain habit" by expecting pain, or finding it emotionally useful, long after its cause has disappeared.

Many of the new treatments for pain focus on self-management. Patients are encouraged to change their attitudes, override pain messages, increase their pain thresholds by means of relaxation and exercise, and avoid the trap of a pain-centered life.

In fact, a sense of control helps to reduce pain. Some hospitals have introduced patient-controlled anesthesia (PCA)—a pump that enables patients to regulate the amount of narcotic painkiller they receive intravenously. As a group, these patients use less painkiller than those who request injections. They feel more in control and less helpless, and use only the amount of medication they need—not more, "just in case." They also have fewer medication-related ailments and resume normal activity earlier.

A sense of control and a positive attitude are essential in mastering pain. Chronic pain may never disappear, but it can be eased—and it's possible to create a life despite it, rather than around it.

the possible complications and side effects with your doctor, so that you can make an informed decision about the treatment.

Maintaining independence goal of treatment

Q. Please give me some encouraging words about lumbosacral degenerative joint and bone disease. It's confined mostly to my back, hips and knees but is rapidly governing my life because of stiffness and chronic pain. I can't have surgical repair, due to my diabetes. Will I continue to deteriorate?

A. I wish I could give you encouragement about the aging process but I cannot. Degenerative joint/bone disease simply means that you are wearing out: The joint spaces are thinning and roughening, the bones are losing calcium and their ability to support your weight. To my knowledge, no one has yet discovered a way to retard these ravages of age.

Nonetheless, much can be done to maintain your independence and relieve your symptoms of pain and stiffness, which are caused by a combination of inflammation and bone/joint stresses.

Anti-inflammatory drugs (Vioxx, Bextra, Celebrex, Naprosyn and others can help you maintain mobility—and, most important, allow you to sleep at night. Also, physical therapy (hot packs, massage, range-of-motion exercises, ultrasonic treatments and so forth) can be very beneficial. You must remain as active as possible in order to prevent weakness, "frozen" joints and muscle contractions.

Surgery is not always the answer, although some forms of joint replacement (notable, hips and knees) produce miraculous results in many patients. Back surgery should, in my opinion, be reserved only for the most severe cases of spinal arthritis in which nerve damage is a complication.

If you have unsuccessfully tried the nonsurgical methods I described, you probably should consider surgery. The fact that you have diabetes is not a contraindication. An orthopedic specialist can advise you about the pros and cons of joint replacement. Look into it. If your local specialist is put off by your diabetes, ask for a referral to orthopedic superspecialists in a teaching center.

Prednisone not likely cause of leg pain

Q. My legs hurt 24 hours a day because of neuropathy caused by prednisone. My doctors can't seem to find a remedy. Zostrix helps temporarily but isn't a final answer.

A. Painful nerves in the legs are not ordinarily attributed to prednisone, a steroid used for many diseases to reduce inflammation, swelling and pain.

I'd be more concerned that your neuropathy might result from the affliction for which the prednisone was prescribed. For example, autoimmune diseases, such as scleroderma, may cause nerve pain—but are treated with prednisone. Are you a diabetic? This disease is associated with neuropathy that can be worsened by steroids, which throw off glucose metabolism. I urge you to return to your doctor and describe your symptoms. He can sort things out and, perhaps, with the help of rheumatology or neurology specialists, identify the cause of your problems.

Zostrix, a cream made from chili peppers, does relieve certain types of chronic pain, but will not, in my opinion, get at the root of your neuropathy.

Self-injected drugs bizarre prescription

Q. About two years ago, my doctor had me self-injecting medication into my butt for severe pain. This helped for about a year but now the pain is back. Moreover, my left foot is now paralyzed. Some doctors say this is permanent, others say it will pass in time. In the past two weeks, I have noticed pronounced weakness in the foot. I now have a dropped foot and cannot walk without a limp. I have no money and am desperate. What can I do?

A. This is a truly bizarre situation.

First off, I'd have to know the cause of your pain. Judging from the sequence of events, you are suffering from continuing spinal nerve damage that could be caused by a herniated disc or some other abnormality in your lower spine. Frankly, I am surprised that your physician apparently failed to test you two years ago, with, at the minimum, X-rays of your lower back. Ideally, you should have had an MRI.

Second, I am shocked that you were prescribed injectable drugs for the pain in the absence of a diagnosis—or, at least, a referral to a spine specialist. A dropped foot is a serious sign of nerve malfunction. Unless the process is addressed and reversed, you are a candidate for a permanent handicap.

To get at the root of the problem, you should see a specialist: a neurologist, an orthopedic surgeon or a neurosurgeon. Don't delay. While you may be financially strapped, you should be able to find appropriate help from a doctor who is more interested in your welfare than in the almighty dollar. Good physicians perform a certain amount of charity work for deserving patients. Make an appointment with a specialist and let me know how events transpire.

Sharp pains on side of face caused by nerve disorder

Q. What is trigeminal neuralgia? Every article I read points to an external stimulus, such as touching my face, as an instigator of pain, yet my own pain worsens when I chew, drink, touch my tongue to a tooth, swallow, cough, sneeze, brush my teeth or shave. I'm now taking Tegretol and wonder if the pain will return once the medication is stopped.

A. Trigeminal neuralgia, called tic douloureux, is a disorder of a nerve on the side of the face, producing sharp shocks of pain that are ordinarily triggered by activity, such a chewing, that may stimulate the nerve. The cause is unknown. Unlike nerve damage from other causes, such as infections and tumors, tic douloureux is not associated with numbness, tingling or loss of sensation.

Some patients appear to be excessively sensitive to any stimulation of the nerve. Thus, your discomfort on sneezing, drinking and coughing is unusual, but consistent with the diagnosis.

Treatment is ordinarily a prescription drug called Tegretol. It usually relieves pain, but must be taken for several months. Customarily, the medication is taken until the patient is free of symptoms. Then it is tapered or stopped. If the neuralgia recurs, further courses of medicine can be prescribed. You need to know that Tegretol can, in rare instances, lead to liver damage and bone marrow depression, so periodic blood tests are advisable. If Tegretol is ineffective, other drugs (such as Dilantin) may be tried. Surgery to cut the nerve is a last resort. I cannot predict whether your pain will reappear after Tegretol therapy. Often it does not.

Painful tailbone may require surgery.

Q. A year or so ago, I fell on my tailbone, injuring it. To this day, any pressure on the area results in a great deal of pain, despite cortisone shots, manipulation and physical therapy. My doctor now suggests removal of the coccyx. Do you agree with him?

A. Injuries to the coccyx, a vestigial bone at the base of the spine, may lead to a chronic pain syndrome that resists nonsurgical treatment.

If you are at the end of your rope and have tried injections, analgesics and other traditional therapy, surgery may be your best option. It is, by and large, curative and is not dangerous because the coccyx lies well below the spinal cord. Follow your doctor's guidance.

Ways to Ease Pain

Acupuncture

In this ancient Oriental technique, fine-gauge needles are inserted at key points under the skin; the needles may be rotated or charged with a small electric current. It's not clear how acupuncture works, but it apparently stimulates nerves that reduce pain perception, releases pain-suppressing brain chemicals and/ or causes non-pain nerve messages to dominate.

Acupuncture is relatively painless and generally requires a series of sessions. Western medicine still views it with some skepticism, but some people have found it helpful in treating such problems as migraine, back pain and muscle aches.

The American Medical Association regards acupuncture as an "experimental medical procedure that should be performed only in a research setting by a licensed physician," and in 25 states, it may be practiced only by a licensed medical doctor. The licensing requirements for acupuncturists vary from state to state. However, the National Commission for the Certification of Acupuncturists has instituted a voluntary certification exam that many states are accepting as all or part of their licensing criteria.

Anesthesia

For temporary pain relief, local anesthesia (or "nerve block") may be used to deaden nerves in a painful area. This treatment consists of anesthetic injections and is useful in treating the acute pain caused by a back injury, neuralgia, bursitis or shingles. However, it isn't a long-term solution: The anesthesia wears off in a matter of hours, and other treatments are more suitable for chronic pain.

Behavior modification

Pain clinics and specialists often help patients to control pain by altering their attitude toward it. Many patients have unconsciously developed a "pain habit": Pain has become their way of life. Over time, they've developed an unusually high sensitivity to pain, or they use pain as a way to control others or make excuses for themselves. Some people derive satisfaction from the medications, treatments and rituals that their pain involves.

Others may use pain as an excuse for narcotics addiction or alcoholism.

In these cases, there may be no physical basis for the pain, which may continue long after an injury has healed—but pain has become a useful habit.

Through behavior modification, patients and their families are taught to change this behavior, adopt healthier attitudes and activities, and stop focusing on (or responding to) pain-related complaints.

Biofeedback

In biofeedback, patients learn how to control involuntary body processes—such as muscle contractions and blood-vessel constriction—that contribute to pain. A biofeedback device is attached to the body and provides sound or visual signs that indicate the patient's relaxation level.

Biofeedback requires training sessions, in which the patient learns how to reach the desired level of relaxation. Portable biofeedback devices are available for home use, but patients eventually learn to relax without monitoring by machine.

Counseling

Many pain complaints are caused by stress or an underlying emotional problem: The pain feels real, but has no physical cause.

Some people may unconsciously deny their emotional distress and transform it into physical pain, which they view as more "acceptable." Others may suffer pain from severe headaches or muscle tension caused by emotional problems. In either case, counseling helps the patient to recognize and manage the real source of pain.

Exercise

Some pain (such as lower back pain) is caused by weak muscles. A physical therapist can teach the patient how to strengthen specific muscles without causing damage or excessive strain.

In addition, some muscle pain can be alleviated by regular exercise, such as swimming, cycling or vigorous walking. This type of exercise stretches muscles, increases oxygen intake, promotes genuine tiredness and triggers the release of endorphins (brain chemicals that counteract pain and give a sense of well-being). Regular exercise also provides a distraction from pain, increases fitness and improves mobility—all of which can help to alleviate pain.

Hypnosis

Hypnosis can ease physically caused pain by blocking pain perception: The patient learns to override pain signals by altering his or her focus and developing a "pain-free" mental state.

Hypnosis doesn't work for everyone, but it can be useful and has no side effects. Contrary to popular belief, hypnosis isn't a form of mysticism or esoteric mind control: It's a medically accepted form of treatment and is practiced by many psychiatrists and psychologists.

Massage

Massage can reduce pain and stress by alleviating muscle tension. It also improves circulation and bombards the body with sensations that interfere with pain perception.

There are numerous types of massage (for example, Swedish and shiatsu); all can be of benefit, depending on personal preference, and most states require that masseurs be licensed. However, medical massage requires special training in the treatment of specific physical problems. To find a reputable medical masseuse, ask for a referral from your physician or a local hospital.

Medication

Several types of medication are used in treating pain. However, medication should be viewed as a short-term solution—a way of "getting over the worst" until a problem is corrected or managed.

Nonnarcotic analgesics are drugs that relieve local pain. They include both over-the-counter medications (aspirin, acetaminophen, ibuprofen) and prescription drugs. They are useful in managing occasional moderate, short-term pain. However, it's unwise to depend on these medications, since continued use can mask pain symptoms that require medical treatment. In addition, some pain problems don't respond adequately to these medications.

Muscle relaxants may be prescribed to alleviate pain from a local muscle injury.

Nonsteroidal anti-inflammatory agents (such as Indocin, Naprosyn and Tolectin) are prescribed to treat arthritis, menstrual cramps, musculoskeletal pain and inflammation. These medications inhibit the body's release of prostaglandins—hormonelike chemicals that contribute to some types of pain.

Narcotics (such as Demerol, morphine and codeine) are available by prescription only. They don't block local pain, but affect the entire central nervous system, have a sedative effect and make the pain seem less troublesome. Narcotics are federally controlled and are addicting; over time, drug tolerance increases and a patient requires ever-larger doses to achieve the same pain relief. Therefore, narcotics should be used only to relieve pain in cases of severe injury, surgery or terminal illness.

Relaxation/Meditation

Meditation, like hypnosis, is a simple way to reduce the physical and emotional stress that contribute to pain. In general, meditation involves progressively relaxing the body, then concentrating on each breath or on some short, neutral word (even "breath" will do), permitting extraneous thoughts to drift by. It's most beneficial if done for a minimum of 15 minutes, twice daily.

Meditation can be self-taught. An excellent book on the subject is "The Relaxation Response" (Herbert Benson, M.D.; William Morrow & Co., 1975/Avon, 1976), which popularized this therapeutic, nonreligious form of meditation. In addition, YM/YWCAs, adult education programs and recreation centers often offer meditation classes.

Surgery

Surgery is helpful when pain is a symptom of an underlying, correctable physical problem. However, surgery isn't recommended—or possible—for every problem. For example, no surgical procedure will alleviate the pain of osteoporosis, polymyalgia, shingles or many types of back pain. (In fact, surgery on the back's complex nerves and muscles can simply complicate the original problem.)

Surgery may be used to sever or section off pain-transmitting nerves in some cases of trigeminal neuralgia (tic douloureux) or severe peripheral nerve damage. However, this is a last-resort treatment, since the severing of nerves damages the patient's ability to function.

Transcutaneous electrical nerve stimulation (TENS)

The TENS device is a battery-powered, portable generator that produces a small electric current. Electrodes are attached to key points on the body, and the current blocks or short-circuits the body's own pain messages; it also may stimulate the production of endorphins (pain-suppressing chemicals). TENS devices are available for home use, and can provide hours of pain relief after less than a half hour of treatment.

TENS is effective in treating chronic pain from sciatica, osteoarthritis, bursitis, migraine and many other problems. However, the device itself is relatively expensive, and some medical plans may not cover the cost. In addition, TENS should not be used by patients who have pacemakers, since the TENS current may interrupt or stop the pacemaker's functioning. (However, TENS poses no danger for those without pacemakers.)

Pain clinics

Pain clinics offer comprehensive treatment of pain and provide the combined skills of many specialist, including anesthesiologists, neurologists, orthopedists, physical therapists, psychiatrists and psychologists. These specialists examine all aspects of the patient's lifestyle in order to diagnose the problem and provide effective treatment. Most pain clinics emphasize self-help techniques, and patients should be committed to getting well: The goal is to manage the problem, not to encourage a "pain habit."

Pain-clinic treatment may require hospitalization or the treatment may be done on an outpatient basis. Most reputable pain clinics are affiliated with large hospitals or medical centers; you can contact the American Society of Anesthesiologists at 520 N. Northwest Hwy., Park Ridge, IL 60068, 847-825-5586, for a list of these clinics. Avoid pain clinics that have no hospital affiliation or ASA listing: Many of these lack the expertise required, and may offer temporary pain relief without examining the full scope of the problem.

24

Skin

—

Bruises and breaking skin may be age-related

Q. I'm 68 and have never been sick in my life. However, for the past year, my skin breaks easily, and I bruise readily. The large, purple spots are unsightly. Can anything be done about this?

A. You are probably experiencing age-related thinning of the skin, which leads to easy injury from trivial trauma. Or you could have a co-agulation problem, as would develop from a low platelet count, the blood cells that are vital for clotting. Or your could have a vitamin deficiency (of vitamin C, for instance) that could cause you to bruise too readily, leading to a tendency for the outer skin to pull away from the deeper layer. Finally, are you taking aspirin? This can cause bruising.

See your physician or a dermatologist for an examination. Age-re-lated skin problems may be helped by creams and lotions; however, other conditions should be addressed by your doctor.

Winter itch annoying but not dangerous

Q. I'm a 77-year-old farmer who stays active, eats sensibly, avoids tobacco and alcohol, and am tormented by severe itching. This occurs only in the winter and involves the skin around my waist—no rash, just itching. It begins in late October, lasts until spring and is not helped by moisturizing creams. Interestingly, last winter my wife and I took off for a two-week vacation in Florida. Within three days after our arrival, the itching disappeared, only to return with a vengeance when we traveled home to New Jersey. Any idea?

A. Without examining you, I hesitate to venture a diagnosis. How-ever, your description of the malady is so characteristic that I'll go out on a limb. You appear to be suffering from a common skin condition called "winter itch." The cause of this is unknown but the affliction occurs only in the winter months and is relieved by warm weather. I recommend that you apply an over-the-counter cortisone cream twice a day to relieve your symptoms. If this ploy doesn't work, I advise you to see a dermatologist for a diagnosis—or, perhaps, a prescription for a more potent steroid cream. Incidentally, winter itch is not a dangerous disorder and is not a hazard to health.

Dry skin? Look to lanolin

Q. I have very dry skin on my face. I would like to apply butter to lubricate my skin and scalp. Will this affect my blood cholesterol?

A. No, it will not. However, I believe that you have more effective options for your dry skin. Butter will not be appreciably absorbed into the skin cells, and—unless you wash it off daily—it could turn rancid, leaving you with a new set of problems.

There are many commercial moisturizing creams and lotions available. If you have unsuccessfully tried some of them, purchase a product that contains lanolin. Lanolin is a great moisturizer and should solve your problem.

Be wary of moisturizing creams

Q. Your advice to people with extremely dry skin conditions is good. However, some folks with persistent dry skin should be alert to the fact that moisturizing creams may contain the very compounds that are causing an allergic reaction. Therefore, if the skin condition persists despite the use of a particular product, the consumer should change brands.

A. Excellent advice. Thank you for your suggestion.

Arizona reader suggests a humidifier

Q. I live in Arizona and was interested in your response to a reader with dry skin. To my surprise, you did not suggest a humidifier. I moved down here from the mountains and, believe me, the colder it gets, the drier. My humidifier dramatically increases my comfort level and helps my dry skin.

A. Good solution. Thank you for reminding me that the desert Southwest can be tough on skin.

Cause of vitiligo remains a mystery

Q. What is vitiligo? I saw a dermatologist who diagnosed me, but didn't have much information to share. Is it dangerous? I had a normal thyroid test; now it seems that my family doctor blames nerves, the sun, weeds and the environment. I have about 10 patches now on my face, chest and arms. Am I doomed for life?

A. This skin condition, which may be seen in conjunction with an underactive thyroid gland, causes patchy depigmentation of the skin. Although there is some preliminary evidence that vitiligo may have a genetic basis, in most cases the cause is unknown. The factors your doctor mentioned probably do not play a role.

Vitiligo does not affect health, but can be a cosmetic embarrassment. For obscure reasons, the disorder may spread and then later regress. Some authorities believe that the singer Michael Jackson suffers from vitiligo.

Treatment consists of cover-up cosmetics or self-tanning products. Remember that areas of vitiligo don't tan; therefore people with this condition must be especially careful not to sunburn, as should any fair-skinned individual.

Skin tags are harmless

Q. What causes skin tags? I know a doctor can cut, burn or freeze them off, but is there any method of removal that can be done by the patient safely at home?

A. Skin tags are just harmless little growths that, with age, can form anywhere on the body. Some patients have had success by tightly tying a piece of thread around the bases of the tags. When deprived of their blood supply, the tags drop off in a few days.

Numerous causes of pressure hives

Q. What can you tell me about pressure hives?

A. Pressure hives are called cholinergic urticaria. These itchy, raised skin eruptions are caused by dilation of small blood vessels (capillaries). The reaction is the result of histamines that are released when pressure is applied to the skins of sensitive individuals. Urticaria also can be caused by stress, allergies or exposure to cold (or heat). People with hives often can control the troublesome breaking out by avoiding the offending factors or by using antihistamines.

Alternative therapy for psoriasis

Q. You have often told readers psoriasis sufferers that the skin disorder is very difficult to treat. Maybe so, but let me share a little secret that may be a blessing.

I suffered from psoriasis for years. Various therapies gave me only temporary relief. Then a friend suggested that I use a dandruff-fighting shampoo as a body soap. No more smelly coal-tar or expensive steroid creams—just plain old shampoo, followed by a petrolatum jelly/vitamin E combination after toweling dry. What a relief!

A. This is new to me but I am passing on your tip to readers in hopes that 1) your remedy will work for others, and 2) I can get some feedback—pro or con—from the public. If your tip for psoriasis-sufferers is half as effective as Vicks VapoRub for toenail fungus, you will be historically held in high regard.

Shingles infections treatable today

Q. Thirty years ago during a routine visit with my doctor, I mentioned I had a slight rash on my lower back. He diagnosed me with shingles and gave me a shot of either vitamin B6 or B12. Two or three days later I had another shot and the blisters dried up and the pain went away. Since then, I've known several people with shingles who have suffered for months and this treatment was never suggested for them. Why not?

A. Shingles, a type of herpes infection of nerves in the skin, causes painful blisters. However, not all patients with this affliction progress to a full-blown rash; some have only a few minor lesions. This is what probably happened in your case, because I doubt the vitamin shots played any role whatsoever in your recovery.

Such shots are completely ineffective in curing shingles. Of course, in the 1960s, there was no treatment for this virus infection, so doctors often felt obligated to give some form of therapy, even if they knew it was ineffective.

Fortunately, today, there is effective treatment for shingles: Acyclovir (Zovirax) when taken in pill form, as early as possible in the course of the disease, will often cure the infection.

Leg ulcers resistant to healing

Q. What causes a leg ulcer and what can be done to get rid of it?

A. Ulcers on the skin of the leg often result from deficient arterial or venous circulation.

In the first instance, not enough blood reaches the skin—usually due to aging. Consequently, minor scrapes and abrasions fail to heal, become infected and enlarge. The diagnosis of arterial insufficiency can be made by a series of tests, including Doppler ultrasound. Treatment includes special dressings, antibiotics—and, possibly, surgery to unclog the artery.

Venous ulcers are more common. In the presence of varicose veins or edema (swelling), stale blood pools in the legs, preventing oxygen and nutrient-rich blood from reaching the tissues. Again, healing is delayed, minor trauma can become infected and ulcers will form.

By and large, venous disease of the lower extremities has a characteristic appearance: bulging veins plus thin and fragile skin. Such ulcers usually respond to elevation, special dressings, diuretics (to reduce edema), elastic wrapping, and other nonsurgical techniques.

Sometimes, operative procedures such as vein stripping or laser surgery may be necessary.

Your family physician can advise you and, when appropriate, refer you to a vascular specialist.

"Nervous sores" common

Q. My mother suffers from what she calls "nervous sores" on her scalp and back. Her dermatologist doesn't think this is unusual, and actually has admitted it is quite common. Please help us understand her problem.

A. In some people, the skin is especially sensitive to emotional upset and stress. Called "neurodermatitis," this harmless condition is relatively common, as your mother's doctor confirmed.

The affliction is marked by periodic outbreaks of a scaly, itchy rash on various parts of the body. The cause is unknown, but neurodermatitis can often be relieved by the combination of counseling, antianxiety medications (such as Ativan or Xanax), and the local application of steroid cream. Ask her dermatologist to coordinate the various aspects of therapy.

Peeling feet an annoyance

Q. For the past five years, from time to time, my feet peel. The situation isn't uncomfortable, but it's annoying. What causes such enormous amounts of skin to peel from my feet?

A. Peeling feet often reflect the presence of a fungus infection, resembling athlete's foot, in the skin. The yeast disrupts the integrity of the skin, causing portions of dead skin (callus) to peel away.

This condition can easily be diagnosed by your family doctor, using skin scrapings that are specially treated and examined in the laboratory.

If a fungus is identified, treatment with antifungal creams, such as Nizoral, should cure the condition.

If no fungus is present in the skin sample, you should be referred to a dermatologist, because skin diseases, such as eczema and psoriasis, can also cause peeling feet and should be treated with other prescription medications.

25

Hair & Nails

Losing hair

Q. I am active and healthy at 53, yet I am losing my hair. What could cause this? I'm too embarrassed to discuss this with my doctor and would value your opinion.

A. You don't say whether you're male or female. It makes a difference.

As men age, they lose body hair—and, obviously, scalp hair as well. This is an inherited characteristic that is probably aggravated by withering of the hair follicles, lessened amounts of male hormone and thinning/drying of the skin.

Women do not ordinarily lose body hair as they age to the extent that men do. (Perhaps because they have less to begin with.) Thus, hair loss in women may reflect physical disorders such as hypothyroidism, anemia or hidden infection.

See your doctor. He has had to deal with far more embarrassing patient complaints than hair loss. Or, if you choose, pass GO and proceed directly to a dermatologist.

Vicks VapoRub for nail fungus

Q. A friend expounded on the effectiveness of Pau d'Arco tea for fingernail and toenail fungus. Is this therapy verified by any medical source, or is it simply an herbal remedy that works?

A. The customary treatment for finger or toenail fungus, an exceedingly common and annoying affliction, has been expensive antifungal topical creams, or even more expensive antifungal pills that must be taken for many days and have the potential for liver damage.

In an attempt to help my readers find a more acceptable alternative, years ago I published a column based on a reader's conviction that soaking the nails in herbal Pau d'Arco tea would cure the fungus. (Steep the tea until it is comfortably hot, then soak twice a day.)

This remedy was, for many readers, a huge success. And I supported it until a new, cheaper and easier alternative was, again, recommended by a reader. (Not the Pau d'Arco one, I should add.)

The revolution centers around Vicks VapoRub, which I have endorsed based on hundreds of positive letters I have received and my own personal experience. (It cured my toenail/fingernail funguses.)

For those readers who want to try this therapy, let me once again repeat how it is use.

First, you must trim the affected nail as short as possible to reduce the "biomass" of the fungus, which infects the growing portion of the nail (behind the cuticle) and enlarges as the nail grows. When I say "as short as possible," that's what I mean. Trim the nail back either by filing a hard, thick nail or by actually cutting the nail as far back toward the cuticle as you can without pain or bleeding. (The un-success stories that I have received usually involve applying the Vicks to a nail that was yellow, thick and deformed—without first cutting the tissue back.)

Once you have reduced the area of the nail as far as you feel comfortable doing, apply Vicks VapoRub twice a day to the nail itself, the cuticle and the toe (or finger). Rub it in well.

If you choose to cover the toes (or fingers) after the application, fine. In my experience, this is not necessary. If the VapoRub is sufficiently massaged, there should be relatively little excess.

The good news is that Vicks is breathtakingly cheap—and safe.

The bad news is that, in advanced cases, the therapy may take months to be effective—and may not be effective at all if the infected nail is thick and yellow. So, be patient. As the nail grows out—incredibly slowly, it seems—the fungus-free portion will appear.

For pennies a day, your problem may be solved, without using tea-soaks or expensive prescription medication.

Fungal infection

Q. My husband's toenails and fingernails are unnaturally convex, woody, thickened, and yellow. The tips of his fingers and toes are red and globular. What could be causing this?

A. Your husband probably has an advanced fungal infection of his nails—or he could be suffering from a circulatory deficiency. In the first instance, he may be helped either by antifungal medication such as Lamisil pills, or, as a cheaper alternative, the application of Vicks VapoRub to the affected nails.

In the second instance, he would need medical attention.

I recommend that he be examined by a podiatrist, who will provide necessary nail care and refer your husband to a physician, if necessary, for examination and testing to determine if your husband has a health issue, such as diabetes or vascular disease, that needs attention.

Ridges on nails

Q. If a person's nails are marked with ridges or lines, what does this indicate?

A. Vertical ridging of the nails affects everybody who enters the ranks of the elderly. Like gray hair and wrinkled skin, nail ridging is inescapable and requires no treatment.

Horizontal ridging of the nails, however, can indicate a nutritional deficiency. If you are young and have newly ridged nails, I suggest a physical examination by a specialist in internal medicine.

Ingrown nails common but painful

Q. I constantly get ingrown toenails in my big toes. Where do they come from, and what should I do about them?

A. One of humankind's most common afflictions, ingrown toenails, are a painful nuisance. I don't know why they occur, but the end result is the same: As the nails grow crookedly into the skin of the toe, they cause pain and inflammation. Intermittent symptoms can usually be controlled by hot soaks and by placing cotton pledgets under the nail to elevate it and keep it from growing in.

In contrast, repeated or chronic ingrown nails need surgery. The procedure, which removes the offending portion of the growing nail, is almost always effective. Therefore, my advice is for you to see a surgeon or podiatrist. Although the simple operation is uncomfortable for several days, it should solve the problem.

Diet & Dieting

Skip the Louisiana fat farm

Q. I've heard of a weight-control clinic in Louisiana that administers a weekly injection of human chorionic gonadotropin. This hormone is supposed to open up fat cells and use them for energy. The clinic also dispenses a thyroid pill and a stimulant to reduce appetite. I'm considering going to the clinic, because I want to lose 30 pounds, but my doctor doesn't have any information on this. Do you?

A. No, I don't. However, I do have a problem with fat farms; you'll surely lose weight but what happens after you leave? You cannot continue hormone injections, thyroid pills and stimulants for the rest of your life. So, if you spend a few hundred dollars to lose a measly 30 pounds and gain back the weight a year later, you've wasted your time and money.

I suggest that you try my (cheap and easy) "no flour, no sugar" diet, increase your exercising, shed a few pounds—then go to Louisiana for some well-deserved, down-home, delicious Creole or Cajun cooking. This is much more fun—and it's more healthful, too.

Low-fat versus low-carb diets

Q. I recently read about new reports indicating that a low-carbohydrate diet is more effective in promoting weight loss than is a low-fat diet. Does this support your "no flour, no sugar" diet?

A. The reports you refer to were published in the New England Journal of Medicine (May 22, 2003). They do indeed show that stout people are more able to lose weight by following a low-carb diet than by using a traditional low-fat plan. This finding supports the value of my "no flour, no sugar" diet.

Obviously, an ideal weight-reduction diet should limit fat intake, too. Unlike the Atkins diet (which is heavy in fat composition), my diet is low in fat—but it is cheap, has variability and is easy to follow. I've received literally hundreds of letters from readers who have had success with my diet. Now, thanks to the new studies, the "no flour, no sugar" diet has sound scientific backing.

No flour, no sugar diet allows for sufficient roughage

Q. For four months, I have been on your "no flour, no sugar" diet, with remarkable results; I have lost more than 20 pounds—and it was easy. I'm committed. However, I've also noticed a tendency to constipation, which I've treated with Senakot. Could the virtual elimination of carbohydrates have led to this bowel problem?

A. In theory, yes. However, if you continue on my diet, you will be consuming appropriate amounts of vegetable fiber, which should aid your evacuation. Try consuming more fluids, especially fruit juices. For the time being, use of Senakot is OK.

Avoid flour and sugar to lose pounds

Q. Recent TV programs have seemed to promote various weight-loss diets such as the South Beach diet, the Atkins diet, and others. Why has your "no flour, no sugar" diet not achieved wide recognition? It worked for me, is cheap and easy to follow, and seems to make a lot of sense for those people who need guidance after their weight loss. Do you have any added advice for keeping weight off?

A. As you pointed out, most weight-loss diets are successful. In the beginning. Problems arise when, after losing unwanted pounds, people are unable to sustain lower weights. There are many reasons for this phenomenon, including diets that are too strict (such as the Ornish diet) or don't provide enough flexibility over the long haul.

This is a major advantage of my diet; people can modify the diet in many ways once they have achieved their goal. For instance, a person rarely has to stick assiduously to the diet. He or she can cautiously begin to consume more carbohydrates in the form of pasta and bread, while continuing to avoid sweets. Therefore, my diet can be "tailor-made" to answer a variety of needs, and that is one of its strengths. Finally, my diet is not particularly restrictive, as is—for example—the grapefruit diet. A person is allowed modest portions of meat, poultry, fish, vegetables, salads and fresh fruit.

I don't know why my diet has yet to achieve national recognition. Maybe that is simply a matter of time. At last count, more than 158,000 people have requested the diet and have had, as far as I know, success with it.

Perhaps the "no flour, no sugar" diet isn't "sexy" enough for talk show hosts. If you know Jay Leno, you might prevail upon him to investigate the issue. The results could well be interesting or even startling.

Forgo honey in coffee

Q. I am trying hard to follow your "no flour, no sugar" diet and have had great success with it.

However, I really need to have a sweetener, such as honey or sugar, in my four cups of coffee a day. I know I should avoid sugar, but is the honey acceptable? Do I have other options?

A. The sugar restriction in my diet includes obvious concentrated sweets, including honey, molasses, cane sugar, maple syrup and corn syrup (commercial sweetener). Other natural sugars, such as fructose and sucrose, in fresh fruits and vegetables, are permitted.

In order to reduce your consumption of calorie-rich sugar products, I suggest that you avoid honey in your coffee, and substitute Splenda, a new calorie-free sweetening agent derived from sugar that should make your coffee more palatable without adding unnecessary calories.

High-fat diet is bad idea

Q. My 60-year-old husband is prone to hypertension. His doctor urged him to eliminate salt from his diet and I carried it further by cutting out lamb, sausage, bacon and high-fat meats. Recently, he developed hypoglycemia. Then his doctor told him to eat butter, sausage, bacon and the like to meet his "fat quotient." Help!

A. I'll simplify this complicated issue by addressing the problems in separate sections.

Salt: Most Americans eat too much salt. However, the mineral is dangerous for only a few—those with high blood pressure. Mild hypertensives can often lower their blood pressure readings by eliminating the salt they add to their diets. I advise such patients to put away the salt shaker (or substitute potassium salt for table salt), and avoid salty foods such as potato chips, pretzels, anchovies and so forth. More stringent salt restriction—such as avoiding processed meats, canned soups and frozen foods—is usually not necessary. You needn't carry the restriction to extremes.

High blood pressure: Often termed the "silent killer," hypertension is a dangerous disease that should be aggressively treated with one or more of the many drugs now used for that purpose. These therapies are so effective that salt restriction may not be necessary, except as a first step in treatment. Perhaps your husband should be taking medicine for his hypertension.

Hypoglycemia: Low blood sugar is a much rarer condition than previously believed. It can be helped by eating several small meals a day and eliminating sugar, alcohol and fats.

I completely disagree with your husband's doctor, who recommended a high-fat diet, because such a diet will do little to improve hypoglycemia and may actually lead to accelerated hardening of the arteries.

I advise your husband to obtain a second opinion from an internist, a specialist trained in diagnosing and treating medical illnesses. He should be able to solve the contradictions that are troubling you.

Medication to lose weight usually ineffective

Q. I have considered taking an over-the-counter medicine to lose weight. The tablets contain phenylalanine. Does this ingredient have any side effects or hazards?

A. Phenylalanine is an amino acid needed for good health. It is plentiful in many foods, including dairy products. It is harmless and will cause no side effects.

If phenylalanine is the active ingredient in the product, you're being taken for a ride; the amino acid will not affect your weight. Read the label again and check out the other components. Many nonprescription diet pills contain phenylpropanolamine, an appetite suppressant that should not be taken by patients with diabetes, thyroid disorders or irregular heartbeats. In addition, the substance often cause jitteriness, nervousness and insomnia.

I discourage the use of appetite suppressants of any kind. They are of temporary benefit at best and do not help people maintain ideal weight. In fact, studies have shown that more than 90 percent of people who lose weight with medication (or in a weight-reduction program) eventually regain the lost pounds within a year or two.

I believe that you would be better off following a diet you can stick to, year in and year out. Start by eliminating sugar, alcohol and junk food. Munch on raw vegetables for snacks. Use sugar-free sweets. Eat modest portions of meat, fish, poultry, vegetables, salads and raw fruit. Exercise regularly. If this plan doesn't do the trick, eliminate products containing flour from your diet. Most people can lose a pound a week and keep off the weight on this simple "no flour, no sugar" diet.

Eighty-seven-year-old's breakfast is just fine

Q. I'm 87 years old and my favorite breakfast for many years consists of dry cereal with skimmed milk and three graham crackers, alternating mornings with a hard roll, lunch meat, a slice of cheese and three crackers. Now I read that cheese and lunch meats have too much cholesterol. Should I make a change?

A. Not on your life. If you have reached 87 with most systems intact, you needn't get off a winning horse. Enjoy your favorite breakfast and look forward to your 90th birthday.

Media alerts help awareness

Q. In my 55 years of life, I've consumed beef tartar, uncooked eggs, water from streams, raw grilled meats, food prepared on unsanitized boards, roasts thawed too long at room temperature, unwashed vegetables, sushi and raw shellfish. Like others in those days who did likewise, I'm still here.

Now all you hear about is people dying from such things, and antibacterial hand washing, wipings and spraying are the rage. Why? Is illness from food poisoning simply more publicized?

A. Food-borne illness is not new, but the patterns have changed over the years. I think that you have been lucky not to have become sick from some of your food choices; I hope that your 55 years have taught you to eat more sensibly.

I believe that the media have played a huge rule in publicizing food-related problems. In large part, this may be just a matter of numbers. If, in the old days, Mom under-cooked a batch of hamburgers and the family became ill for several days, the event wasn't news; maybe the only people to learn of this were the neighbors. Now, however, if the folks at a church picnic get sick from bad mayonnaise, or a bunch of kids get a bug from contaminated burger meat at a fast-food restaurant, these events quickly become public knowledge. Consequently, all of us are now more alert to the problems of public food poisoning and, I hope, are more prudent about how what we eat is prepared and served.

Calories, not thyroid, cause of weight gain

Q. I'm female, 51, and overweight. Despite periodic dieting, I've been unable to trim down. I take Synthroid, and my last thyroid blood test was normal. Could there be a connection between the medication and my obesity?

A. Unlikely. You were probably prescribed synthetic thyroid hormone replacements to correct an underactive thyroid gland. If your blood tests show that you are receiving the proper dose of medicine, you can ignore the thyroid gland as a cause of your weight problem. Ordinarily, an underactive gland does not cause obesity, although this has been a popular theory in the past.

Most cases of overweight are cause by too many calories in the diet. More precisely, people gain weight when their caloric intakes exceed their caloric requirements; those calories not burned for energy are stored as fat.

Granted, some obese people have a very low metabolism and require fewer calories than normal. But most overweight persons can lose weight by following a sensible, low-calorie diet.

Ask your doctor to refer you to a dietician and regularly monitor your progress. Or consider any of the popular diet plans, such as Weight Watchers or Slim-Fast.

Drastic change in eating habits needs investigation

Q. My husband and I have been married for more than 50 years and he has always eaten sensibly, until now. For the past year, he has craved sweets in any form—chocolate, cookies, cakes, candy—you name it. He is steadily losing weight, and I'm concerned. Should I be?

A. Any drastic change in dietary preferences, especially in the presence of weight loss, should be investigated. In my opinion, your husband needs to address this situation with his doctor. I am particularly concerned that, despite a superfluous consumption of calories, he is losing weight. Such an unexplained and unexpected result could be caused by a serious ailment, such as hidden cancer or a glandular disorder. Encourage your spouse to seek medical attention.

Moderation in all things

Q. I like good food, including desserts. However, I've read that sugar

"Natural" Weight-loss Aids Are Just as Ineffective, Gimmicky or Unsafe as "Unnatural" Ones

The only natural reducing aids are less food and more exercise. Most fad-supplement regimens recommend highly restricted diets, which are the real reason for any weight loss.

Some "*diet teas*" are "dietetic" only because (like all plain teas) they're calorie-free. Others contain diuretic or stimulant herbs, which have no weight-loss function and can be harmful in large quantities.

Fiber doesn't promote weight loss or speed food through the system. It does give a sense of fullness—but fiber foods have the same effect.

Glucommannan (konjac) and *guar gum* are vegetable fibers that expand and become gel-like in the stomach, allegedly decreasing appetite. Glucomannan can cause digestive problems; if it expands in the throat or esophagus, it can cause choking, obstruction and asphyxiation.

Grapefruit doesn't increase weight loss or metabolism. Many grapefruit-diet pills contain phenylpropanolamine (PPA), an over-the-counter stimulant that can cause anxiety, hypertension and palpitations.

"*Growth-hormone releasers*" are amino-acid compounds that are said to increase metabolism and burn fat. They don't, they're expensive, and they can be harmful.

Herbal diet formulas usually contain vitamins, minerals and stimulant or diuretic herbs—none of which has anything to do with weight loss.

Kelp, lecithin, B6 and cider vinegar may be the most popular, peculiar and unpalatable of "diet aids." They also have no basis in scientific fact: Kelp doesn't stimulate metabolism; lecithin doesn't mobilize fat; B6 has mild diuretic effects, but can cause numbness and nerve damage; and cider vinegar is simply vinegar.

Lipotropic substances prevent fat accumulation in the liver, but do not promote weight loss.

Meal-replacement liquids are variations on liquid protein crash diets. They don't alter eating habits that lead to overweight, and they can cause imbalances, deficiencies and constipation.

Spirulina, a type of algae, hasn't been proven to suppress appetite. (Its only feasible use is as a protein source for developing countries.)

Starch blockers were banned by the FDA until they could be proven safe and effective—and there's no proof yet. These bean derivatives don't block starch digestion and calories, but can cause serious digestive problems.

is not good for me. What is the most sensible approach to sugar in the diet for people who have no health problems whatsoever?

A. Moderation.

Bizarre diets are unhealthful

Q. A man and his wife who are close friends of mine are trying to live on vitamins only—no food to speak of. Only when extremely hungry do they make a sandwich or order in fast food or a pizza. Vegetables, meat, fish and fruit are basically avoided. Isn't this practice an open invitation to nutritional deficiencies? They refuse to accept this view.

A. A diet made up merely of vitamins with periodic binge-eating will probably not satisfy their nutritional requirements in the long run. While I hesitate making any specific predictions, a diet that is nutritionally deficient could, sooner or later, adversely affect your friends' immune systems as well as contributing to a variety of ills such as anemia and heart disease (from inadequate protein intake). While the couple may not listen to you, show them my response to your question, or—better yet—urge them to review their dietary patterns with a physician.

Binge-eating/dieting cycle is unhealthy

Q. I'm a compulsive over-eater. Does dieting to control weight followed by binge-eating have any effect on my overall health?

A. Recent studies have shown that overweight people who lose and gain weight cyclically are at greater risk of health problems (such as heart disease) than are stout folks who maintain constant weights.

Therefore, unless you're so motivated to lose that you're willing to stick to a consistent diet, I recommend that your swear off the binge-eating cycles. You'll feel better about yourself and life will certainly be less complicated for you.

Check with your doctor about this to make sure that you don't have an undiagnosed ailment, such as diabetes, that may be contributing to your problem. Also, because of your addictive pattern of eating, you might consider counseling.

Compulsive overeating is a form of substance abuse.

Drink high-caloric supplement to gain weight

Q. I am 85, active, eat normally and have gone from a stable weight of 170 to a skinny 135. Nonetheless, after extensive testing, my doctor cannot pinpoint the cause. I'm literally fading away. Any suggestions?

A. Yes. As people reach their 70s and 80s, they often lose considerable amounts of weight. The causes for this are complicated and, in an otherwise healthy adult (without an underlaying disorder such as a hidden cancer), may be difficult to identify. Older folks tend to lose muscle mass. Their metabolic rates change. They may actually eat less than they did at younger ages.

What you need is more calories in your diet. I suggest that you purchase a high-calorie protein supplement drink, such as Ensure, Carnation Instant Breakfast or others, and consume one or two servings of it, in addition to your regular meals. Drink a supplement in the evening, and—perhaps—a second one in the afternoon. Such a ploy may more than double your caloric intake at no risk and little cost. With this strategy, I'd be surprised if you failed to gain back several pounds.

27

Vitamins

Too much of some vitamins can be dangerous

Q. Is there such a thing as vitamin abuse? I am concerned about a relative who may be using vitamins in excess.

A. Some vitamins can, indeed, be poisonous in large doses. The most notorious are the following:

• Vitamin A is contained in meat and fish products, as well as in many fruits and vegetables. It is necessary for normal vision and healthy skin and bones. The recommended dietary allowance (RDA) is 5,000 international units a day. Supplements above 25,000 units a day will lead to serious consequences, such as anemia, loss of appetite, poor vision, bone pain, mouth ulcers and many other complications.

• Vitamin D is found in fish and eggs. Milk is often fortified with D. The vitamin is vital for normal bone metabolism (a deficiency causes rickets and will aggravate osteoporosis). The RDA is about 200 international units a day. Excess quantities (above 1,200 IU) are associated with weight loss, nausea, headache, fatigue, anemia, kidney damage and other consequences.

• Pyridoxine (vitamin B6) is available in nuts, grains, meat and fish. It is needed for normal nerve functioning. The RDA is 2 milligrams daily. Modest doses (5 mg) may block the beneficial effects of L-dopa, a drug used to treat Parkinson's disease. Higher doses (2,000 mg) can lead to unsteady gait and numbness of the feet.

• Vitamin C is plentiful in fruits and vegetables. It is a necessary component of many metabolic reactions, including wound healing, blood formation and healthy teeth and gums. The RDA is 60 milligrams. Doses above 2,000 milligrams a day may lead to diarrhea, kidney stones, joint pains, rash, iron overload and other complications. Vitamin C has not been shown to protect against the common cold.

Is B12 a safe vitamin supplement?

Q. Please discuss the vitamin B12.

A. Vitamin B12 is critical for the life processes in the body's cells (the synthesis of RNA and DNA). It also stabilizes nerves (by maintaining insulation around them), functions as a key constituent in the manufacture of blood cells, and helps maintain normal growth in children. The recommended dietary allowance is about 3 micrograms.

B12 is derived from animal sources; meat, eggs, fish, and dairy products are rich in this vitamin. For this reason, strict vegetarians should take B12 supplements orally.

In order for the vitamin to be absorbed into the body, a chemical (known as "intrinsic factor") must be present in the stomach lining. For unknown reasons, some people lack intrinsic factor.

Therefore, despite a well-balanced diet (or oral supplements of B12), they will eventually develop B12 deficiency, leading to a serious blood disorder called pernicious anemia, which is often associated with depression and with tingling, numbness and weakness of the extremities. Pernicious anemia, which is not related to iron deficiency, is readily, safely and inexpensively treated with monthly injections of B12.

For years B12 was considered by most physicians to be a harmless placebo. Vitamin shots were routinely administered to perfectly healthy people who suffered from lassitude, fatigue and a loss of stamina. In many instances, the injections were successful; patients believed they worked—and they did. But this was due to the placebo effect, not to any consequences of the vitamin itself.

Vitamin B12 is virtually nontoxic: Up to 10,000 times the RDA has been given to patients without ill effects. (The excess simply passes from the body in the urine.) Nonetheless, most experts recommend that B12 injections be reserved for those patients in whom a bona-fide deficiency exists, a situation readily diagnosed by a blood test.

A medical history that contains the clue

Q. I have a complicated problem.

I am a woman, 54, in good health except for neuropathy in my legs. This has been present for at least 15 years, but my doctor assured me it was early menopause. I experience pain, tingling and numbness in my legs; now I am also somewhat weaker than before. I have received cortisone shots for bursitis, prescription drugs (such as Neurontin) for pain, anti-spasmodics, physical therapy, and numerous nerve tests. I don't have diabetes, thyroid problems or Lyme disease, but I am slightly anemic and my red blood cells are too large.

I've been referred to an orthopedist (no help), a neurologist (a waste of time) and a rheumatologist (I was told of fibromyalgia, but no treatment).

Last summer, I began having muscle spasms in my neck, was told of osteoarthritis and spinal stenosis, and was referred to a neurosurgeon whom I have yet to see. But no one has been able to discover why I am so easily fatigued, suffer from constipation and a sore tongue, have unexplained weight loss and feel awful. I've been told that neuropathy is difficult to diagnose. Can you?

A. I believe that you, not I, have made the diagnosis. In your letter, which I have shortened because of space restrictions, you describe your symptoms and experiences. But, hidden away in your medical history, is a pearl of information that I think explains your symptoms and leads the way to therapy: your anemia and the fact that your red blood cells are enlarged.

Called megaloblastic macrocytic anemia, this condition is the result of inadequate levels of vitamin B12 and/or folic acid in your system. This can result from dietary inadequacy or from a disorder called pernicious anemia, in which your body is unable to absorb and use vitamin B12. This affliction may lead to the very symptoms you describe, especially the fatigue, sore tongue and neuropathy (malfunction of the nerves in your extremities).

In my opinion, you should return immediately to your primary care physician for further blood tests (especially B12 and folic acid levels) and, perhaps, a bone marrow exam or something called a Schilling test. If, as I suspect, your problem is a vitamin deficiency, you can be cured by supplemental B12/folic acid therapy.

Vitamin shots unlikely cause of rash

Q. Because I have pernicious anemia, my doctor gives me monthly B12 shots. Recently, however, I've developed an unbearable itchy rash on my legs. Could the shots be to blame?

A. Pernicious anemia is caused by the lack of a substance called intrinsic factor in the stomach. Intrinsic factor permits vitamin B12, an essential element, to be absorbed from the diet. Without adequate amounts of B12, patients develop anemia, severe nerve damage and profound mental changes, including dementia.

The most satisfactory method of treating this disorder is to administer supplemental B12, usually in the form of injections, which "bypass" the need for intrinsic factor.

I have never heard of B12 shots causing a rash. Usually, these inexpensive injections are completely safe—so safe, in fact, that most patients can easily be taught to self-administer them, much as a diabetic gives himself insulin.

I suggest that you be examined by a dermatologist, who will diagnose the cause of your rash and prescribe therapy.

Vitamin C unstable

Q. I know that vitamin C is destroyed by heat, sunlight and air. Is there any left in frozen, canned or bottled juice?

A. Because vitamin C is, as you mentioned, somewhat unstable, companies that process orange juice and other products take special pains to preserve it. The vitamin is not affected by freezing. Cans keep out light. Bottle juice is vacuum-packed to seal in freshness.

The primary problem with orange juice is its tendency to lose vitamin C once out of its original container —when the juice has, for example, been reconstituted and left open to the air or put in the refrigerator. Therefore, for maximum benefit, processed orange juice is best when not stored after opening. Of course, the most effective container is the orange skin itself; perhaps this is why fresh-squeezed orange juice remains the gold standard for us juice-lovers.

Taking Coumadin? Be wary of vitamin K

Q. I recently read an article saying that vegetables containing vitamin K should not be eaten by people on Coumadin. Is this true and should I, as a Coumadin user, deny myself these vegetables?

A. Vitamin K is necessary for proper blood coagulation. Drugs, such as Coumadin, interfere with vitamin K metabolism. Thus, the treatment for Coumadin-overdose is vitamin K.

In addition, small amounts of the vitamin (in the diet) often neutralize the beneficial effect of the prescription anticoagulant.

Natural vitamin K is present in leafy green vegetables, such as spinach, broccoli, cabbage, lettuce, and turnip greens. In people taking Coumadin to prevent blood clots, stroke and heart attack, these vegetables may alter the effectiveness of the drug, making proper dosage control (with a blood test) almost impossible.

Therefore, most experts caution Coumadin users to limit or avoid ingesting vegetables rich in vitamin K. Actually, if you ate such vegetables every day, your doctor could probably adjust the dose of Coumadin (based on a blood test) relatively easily. Problems arise because patients don't eat such vegetables every day; consequently, the effects of the vitamin vary, leading to potentially serous medical consequences, such as hemorrhage.

Although you should ask your doctor about this, I recommend that you minimize your consumption of vegetables with contain vitamin K.

A little sunlight will do ya

Q. Can the vitamin D benefit of the sun be obtained through windowpanes?

A. No, it cannot. In the body, vitamin D is activated by ultraviolet radiation, which is filtered out by window glass. This is why it's impossible to tan through a window.

On a positive note, very little unfiltered sunshine is required to activate vitamin D for metabolism; 20 to 30 minutes of sun exposure a day (even in winter) will suffice.

Vitamin side effects can be bizarre

Q. I just had to write to let you know how much your column has helped me.

For the past two years, I've struggled ineffectively with profound fatigue; at times, I literally could not get out of bed in the morning. Moreover, I had an irregular heartbeat that I thought was the cause of my problem. My doctor told me that my heart was probably not functioning to its full capacity. She prescribed propranolol, which slowed by pulse to 40 beats a minute. I felt worse, so I stopped the drug.

Then I read your response to a reader who wondered about the dangers of high-dose vitamin E. You mentioned that vitamin E can cause fatigue and an irregular pulse. I had been taking 1000 IU of E, so I cut back to 60 IU, which is included in my regular multivitamin pill. Within a few weeks, the fatigue had lifted and my pulse was regular and strong. I'm due to see my doctor next month and I can't wait to share my experience with her. Thanks to your advice, I am a new woman.

A. On occasion, people do experience unusual and rare idiosyncratic reactions to drugs, vitamin supplements and herbal remedies. Such appears to be your case. Thank you for your compliment. I am glad I could help you. The issue you raised certainly emphasizes what I have stated many times: Patients must tell their physicians of any drugs, herbals or supplements they are taking. And it never hurts to discontinue or reduce such compounds in the presence of unexplained symptoms.

I don't mean this to critique your doctor, but I believe she should have tested you with a cardiogram, a cardiac ultrasound and—possibly—a Holter monitor and a stress test before she shared her impression that your heart was not functioning to its full capacity. This type of serious diagnosis must be supported by appropriate cardiac testing. In addition, when your pulse rate fell from the medication, she might have properly chosen to refer you to a cardiologist for a second opinion.

In any case, I'm sure she will welcome your comments (and improvement) as continuing medication education, and you can bet that she will question future patients with fatigue and pulse irregularities about their vitamin consumption.

Is antioxidant therapy helpful?

Q. I've been told that antioxidant vitamins will help protect against cancer, unplug arteries, and treat hypertension and asthma. What are antioxidants? Should I be taking them?

A. During normal metabolism, the body produces chemicals, called free radicals, that can damage tissue and, some experts claim, lead to cancer and heart disease.

Therefore, there has been a lot of interest in developing compounds to block free radicals before they can do harm. Such compounds are the antioxidant vitamins E, C and beta carotene.

Despite an initial flurry of enthusiasm, medical studies have failed to prove that vitamin C and beta carotene exert any substantial health benefits when taken in large quantities to prevent cancer, heart disease, hypertension, asthma or any other affliction. (The final word is still out on vitamin E.)

The Best Advice

Food is the best source of nutrients, and nutrient deficiencies are unusual. A daily multivitamin provides insurance, but additional supplements can upset the body's balance. Despite this, the "natural" remedy/supplement trend is booming, and it's hard to tell fact from quackery.

Many supplements can interfere with prescription medications, exacerbate illness, or have harmful side effects. Most are safe in small amounts but many people take more than one supplement or take large doses, wrongly assuming that "more is better" and that "natural" remedies are harmless. Get nutrition advice from legitimate sources: Check credentials, or ask your physician or the American Dietetic Association for a referral.

See a physician about chronic symptoms: Don't treat them yourself, and don't use supplements or "natural" remedies if you're ill or take prescription drugs.

Most nutrition experts emphasize that people can obtain adequate amounts of naturally occurring antioxidant vitamins by eating wholesome, well-balanced meals, especially those containing vegetables, fruits and grains. Therefore, assuming that your diet is adequate, you don't need antioxidant supplements.

Some people, however, choose to take modest doses although such supplements are probably not necessary.

28

Alternative Therapies

A perspective on herbal remedies

Q. Your frequent dismissal of herbal therapy is a sad testimonial. I think you do a great disservice to your readers and physicians who, in the spirit of true medicine, are open to herbal treatments. So much more healing could be accomplished if practitioners of Western medicine were willing to embrace all avenues to better health.

A. Although many people endorse nontraditional treatments, herbal therapy really has no place in the modern treatment of serious diseases.

Scientists are actively investigating herbal remedies (and have found some that appear to be somewhat effective; see sidebar). In the main, however, most are not useful. As I have repeatedly written, there is a major problem with the purity of these preparations and the accuracy of the dosage. For example, some Asian anti-arthritis herbal remedies actually contain cortisone drugs, but this fact is not listed on the label, as it should be. And many herbals contain far more (or significantly fewer) active ingredients than the labels testify, so there is clearly no quality control in their manufacture.

My position is this: be cautious. This is not to say that it's impossible that undiscovered herbs may hold promise, but—to date—herbal therapy for serious diseases is not appropriate. As you know, many miraculous drugs have an herbal basis, most notably digitalis (from foxglove) and morphine (from the opium poppy). And, I am certain, we will see great strides made in purifying useful drugs from natural sources in the future. However, most experts doubt that people's health will improve as a result of herbal therapy, which—in numerous instances—can be harmful or downright poisonous. For instance, comfrey, germander, willow bark and ma huang have been reported to cause life-threatening side effects.

Rather than relying on herbs, patients with symptoms should be examined by their doctors.

Herbal remedies aren't proven but seem to be helpful to some

Q. When I read your columns, I am often curious why medical doctors fail to mention herbal treatments. I've been taking an herbal remedy for the symptoms of menopause, and am well-satisfied. After the first week, my night sweats and hot flashes disappeared. Please don't downplay phytoestrogens.

A. OK, I won't. The reason that herbal remedies are not generally recommended by the medical profession is that the compounds are usually ineffective and many have major problems in purity and quality, according to medical authorities. Most women pass through menopause relatively uneventfully, except for moodiness and hot flashes.

For those women who suffer more severe symptoms such as heavy bleeding, hormone replacement therapy, prescribed by a physician, is more appropriate.

However, as I have stated before, you can't argue with success.

Therefore, if phytoestrogens have helped you, all well and good. Continue with the therapy. I have no information that the practice could be harmful.

Herbals not good cancer therapy

Q. My father has stomach cancer that has not responded to surgery or chemotherapy (which made him sick). I want him to try herbal supplements. Could they hurt him?

A. Probably not—but they won't do much good either. I suggest that you pose this question to your father's oncologist. Speaking bluntly, it seems to me your father has advanced cancer that, at this point, is untreatable by conventional means. So, what harm is there in turning to alternative medical options? But before taking this action, you should run it by the cancer specialist, who may have other, more effective options.

Herbal Remedies—
the Good and the Bad

Herbal remedies are the fastest growing diet supplement in the United Sates, reaching almost $4 billion in annual sales. Gingko, St. John's Wort, and ginseng are the top sellers.

There is a significant and dangerous interaction between herbals and traditional medications, of which every consumer must be aware.

Gingko is the oldest living tree species and dates back about 230 million years, even surviving atomic blasts at Hiroshima and Nagasaki. No wonder it enjoys a rich heritage of medicinal usage.

Gingko extract is marketed primarily for vascular insufficiency. Studies have shown that it increases the utilization of oxygen and glucose by the brain and encourage improved circulation. Also, it may stabilize or improve cognitive brain function in patients with dementia, including Alzheimer's disease. Finally, it may be effective in treating depression and impotence.

The usual dose of gingko biloba is 120 to 160 milligrams a day; up to 240 mg have been used. More than six weeks may pass before the drug produces results. Side effects include low blood sugar, headache and palpitations. Because gingko affects the blood's "stickiness," it must be used very cautiously in patents who simultaneously take aspirin, Coumadin or heparin; moreover, the remedy should be stopped at least a week before elective surgery.

Finally, gingko may have inhibitory effects on the liver's cytochrome P450 enzyme system leading to the possibility of toxicity from other, prescription drugs that are metabolized by the same pathway.

St. John's Wort was used in the past to ward off evil spirits. Now it is achieving international recognition in beating depression, a very modern evil spirit.

The remedy contains at least 10 pharmacologically active constituents, some of which are identical to the ingredients in prescription antidepressants. In short, St. John's Wort inhibits serotonin uptake in the brain, making it at least as effective as standard prescription medicines for treating depression.

The usual daily dosage is 900 milligrams; the remedy may take up to 12 weeks before it produces effects.

Like gingko biloba, St. John's Wort affects the cytochrome P450 liver-enzyme system, resulting in serious drug interactions with many pharmaceuticals, including antidepressants, protease inhibitors (in AIDS patients), cyclosporine (for organ-transplant patients), digoxin—even birth control pills. In fact, the potential danger of combining St. John's Wort with prescription antidepressants is so significant that authorities insist that such dosing be avoided or undertaken by an experienced practitioner.

Ginseng has been part of traditional Chinese culture for more than 2,000 years. Interestingly, almost the entire crop of American ginseng is now exported to China.

The herb has several effects, including the ability to increase energy, help cope with stress, enhance intellectual performance, improve the immune system and reduce blood sugar levels. It can also delay clotting and, therefore, should be discontinued at least a week before any surgical procedure. Side effects include nervousness, insomnia, headache, and hypertension—so it should not be used in patients with chronic anxiety or bipolar mood disorder. Ginseng is not substantially metabolized by the cytochrome P450 system, so drug interactions are rare.

The major safety concern with the product—indeed, with all herbal remedies—is consistency. Because these compounds are not subject to Food and Drug Administration supervision, the concentration of ingredients can vary widely from batch to batch, as much as 36-fold with ginseng capsules and liquid. This means that consumers may be markedly under-dosed with some pills but dangerously overdosed by others.

Garlic has been used as a medication for more than 5,000 years. This remedy is experiencing a resurgence. The supplement may be effective in lowering blood cholesterol and triglyceride levels, reducing high blood pressure, improving arterial elasticity, fighting inflammation and protecting against cancers of the colon, stomach and prostate gland. Topical garlic cream may kill fungus infections of the skin.

Because garlic also prolongs blood clotting, patients taking anticoagulant medication, such as Coumadin, must be closely monitored. Garlic can also interfere with certain medications.

Although the herb is ordinarily free of side effects, large doses can lead to stomach upset, rash and—in rare instances—allergic shock. As a general rule, any garlic preparation that is odorless is probably worthless.

Echinacea is an herb contained in the common North American wildflower called the purple coneflower. The supplement has been shown to reduce the inflammatory response, much as cortisone does, as well as to fortify the immune system. Although it does not prevent colds and upper respiratory infections, echinacea may limit the severity and duration of these common ailments. It may also be useful in treating urinary infections and vaginal yeast infections.

The usual dosage is 300 milligrams three times a day. Side effects are unusual and consist primarily of allergic reactions; hence, people who are sensitive to plants and flowers (ragweed, daisies and so forth) should avoid echinacea.

Saw palmetto: Extract from these berries appears to be effective therapy for prostatic enlargement. In fact, it may be as effective as the prescription drug Proscar.

Saw palmetto rarely causes side effects (at a dose of 160 mg twice daily), but occasionally may be associated with nausea, vomiting, diarrhea or constipation.

Grape seed extract: The effective ingredients are procyanidolic oligomers (PCOs), which are also found in cranberries, blueberries, black currants, green and black teas and red wine.

PCOs act as antioxidants; they scavenge so-called "free radicals," products of metabolism that are associated with vascular diseases and ill health. Thus, grape seed extract (an inexpensive source of PCOs) is often helpful in treating venous insufficiency, capillary fragility, diabetic retinopathy and macular degeneration. PCOs may also improve night vision in heathy people.

For standard antioxidant support, the usual dose is 50 mg a day. However, when used for specific therapeutic purposes, the dose of grape seed extract is increased to 150 to 300 mg a day. No adverse reactions have been reported.

Kava: Used for centuries in the South Pacific islands, this herb has several effects, not all of them beneficial. It relaxes muscles, reduces pain, prevents seizures, lessens anxiety and the symptoms of early menopause and helps insomniacs to sleep.

Unfortunately, there is the very real potential for serious liver injury. This side effect has been reported so often that the Food and Drug Administration recently issued a warning to health care professionals advising them to inform their patients of the risks and to report any kava-induced liver injury. The FDA does not recommend the use of kava and lists the following label-names of the product: Ava, Ava pepper, Awa, kava root, Kava-Kava, Kawa, Kavapepper, Kawa-Kawa, Kew, Sakau, Wurselstock, and Yangona.

Evening Primrose: The ninth bestselling herbal preparation is believed by some patients to be an effective antidote for premenstrual syndrome and cyclic breast pain. In addition, evening primrose oil has shown promise in reducing the signs and symptoms of rheumatoid arthritis and may help treat diabetic neuropathy.

Some studies have shown a beneficial effect on attention deficit disorder.

The usual dosage ranges from 540 mg to 6 grams a day. Evening primrose should be taken with food to enhance absorption; benefits may not be seen for several months. Adverse reactions include nausea, indigestion, abdominal cramps and diarrhea. The supplement is contraindicated in patients who are pregnant, have a seizure disorder or suffer from schizophrenia.

Aristolochic acid: Widely present in many Chinese herbal preparations for weight loss, this compound has caused kidney failure in more than 100 women. It is known to be nephrotoxic (damaging to kidneys) and is also associated with urinary tract cancers. Despite these dangers, the FDA has no authority to ban the product, which continues to be detected in botanical products exported to the United States.

Goldenseal: This is now an endangered species because its popularity as an herbal antibiotic led to overharvesting. It is now cultivated as a cash crop in the state of Washington.

While it is true that extracts from the plant do have documented antibacterial properties, most authorities believe that goldenseal is so poorly absorbed form the gastrointestinal tract that it could never reach therapeutic levels in humans. The herb has, however, been shown to be effective in treating infections with giardia, an intestinal parasite, and throat inflammation (probably because of direct contact with the sites of infection).

It does not effectively prevent or treat colds, despite extensive marketing campaigns to the contrary; nor does it mask the presence of illegal or controlled substances in the urine.

The usual dosage is 250 to 500 milligrams three times a day; goldenseal can also be made into a tea.

Side effects, although uncommon, include hallucinations, irritability, stimulation, and—in rare cases—heart toxicity. In addition, the remedy may interfere with the cytochrome P450 liver enzyme system that usually degrades many prescription drugs. Thus, goldenseal could, at least in theory, set the stage for significant drug toxicity.

Finally, because goldenseal products are costly, they have been adulterated with other compounds, so the consumer may not be getting what he is paying for.

Cranberry: Along with the blueberry and the Concord grape, the cranberry can honestly claim a North American heritage, stretching back for centuries. Native Americans used the fruit for food and dyes, as well as for treatment of arrow wounds.

Modern scientific studies have confirmed that cranberry juice is effective in preventing and treating urinary infections in both men and women. It also may help patients with peptic ulcer, control gum disease, lower blood cholesterol levels, and—in some cases—improve the outcome of certain cancers.

There is no uniform dosage, but excess consumption may lead to acid stomach, diarrhea and kidney stones.

Valerian: Medically, the root stock of this plant has been used as a sedative, sleep aid, pain reliever and antioxidant product. It has been a popular herbal remedy for at least five centuries.

Its successes are apparently the result of several oils contained in the plant. Medial studies have clearly shown that valerian, when taken on a regular basis, is an effective sleep aid, without the "hangover" effects of grogginess and poor concentration that may accompany prescription sleeping pills.

The usual dose is 2 to 3 grams of dried herb made into a tea and taken about an hour before bedtime.

Although valerian appears to be safe, rare cases of liver toxicity have been reported. The product, like so many others, affects the cytochrome P450 system; thus, drug interactions are potential hazards. Patients taking valerian should avoid driving or operating heavy machinery for a few hours after ingestion.

Herbal remedies appear to be gaining popularity for treating a multitude of disorders. However, caution is still appropriate. Many countries, notably Germany, have laws regulating the purity of botanical supplements; such compounds are considered similar to prescription drugs. Not so in the United States, where such supplements are neither tested (for constituents, safety, or efficiency) nor monitored. Consequently, there is a distressing absence of standardization. What you think you're getting may be more, less or different from what you are truly getting.

If I were to define the reluctance most physicians have in recommending herbal products, it would be precisely this: There is no quality control whatsoever. Foreign companies that compound and export these products can—literally—put anything they choose on the labels—or, worse, add ingredients, such as cortisone, without informing the purchaser.

Most doctors, whose patients take herbal supplements, would welcome American companies into this market and would rejoice if there were a strict consistency in the products' ingredients. Until then, buyer beware.

Herbals are ineffective breast-enhancers

Q. After having had three babies in a relatively short period of time, my body has been "out of sorts." In particular, my breasts are small and saggy. I've been considering breast enhancement with herbal pills. This seems a lot easier than undergoing breast implants and, I guess, because the therapy is "herbal," it must be safe. What do you think?

A. Taking a pill to enhance breast size is a seductive concept. But it doesn't work. This technique, although aggressively advertised, is useless. Moreover, the label "herbal" on a product is neither a guarantee of safety nor of effectiveness. As you know, herbal remedies are not considered by the Food and Drug Administration to be medicines; they are "dietary supplements." As a result, such compounds are not certified for purity, consistency of ingredients or supposed benefits. As I have repeatedly stated, such remedies should be taken with a tablespoon of skepticism, if at all.

While I have vowed to keep my readers informed of new information—both pro and con—about herbals, breast augmentation pills have yet to achieve any degree of scientific validation. Save your money.

Also, I urge you to rethink your concern about breast size. Many slim women discover, to their dismay, after pregnancies, that their breasts have unavoidably become smaller and more lax. This is a normal consequence of childbearing. If you feel comfortable with yourself as a wife and mother, you can confidently ignore breast changes. No one in his or her right mind expects young mothers to have the idealized shape promulgated by the aggressive and unrealistic advertising that is so popular in our culture. These ads customarily show nubile, young ladies with "perfect" figures—an unobtainable goal for women whose orientation has changed from catching a man to assuming the responsibilities and accepting the consequences of motherhood.

On the other hand, if for whatever reason you truly need larger and perkier breasts, plastic surgery is the logical solution. This is really a very personal decision. But, in any case, herbal pills are not the answer.

Glucosamine/chondroitin to relieve muscle soreness?

Q. After 20 years of working on my feet, the muscles in my legs have begun to hurt. Over-the-counter meds don't help much. My friends tell me to try glucosamine/chondroitin. What are your thoughts?

A. This health food product is marketed to help rejuvenate age-related joint disorders and, in some cases, it appears to help. However, it is not appropriate therapy for muscle ailments.

I suggest that you discuss this with your family physician, because you could have an affliction, such as Lyme disease or polymyalgia, that should be treated with more conventional therapy. Also, recent reports have confirmed that the purity and consistency of the product varies considerably.

L-carnitine not effective but not harmful

Q. I've read that 250 to 500 milligrams per day of carnitine will improve heart muscle function, lower body weight and cholesterol level. I dropped 15 pounds in two months and lowered my cholesterol level in one month. Does it really work, or am I being misled?

A. Don't believe everything you read; examine the source. I believe you have been misled by claims about L-carnitine, a substance necessary for the transport of certain fats to the cells. Carnitine is widely distributed in most animal foods, such as red meat and dairy products.

Moreover, humans are capable of manufacturing all the carnitine they require; therefore, deficiencies do not occur, except in newborn infants, who cannot make enough and who should be breast-fed. (Many infant formulas do not contain carnitine.)

No benefits have been identified from carnitine supplements, and no toxicity has been reported.

I suspect that your weight and cholesterol level dropped because you have been eating fewer calories and less fat. Since you are benefiting from your diet (and extra carnitine will not harm you), I suggest you continue your present program.

Iron therapy should not be routine

Q. Because I feel run-down, I talked my doctor into giving me a prescription for iron pills. When I checked with the pharmacist, he told me to pick the exact same thing over-the-counter at half the price. Besides paying the doctor $85 for an office call, I have found that many times I can get the same medicine more cheaply over-the-counter. Any comments?

A. Iron, a mineral necessary for the normal production of red blood cells, may be dangerous. Excess quantities can cause liver and heart disorders. Also, some people suffer from inherited iron-storage disease, which they may not know they have. Iron supplements can be highly toxic in such individuals. Therefore, folks should not take extra iron unless there is a bona fide medical reason, such as iron deficiency anemia, for doing so.

Consequently, I discourage patients from self-medicating with over-the-counter iron remedies. Many people who feel run-down and tired may choose to take iron pills. This can lead to health problems if iron deficiency is not the cause of the symptoms.

I hope the $85 you paid your physician included a blood test for anemia. If not, you were ripped off by the doctor, who should know better than to prescribe a potentially hazardous substance without first testing you.

Having said this, I admit that I will, on occasion, suggest a patient use iron without formal testing. For example, if a woman with excessive menstruation calls me to complain that she recently had a exceptionally heavy period and feels dragged out, I'm likely to order iron supplements to replace the mineral she lost from her bleeding. However, such a situation is the exception, not the rule.

Finally, I'd like to add that medicines purchased without a prescription are every bit as good—although not usually as strong—as their prescription counterparts. So, if your doctor recommends a certain remedy that you can obtain more cheaply over-the-counter, fine. The important consideration is that you and the physician are working as a team: He or she suggests a medicine and you obtain it at the best price you can, providing it meets the quality and type that was prescribed.

Obviously, this is a far cry from the person who abhors medical attention, preferring instead to purchase one drug after another, smorgasbord-style, in an attempt to solve a perceived problem. In essence, this constitutes practicing medicine (on one's self) without a license— not a good arrangement.

Alternative therapy for diabetes: not effective

Q. Will lecithin and chromium lower the blood sugar level in a diabetic?

A. No. The high blood sugar that characterizes diabetes can be lowered only by one or all of the following methods: strict dieting, weight loss (for obese patients), exercise, oral medication or insulin injections (for severe diabetes).

Lecithin is not classified as a vitamin, despite the claims of the health food industry. The body can manufacture it. High doses of supplemental lecithin have not been shown to possess health benefits.

Although chromium (a trace mineral needed to maintain normal blood sugar levels in conjunction with insulin) is essential for metabolism, it is plentiful in most foods, including meat, cheese, grains, eggs and fresh fruit.

Therefore, chromium supplements are not required. The recommended dietary allowance is 50-200 micrograms, an amount readily available in a well-balanced diet. Chromium poisoning occurs at doses above 50 milligrams a day and causes liver and kidney damage.

Vicks VapoRub for toenail fungus

Q. I'd like to share a simple and inexpensive method to cure toenail fungus.

I was told that Vicks VapoRub spread on the affected nail twice a day (for several months) would cure the condition. Of course, I was skeptical—until I learned that a prescription drug to cure the problem would cost $800. So I gave it a shot. Within a month, I noticed the fungus disappearing, replaced by healthy nail tissue. I was so impressed that I urge my husband to try it. (He chose the generic equivalent, which is cheaper.) He had the same success. Please pass this on to your readers. My family doctor had never heard of this treatment, and a podiatrist dismissed the technique with the comment: "It won't work." Well, I'm here to say it does work, and I am at a loss to explain why medical professionals are not familiar with it. What do you think?

A. This is a revelation to me, as it must be to many practitioners. However, as I have stated before, you can't argue with success, especially if the cure is as safe and inexpensive as generic VapoRub.

If I know my readers at all, some of them will try your stunning therapy and report back to me about success—or failure. I'll publish a follow-up after I hear from them. Thanks for writing about an antidote to a universal and annoying problem.

More on Vicks for nail fungus

Q. When I read of your twice-daily application of Vicks VapoRub for toenail fungus, I thought it was another myth. But, because the cost was so reasonable, I gave it a try.

I am now halfway through a jar of Vicks. Initially, after two weeks of treatment, I noted definite improvement. One nail that was thick and partially separated from the nail bed is growing out firm and clear. The effects of Vicks are astonishing and I can eagerly endorse the therapy based on my personal experience.

Is there more than one type of toenail fungus? My doctor says that pills are the only answer and that topical products are useless.

A. I suppose that there are different types of fungus that can attack the nails, but this is not the important issue. The key element is to reduce the infected portions of nail as much as possible, by trimming, clipping or filing the yellow, thickened nail and removing as much of the fungal debris under the nail as you can. Then, as the nail grows out, continue to trim away the affected portion.

While the Vicks treatment takes months to be effective, it is cheap and easy—certainly safer than expensive prescription pills that can cause liver damage and other consequences.

When a reader first wrote me about this remedy, I—like you—thought it was another myth, but I tried it anyway, with astounding success. Doctors almost never experiment on themselves by using the medications they prescribe for patients. So here is an example of an old gaffer who did. It worked for me, and—judging by the positive mail I have received—it works for others as well. Remember the key element: clean away the nail. And be patient.

Nicotine patch effective for Parkinson's disease

Q. I was intrigued by your column about the benefits of nicotine in patients with Parkinson' disease. Where did you find this information?

A. In the Sept. 23, 2000, print edition of *The Economist.* The article describes the benefits of the nicotine patch in alleviating the symptoms of Parkinson's disease, Alzheimer's disease and Tourette's syndrome. The effect is so striking that at least one drug company (Abbott Laboratories) has begun trials with a similar compound called ABT-418. Doctors hope that future research will lead to an antidote for these diseases. In the meantime, the nicotine patch, which is available without a prescription, appears to be a reasonable substitute.

Melatonin sets sleep clock

Q. What is your opinion of melatonin as a sleep aid? I frequently travel on business across several time zones and have difficulty adapting my sleep habits. Would melatonin help? Is it safe?

A. The human sleep cycle, a form of biological clock, is largely governed by the interaction between light and naturally produced melatonin (formed in the brain). At times when melatonin levels are high, we sleep; once the melatonin is reduced (by exposure to light), we awaken.

This substance, which is classed as a dietary supplement and does not require a prescription, is safe and available in pill form.

Although melatonin is not consistently effective as a sleep aid in the general population, it is exceedingly useful for pilots, travelers and other people who must frequently adapt their sleeping habits to changes in time zones. I suggest that you try the product, according to the manufacturer's directions, on your next business trip. The melatonin should reset your biological clock and enable you to overcome your problem of insomnia.

Magnetic therapy does not relieve pain

Q. I put magnets on my neck for pain. If I don't apply them to my toes, my feet swell up and get numb. Should I seek medical attention?

A. Only if you're willing to accept the doctor's view that magnetic therapy has not been shown in a single reputable medical study to provide any health benefit at all.

I suggest that you involve your family doctor in making a decision about how best to approach your problems of neck pain and swollen feet. From your very brief description, I assume that you have neck pain that could be secondary to arthritis and foot swelling that is caused by fluid retention. Are we dealing here with benign osteoarthritis, or should chronic heart failure (a cause of ankle swelling) also be considered? Your doctor can sort out these issues.

Home remedy for chapped hands

Q. What can I do to treat the constant cracking of the of the skin on my hands? Is there some way I can prevent this?

A. When the skin on the hands dries out, as is likely to happen in winter, painful cracks can appear. These lesions can be quite deep and difficult to treat. The problem is worsened by hand washing, which further removes natural skin oils.

I suggest that you try using a hand cream regularly. There are several effective brands, especially those containing lanolin, a natural lubricant.

As an alternative, many consumers swear by an old, country remedy called Bag Balm. I have been told that applying the product liberally and leaving it on for several hours (for example, at bedtime) and covering the hands with gloves (fabric, not plastic) to protect bed linens, may notably improve the situation. The product is available in most agricultural supply stores, such as Agway, and in some pharmacies.

'Home, home on the range' approach to various conditions

Q. I read your column on athlete's foot. I, too, suffered this while growing up, and my mother treated it by having me stand barefooted in fresh cow manure. I know this sounds pretty farfetched, but it really works. Maybe your readers can find relief this way.

A. Thank you for your suggestion—I think. I don't know how many of the urban and suburban public would be willing to try your remedy. Perhaps more than I predict. From your brief description, however, I wonder if there might not be some distressing social consequences of standing in cow manure. But that could be a topic for a future essay.

By the way, what on earth do you do while standing in cow manure? Look around and wonder about who's watching you? Meditate about what you did wrong to deserve this? Memorize the Gettysburg address? Make a mental list of all the demagogues and dictators actively supported by the U.S. government?

Also do you have to stand in the stuff for it to be effective? Why can't you sit down and wiggle your toes in it? If so, what would be the most appropriate reading material to pass a few glorious minutes while you perch on a stool with your feet ankle-deep in cow plop? All this for a 10-cent case of athlete's foot? What about jock itch? I could go on, but I won't. Let me shift gears.

I knew I would be in for some interesting mail when, several months ago, at the conclusion of answering a reader's question about using the veterinary skin ointment Bag Balm on chapped human hands, I requested information about the use of other veterinary products on people. I was deluged with letters. Therefore, I'll take some time now to share with you some of the responses I received.

Several readers mentioned how effective hoof hardener is for brittle nails. "Straight Arrow" was a popular brand. It costs about $8 for a 2-pound can. This is a deal, folks.

Hoofsaver (probably related to the above compound) was touted as a great cure for rough heels. When massaged into toenails and dry, cracked skin of the feet, the product produces astounding results.

Phillip's Corona Ointment, which supposedly has multiple uses on the farm, cures diaper rash and, some readers claim, any kind of chronic skin irritation caused by urine or perspiration.

Clean kerosene works as an antiseptic for cuts and abrasions.

OrthoSoap, which is used to wash livestock, comes in gallon jugs. It's great for laundering sweaters and makes an efficient, inexpensive shampoo. (Don't ask me to verify this; I'm merely passing on information.) According to one reader, OrthoSoap is often used in commercial dry-cleaning establishments to hand wash delicate fabrics.

My favorite response came from a horse-breeding family in Colorado. I guess some horses are worth more than humans, in dollar amounts. Therefore, horses have a whole line of cosmetics that are believed to be a effective as products for humans at a fraction of the cost. Shampoos and hair conditioners are, it seems, as appropriate for a woman's mane as for the pampered thoroughbred. In fact, out West, some beauty parlors are using equine cosmetics. "Soft and Silky," "Mane Tamer" and "Silk Shine" are popular items that can be purchased by the case for far less than the familiar human equivalents. The horse breeders concluded that these products "don't make a stallion a better sire, a mare a better brood, or a gelding any better a riding horse." But they look better, and who knows what marvelous repercussions could befall a woman with the horse sense to shop from veterinary salesmen, rather than pay the department store markup?

Finally, Bag Balm really does cure chapped, raw, cracked skin. After all, generations of cows swear by it.

Mexican cancer clinic a success?

Q. While I regularly read your column and generally agree with what you say, you badly stubbed your toes when you recently criticized Mexican cancer clinics.

I'm a retired engineer who was diagnosed with metastatic cancer 18 years ago. I refused chemotherapy, radiation and surgery because I didn't want to feel sicker than I already was. Instead, I signed into a Mexican cancer clinic, where I underwent concentrated therapy, including diet modification. (My local oncologist had said: "You might as well go to Disneyland as to think diet will help with cancer.")

Now, 18 years later, I am happy and healthy. No sign of cancer. Before you pan alternative therapies, you ought to check out whether some are truly useful. Mine was.

A. While I am delighted to hear of your victory over cancer, I am not as quick as you are to give credit. As I've written many times before, there are documented cases of "spontaneous cure" from almost any disease, cancer included.

Although it's tempting to credit your Mexican doctors with such a stunning success, something else may have been going on. This is the reason well-controlled, scientific experiments are such a vital part of medical progress. Testimonials just don't cut it, I'm afraid.

If the Mexican clinic is really on to something—and they may well be—they owe it to the medical community to publish their findings and methods. Only then can their approach be fairly and impartially judged by their peers.

Such a breakthrough in cancer therapy is the dream of every research scientist. Why, then, don't the Mexican doctors publicize their techniques so that humanity as a whole can benefit? Or do they prefer to rake in the tourist dollars, rather than being "up front" about joining the battle against cancer?

Cayenne pepper for hypertension?

Q. For more than two years, I've been on prescription medicine for hypertension with fair results: I averaged about 150/90. Recently, I read about cayenne pepper as alternative therapy. I tried it. Within two weeks, my BP was 140/80. What is your opinion about this therapy?

A. I have no experience with cayenne pepper for hypertension, but I am impressed with your success. A blood pressure of 150/90 is, indeed, too high. The fact that you seem to have brought it down by using cayenne is noteworthy.

As a general rule, herbal remedies are not particularly effective in lowering blood pressure; prescription drugs are superior. I advise you to bring your observations to your doctor's attention. He should carefully monitor the situation.

Having said this, I want to emphasize that many hypertensives can achieve enormous benefit (without expensive drugs) simply by modifying their lifestyle. For example, exercise, meditation, stress counseling, salt restriction, weight loss, reduction in alcohol consumption and calcium supplements are valuable non-drug therapies for lowering blood pressure. If the cayenne works for you (and is approved by your physician), I see no reason you shouldn't continue to take it. But also pay attention to the "natural" remedies that I mentioned.

Oxygen offers remedy for leg sores

Q. As a nurse working with elderly patients, I've been pleased to see how often you address the issue of stasis ulcers (leg sores), using both traditional treatment as well as new and innovative therapy. Let me tell you my own secret: oxygen. This simple remedy really works.

Secure a plastic bag in place (top and bottom) over the ulcer. Then, through a small hole, infuse oxygen for about 15 minutes a day. Within a short period, no more ulcer!

I've tried this technique many times over the years, always with success. Doctors are not familiar with it but this doesn't surprise me; they never listen to nurses anyway, even though we are with patients for many more hours than they are.

A. OK, I'm listening. More important, I'm publishing this as a tip to patients and practitioners alike. The method makes sense, because stasis ulcers are the result of too little oxygen reaching the skin, which eventually breaks down and ulcerates. Therefore, treatment with local, high-concentration oxygen—a cheap and easy alternative to other therapies—is appropriate. Thank you for writing, nurse.

Vitamin C therapy has its limits

Q. You should do more research before you give out false information about vitamine c it has been proven over 50 years ago that all animals except humans, ape family, guinea pigs all produce their own vitamine c. there is no over dose except diarrhea when a large amount is taken with out working up to it. it is very necessary to keep the arteries clean and strong and will prevent all the by pass surgery that is going on at this time and would cut death from heart attacks by at least 90 percent at least 5 to 6 grams are required to do this I know a lot of Drs. Taking 15,000 to 20,000 mg per day check it out hope you can be truthful about this

A. First of all, I am publishing your letter exactly in the form that I received it. Let me say that I don't pay much attention to letters that are incoherent, poorly written and defy the rules of English grammar, spelling and punctuation. I'm not sure which of the species of non-ascorbic acid producers you are in, but your conclusions about megavitamin therapy with C are incorrect.

It has not been proved to reduce arteriosclerotic plague, lower serum cholesterol or keep arteries healthy. Although relatively safe in large doses, vitamin C has been reported to cause diarrhea, interference with pregnancy, alteration of copper metabolism, increased iron absorption, kidney stones, damage to tooth enamel, and diminished resistance to bacterial infections.

If you are broad-minded enough to want further information, I suggest the following two resources.

—*Vitamins and Minerals: Help or Harm* by Charles Marshall, Ph.D. (Lippincott Williams & Wilkins Publishers)

—*Popular Nutritional Practices* by Jack Yetiv, M.D., Ph.D. (Popular Medicine Press)

Bee pollen is for the bees

Q. Within four hours of taking one tablespoon of liquid bee pollen, I experienced increased energy and mental alertness. With regular use, over several weeks, I noticed fewer incidents of illness, a feeling of well-being and improved sexual enjoyment. Unfortunately, I have had to stop buying bee pollen because of the cost. My health insurance will not cover it, even though it improved my life tremendously.

You claimed that no "reputable" scientific studies have confirmed the benefit of bee pollen. I would wager, however, that you considered only medical field studies. Sadly, the medical profession avoids studying the health benefits of herbs and other alternative therapies.

Please use your column to disseminate sensible information. Don't just spout scare tactics to keep people dependent on unnecessary pharmaceutical drugs that can only be prescribed by you and your buddies.

A. To quote Yogi Berra, this is deja vu all over again.

If a pharmaceutical company, through research and development, discovers a new drug, the compound must undergo a rigorous set of studies to prove its effectiveness and to define its dangers and side effects. Why, then, are not the manufacturers of herbal remedies held to the same high standards? Because such products are usually classified as dietary supplements, not medications. This playing field is not level. Bee pollen—along with aromatherapy, homeopathy, reflexology, and other unproved alternative treatments—is not dangerous, but is nonetheless ineffective. When manufacturers of bee pollen rigorously test the product in a valid, double blind study and can prove that the pollen is associated with clear-cut health benefits, I'll change my tune, support the claims and publish an update for my readers. Until then, reader, I'll continue to advise against using bee pollen for any reason other than pollinating plants. This issue has nothing to do whatsoever with scare tactics or my buddies.

Your "improvement" from taking been pollen is probably a placebo effect. As many as 20 percent of people will note substantial benefits when given an inactive substance if they believe the substance is beneficial.

I try to offer sensible advice in this column. And nothing seems more sensible to me than urging people not to waste their hard-earned money on alternative therapy scams, the sole purpose of which is to separate the sucker from his buck.

Hydrogen peroxide ear-cleaning is harmless

Q. I read in your column that using hydrogen peroxide is a way of cleaning the ears of wax. So I tried it. It works, but has side effects. Within a week I suffered from a painful ear infection. Now I've wised up: It's better to put up with the wax than to have an infection. Please notify your readers of this.

A. The human ear canal is composed of three portions: the external ear canal, the middle ear (which contains the mechanism of hearing) and the inner ear (that houses the organ of balance and other nerves).

The external ear canal, which produces cerumen ("wax"), is separated from the middle ear chamber by the tympanic membrane ("eardrum"). Therefore, it is virtually impossible for infection in one region to spread to the other; cleaning out cerumen ordinarily does not affect the middle ear—although the process can, of course, irritate the tympanic membrane.

Putting a half a capful of peroxide into the ear canal will not infect the middle ear (unless there is a hole in the eardrum). Middle ear infections are caused by microorganisms that enter the chamber from internal sources, through the Eustachian tube (the vent that pops during pressure changes, such as those connected with flying or underwater diving).

I believe that your peroxide therapy bore no relation whatsoever to your middle ear infection. Ordinarily, such therapy is totally devoid of complications and side effects. Nonetheless, to be on the safe side, you should run this by your family physician who should, at the very least, check you for a perforated eardrum.

Is honey useful treatment for burns?

Q. Two years ago, I fell against a hot wood stove, severely burning my forearm. I immediately applied honey to the burn, with the result of fast healing, no pain or scarring. I've also treated skin ulcers this way. Is there something to these findings?

A. If it works for you, there must be something to it—although I must admit it sounds pretty far out. Burns are uncomfortable because sensitive nerve endings are damaged; the pain my be worsened by exposure to air. This is the reason doctors usually recommend that blisters be kept unbroken; the lymph fluid in a blister protects the sensitive tissue beneath until healing has had a chance to get started.

I suppose that a coating of honey might similarly insulate a burned area. In addition, the high content of sugar in honey could, I imagine, effectively diminish bacterial growth, thereby protecting a wound or burn from infection.

As you may have guessed, my conjectures about your sticky problem have no scientific basis. But I'm trying. Valiantly. For all I know, honey may be superb therapy for burns and skin ulcers in primitive cultures; it isn't in ours. Perhaps this is a topic that should be addressed. We could certainly learn a great deal from other civilizations, both old and new.

I recommend a book *Native Harvests* by Barrie Kavasch (Vintage) that describes recipes and botanicals of the American Indian. In particular, the section on wild medicines is fascinating. Numerous Indian tribes used clovers, comfrey, valerian and yarrow in soothing salves to treat burns. I do not know whether honey made from the flowers of these plants might contain medicinal remedies, but such a possibility exists. The Native American culture, at the time of the European invasion, was a proud, efficient, multi-tribal, successful and honorable conglomeration of nations. Even after we whites treated them so abominably, they may still offer us some traditional cures. Check out the book.

Lecithin for high cholesterol?

Q. Will lecithin help the cholesterol in one's blood? Some people claim it brings the count down.

A. Unfortunately, there are no valid scientific studies supporting the claim that lecithin lowers serum cholesterol. Lecithin and cholesterol often coexist naturally. However, the only effective ways of lowering blood cholesterol are to reduce dietary fat and, in some instances, to use medication to reduce intestinal absorption of cholesterol.

Soundwaves to relax muscles

Q. Is ultrasound safe to use in treating muscle spasm? Under what conditions, if any, might such treatment be harmful?

A. Ultrasound consists of the administration of high-frequency soundwaves to tissues. If the bounce-back is recorded, a sonogram picture can be obtained. This test is particularly useful in the evaluation of pregnancy, cysts and gallstones. When the soundwaves are beamed into a spastic muscle (and no bounce-back is recorded), the ultrasound may produce muscle relaxation. Therefore, the technique is a useful adjunct to other methods used by physiotherapists.

I cannot think of an instance in which properly applied ultrasound physiotherapy would be harmful. If, after a reasonable length of time, there is no improvement, the practitioner would presumably investigate other methods of treatment.

Cornstarch safe replacement for talcum powder

Q. I use cornstarch as a dusting powder and have been very pleased with the results. Now I am concerned about whether inhalation of pure cornstarch can cause an accumulation in the lungs like coal dust or asbestos particles. Since it is corn-based, can it be absorbed by the body and disposed of as waste?

A. Cornstarch is a digestible substance, unlike asbestos, silica and talc. Therefore, it will not cause lung damage or respiratory disorders when used appropriately as a dusting powder.

Obviously, as with any inhaled vapor or dust, you should minimize your exposure (by not breathing in excessive quantities of cornstarch). However, when used prudently, this product is safe and, as you've discovered, quite effective as talcum powder.

Garlic has health benefits

Q. Does garlic have any health benefits?
A. Yes, it does.

Garlic, an herb known for more than 5,000 years, was believed by the ancients to have healing powers. In many societies, garlic was used to treat infections, cough, poisoning, snakebite, poor digestion and circulatory problems.

Spurred on by anecdotal reports of the benefits of garlic in preventing heart attacks (in many countries, notably Italy), modern scientists have conducted studies to determine if the herb possesses health benefits. The findings confirm that, indeed, garlic has two major attributes: reduction of serum cholesterol and prolongation of blood coagulation.

The active ingredients in garlic are unstable sulfur compounds, mainly alliin, which are odorless and tasteless. When fresh garlic is crushed, alliin is converted to allicin by the action of the plant enzyme allinase. The resulting substance is pungent and highly reactive, but decays in about 48 hours into disulfide and sulfunic acids, the primary constituents of garlic oil.

> 66 *Unfortunately, there are no valid scientific studies supporting the claim that lecithin lowers serum cholesterol.* 99

Dried garlic powder contains both the oily sulfides and unconverted alliin. This product is considered to have medicinal properties equal to those of fresh garlic, without the odor. Dried garlic pills are the most popular over-the-counter remedy in Germany; they are rapidly becoming used worldwide. Most studies on garlic have used the dried powder.

European investigators have discovered that this substance lowers serum cholesterol levels by as much as 12 percent; the higher the level, the greater the reduction. In addition, elevated serum levels of triglycerides (the other major blood fat) can be reduced by more than 15 percent. While these effects are not as significant as the reductions produced by prescription drugs, such as Lipitor and Zocor, the fact that any reduction occurred at all is intriguing.

Further studies have documented that garlic has a significant anti-platelet function. By preventing these tiny blood cells from sticking together, garlic acts to slow blood coagulation, thereby lessening the possibility of heart attacks and strokes. The herb also encourages arteries to dilate, which improves blood flow to various organs. In this manner, it appears similar to many prescription medications, such as calcium channel blockers.

The practical, medical implications of these findings are, as yet, unclear. However, some authorities are convinced that future studies will prove garlic to be an inexpensive and safe adjunct to therapy which prevents cardiovascular diseases, even though the herb has not been shown to reduce high blood pressure, a claim frequently made by health-food aficionados.

Nonetheless, garlic appears to have definite—albeit small—health benefits. To me, it's comforting to learn that, unlike so many foods and flavoring agents, garlic is not only safe but is probably a necessary component in a healthful diet. While it may be many years before processed garlic finds a niche in our everyday eating habits, I'm going to be on the cutting edge of any new discoveries. I plan to surrender to my dietary delights and ignore the obvious (odoriferous) consequences of my commitment. Pass the pesto, please.

Supplemental chromium not shown to have health benefits

Q. I'm not interested in what you have to say, ever since you stated that there are no medical studies showing that chromium picolinate has any health benefits. Haven't you ever heard of alternative medicine? Our diets lack chromium because our farm soils are depleted of vital minerals. I was overweight until I started eating a brand of health food (containing chromium). Now I've lost 10 pounds, stopped eating my husband's leftovers and feel great!

A. No reputable scientific studies have shown that supplemental chromium leads to any health benefits. When such a study is published, I'll update my readers. A balanced American diet contains adequate amounts of the mineral, which is necessary for proper insulin metabolism. If you choose to take supplemental chromium, be my guest, but I cannot, in all honesty, endorse such an option for the general public, based on the current information available.

Tea does not protect against stroke

Q. I've heard that people who are tea drinkers seldom, if ever, have strokes. Are there components in tea that are responsible? Since I prefer to avoid beverages that contain caffeine, I would like to find a substitute—unless, of course, caffeine is the magic anti-stroke ingredient.

A. I am not aware of any valid studies showing that tea drinkers are immune to stroke. There is no sound scientific evidence proving that this beverage protects against disease, heart disorders or cancer. Nonetheless, recent reports from Asia indicate that green tea may well have some health benefits. At this point, I am awaiting confirmation of these data.

For now, I advise you to continue drinking tea if you like it, not for any supposed health issues. Because many standard teas do contain caffeine (which does not improve health), you may wish to switch to non-caffeinated, herbal teas.

Coca-Cola ineffective cold fighter

Q. I have a difference of opinion with a beloved aunt who is convinced that Coca-Cola syrup is a vital method of treating the common cold when her children get sick. Apparently, the use of this syrup was very popular years ago, but the medical professionals I've spoken to have never heard of it and cannot understand how it would work. In spite of this, my aunt continues to administer Coke syrup to herself, her children and an aging dog. Is there any validity to this?

A. Decades ago, Coca-Cola contained cocaine, a narcotic that—despite its dangers—produced positive side effects, such as sedation, cough suppression and pain relief. In those bygone days, there was pitifully little else available to remedy the symptoms of upper respiratory infections, so Coke syrup was, for a while, an accepted therapy.

Modern Coke syrup is basically sugar water with coloring and caffeine added; it contains no narcotics. Consequently, it has little or no medicinal value. I believe that your aunt and the children would achieve more satisfactory results by using one of the many over-the-counter cough and cold remedies. As far as the dog is concerned, I pass.

Soap for leg cramps?

Q. You asked to hear from readers experienced with the soap cure for leg cramps.

Let me begin my answer by saying that I am a college graduate and a professional scientist who is naturally skeptical of unproven treatments and cures.

However, I do have chronic obstructive pulmonary disease (COPD) and check in periodically with the related Web sites (such as www.copd-international.com) to check on recent updates. For decades, I have been troubled by leg cramps that disrupt my sleep five to 10 times a night. All the standard therapies, including quinine pills and massage, have been ineffective. Several people on the Internet have touted the soap cure: a bar of soap placed under the mattress cover near my legs.

Did this sound ridiculous? You bet. But I gave it a try. Did it work? Yes, indeed. I haven't had a cramp since. The proper technique is simple. Unwrap a fresh bar of soap (don't use Dove or Dial) and discard the wrapper. It doesn't need to be a huge, bath-size bar; even the small bars common in hotels work for most people. Then place the unwrapped bar directly under the bottom sheet or on the bed where the legs are usually located. That's it. Some people may need to rub the legs with an extra bar of soap, but, in most instances, this is not necessary. The cramps are gone. Why? I haven't a clue.

A. Nor have I. But I am publishing your letter—which is one of dozens I have received since mentioning the soap cure for leg cramps—because the therapy is, apparently, an effective preventive for a common human malady. In such circumstances, we probably don't need an explanation of how the technique works, but it does. Thanks to you, and other readers, for writing.

Ladies Only

Breast reduction surgery may help

Q. I have had extraordinarily large breasts since my teens. I was a 38C until my early 40s, when my breasts progressively enlarged to a 44C. Now I'm in my 60s, with heavy, pendulous breasts that inhibit my breathing, cause extreme shoulder discomfort and are an embarrassment, because I am 4 feet 10 inches tall and weigh 120 pounds. I don't believe that breast reduction surgery would be right for me. Can I get help through hormone therapy?

A. Probably not. I am not sure why breast reduction is not appropriate for you. Ordinarily, large-breasted women who have symptoms such as yours can easily be cured by this simple procedure. The operation is safe, easy and can usually be covered by insurance if there are compelling physical reasons for surgery, in contrast to a purely cosmetic concern.

I suggest that you review this situation with your gynecologist. He or she may suggest that you consider other options. However, in my experience, the most satisfactory solution to breast-related breathing difficulties and shoulder pain is to have the excessive breast tissue surgically removed.

Monistat for yeast infections

Q. Do you recommend Monistat cream for treatment of vaginal infections?

A. Only if the infection is caused by a yeast. Monistat (miconazole) cream and vaginal suppositories are an effective treatment for yeast (candida) vaginitis. However, Monistat and similar antifungal agents are not appropriate therapy for other types of vaginal infection, such as bacterial vaginitis. Therefore, before beginning treatment, doctors usually attempt to identify the source of the infection by examination and smears/cultures of the discharge, which always characterizes the disorder. Once the offending agent has been identified, appropriate therapy can be prescribed.

That's the standard medical approach. Let me suggest an alternative, which may be more useful for you.

If you have a history of yeast vaginitis, are a diabetic or are overweight, have been using antibiotics, or note that your vaginal discharge if painful, "cheesy" and malodorous, you probably have candida. In such circumstances, I recommend Monistat. This is available without a prescription.

On the other hand, if your answers to the above questions are "no," you should check with your family physician or gynecologist.

Estrogen cream may be the answer

Q. Please comment on atrophic vaginitis.

A. The vaginal lining requires the female hormone estrogen to remain moist and elastic. When a woman's estrogen level declines during and after menopause, the vaginal wall becomes inflamed and atrophic (thin, dry and less healthy). This can make intercourse difficult or impossible. In addition, there may be a slight discharge with an unpleasant odor.

Although the problem can be partially overcome by using lubricants during intercourse, what is really needed is estrogen.

Until recently, women with atrophic vaginitis were prescribed estrogen pills or patches. However, because of current studies showing that hormone replacement therapy increases the risk of certain cancers, HRT has fallen out of favor.

Many specialists have now adopted a compromise: estrogen cream applied daily to the deficient tissues. The cream is not associated with cancer-risk and will often improve the vaginal symptoms after as little as a week or two of therapy.

Atrophic vaginitis is not so much a health problem as a gigantic nuisance. Ask your primary care physician or gynecologist about prescribing topical estrogen cream.

Hysterectomies unavoidable?

Q. Are hysterectomies absolutely necessary? My menstruation ceased a year ago; I have no problems with bleeding or cramping. I do have small fibroids that don't give me any trouble. I am completely healthy. So why, then, does my general practitioner urge me to undergo surgery?

Looking One's Age Is OK

Q. With respect to your column about accepting aging and not using plastic surgery to look young, I take issue. You must not be aware of reality. If we look old, we women are discriminated in the work force. We won't be hired for a position, even if we are qualified, if we are in competition with someone who is young and pretty. On the other hand, as men age, they are said to look "distinguished."

A. You quite properly remind me that the work force, despite having come a long way in the past 20 years, is still sexist and elitist. I view this as abhorrent, but people are people, and life isn't always fair.

The purpose of the column (on accepting aging as inevitable) was to point out that creams, pills, lotions, Botox, hair coloring, plastic surgery and other cover-ups do nothing more than that—cover up. Don't you think that prospective employers will see through these techniques? The boss sits there—with a paunch and gray hair combed over the top of his bald head—looking at your application. He notes your birth date and then glances up, with surprise, to view a wrinkle-free woman in a mini skirt, with mahogany hair. Ouch! Wouldn't you come across better in a more natural mode? A confident, qualified, smartly dressed, engaging, gray-haired, no-nonsense, articulate and experienced woman could skate circles around a younger candidate.

I cannot believe that age, if handled gracefully, is a negative factor in the workplace. Yes, there are exceptions, I am certain. But, I sure as heck wouldn't want to take a job where my employer was primarily obsessed with youth. Wisdom and experience count. In my opinion, the process of aging should be acknowledged and dealt with, not covered up by phony means that are all too evident to the observer.

P.S. Aging men do not always appear as distinguished as they think they are. This is a power issue. Who's gong to tell the boss he looks like a twerp with dyed red hair, a size 18 neck, a heavy gold necklace, tinted glasses and a beer belly?

A. Hysterectomy (removal of the uterus) was a commonly performed operation in the past. Women underwent the procedure for a variety of reasons, some valid (such as cancer), some questionable (such as contraception). Today, fortunately, the rate for hysterectomy is far lower than it was previously, because alternative therapies are available and women are much less likely to undergo unnecessary surgery that is urged solely at the discretion of their male doctors. (If you're reading gender issues into this, you are correct. Such issues were a major problem for women in past generations.)

I do not know why your primary care physician has advised surgery. You do not seem to have a compelling reason to do so. Based on the limited information you supply, I'd have to conclude that surgery may not be appropriate or necessary in your case.

Nonetheless, your doctor may have a specific reason, which he has yet to share with you, for encouraging the operation. Thus, in all fairness, before criticizing your doctor for being too aggressive, I advise you to discuss the situation with him. However, even if he remains adamant, you should still obtain a second opinion from a gynecologist, the specialist who would actually operate on you.

In my view, hysterectomy is far from necessary unless uterine cancer is present or a woman experiences repeated episodes of uncontrolled bleeding. Fibroids, benign uterine growths, are exceedingly common, may disappear on their own, and—as a general rule—do not constitute an indication for hysterectomy.

Bartholinitis always painful

Q. Please inform me about the Bartholin's gland. What happens if it gets inflamed? Can long-term problems lead to cancer?

A. Bartholin's glands are two small nests of tissue located at the vaginal opening. They provide lubrication. They are also subject to two relatively common disorders: cysts and infection.

Bartholin's cysts result from blockage of the glandular openings. The glands fill with clear fluid and distend, causing a lump that is sometimes painful. At times, the swelling can be quite noticeable and may interfere with sexual activity. However, these cysts do not ordinarily require treatment unless they grow large or become inflamed.

Bartholinitis is infection of the glands. This may or may not follow cyst formation. The condition is always painful, can lead to large abscesses or may enlarge to produce fistulas (abnormal openings) between the Bartholin's glands and the surrounding tissue, such as the vagina or anus. Antibiotics are required for treatment.

In severe cases—or in patients who experience repeated infection and cyst formation—the abscesses have to be drained. The preferred operation is called marsupialization. The surgeon opens the infected area and exposes the gland. This forms a small sac that does not close over and, therefore, prevents the accumulation of cystic fluid and/or infected material.

> 66 Today, fortunately, the rate for hysterectomy is far lower than it was previously, because alternative therapies are available and women are much less likely to undergo unnecessary surgery that is urged solely at the discretion of their male doctors. 99

Cardiologist not required

Q. I have a painless growth that fills my entire vagina. I'm post-menopausal. What sort of specialist should I see?

A. Well, you don't really need a cardiologist, I guess. Seriously, this question's answer seems to me to be self-evident. You need a gynecologist. Although your "growth" could, in theory, be a tumor, it's more likely to be an innocuous condition, such as a uterine prolapse. Many years after having borne children, a woman may experience a "dropped uterus." Deprived of is supporting tissue, the womb may sag into the lower pelvis and, in advanced cases, actually begin to protrude through the vagina. This is more a nuisance than a serious health matter and can be easily repaired surgically.

Because your problem involves your reproductive tract and you need a diagnosis (and treatment), I believe that a gynecologist is your best resource.

Is estrogen treatment unwise?

Q. At menopause, I was prescribed the estrogen patch. This led to a low-grade malignancy in my uterus, requiring a hysterectomy. Now my doctor wants me to take Provera along with the patch, but I'm not sure why.

A. Neither am I.

The use of estrogen (without Provera) in a woman with a uterus is associated with a statistical risk of uterine cancer. Provera reduces this risk but is associated with continuing monthly bleeding.

Once a woman has had a hysterectomy, the benefits of Provera fall to zero. In such cases, using estrogen alone is acceptable and will reduce the risk of heart disease, help prevent osteoporosis and improve sexual functioning. Therefore, a woman without a uterus can safely be prescribed estrogen alone.

However, your case is somewhat unique. I am not at all sure that you, having had cancer, should take any female hormones. Estrogen may stimulate uterine cancer cells to grow.

While I'm sure that your gynecologist removed all the malignant tissue and you are now in good health, it is possible that before the hysterectomy, a few undetected cancer cells may have spread to the lymph glands in your pelvis.

In this situation, taking estrogen could be akin to pouring gasoline on a fire. Although I am not a gynecologist, I am uncomfortable enough about your continued use of estrogen (with or without Provera) to urge you to seek a second opinion from another gynecologist.

Perhaps I'm just being fussy and overcautious, but I don't recommend that women with a history of uterine cancer take estrogen, any more than I would advise a man with a history of prostate cancer to take male hormones. The risk of stimulating hidden cancer cells is just too great.

Barbiturates for menopause?

Q. Why are doctors so secretive? I recently asked mine why he prescribed Butisol elixir and he replied that it would relieve my hot flashes. After researching this on the Internet, I discovered that this is a barbiturate that will make me sleepy. True, I have trouble sleeping, but this is because of my hot flashes. And I am constantly fatigued. I feel he has done me an injustice.

A. I agree. In my opinion, doctors owe patients explanations about prescription drugs, especially those—such as barbiturates—that have a definite potential for abuse or addiction. I think your doctor could be severely criticized for not leveling with you.

Moreover, barbiturates are not appropriate therapy for the symptoms of menopause, which you appear to be experiencing. If you need treatment for this, estrogen replacement, under the guidance of a gynecologist, would be preferable. I say "if" because hot flashes do not indicate ill health. Many women choose to "ride them out" and get through menopause without drug supplements. The gynecologist can advise you, especially if you are at risk for osteoporosis, which can be treated with hormones.

Also, I recommend that patients not take medicine until the prescribing doctor has reviewed and explained the various side effects and potential consequences.

If you have been taking Butisol for several weeks, I advise you not to discontinue it abruptly. To do so might place you at risk for withdrawal symptoms, such as seizures. It's preferable to reduce the dosage by half each week; when you're down to a half teaspoonful a day, you can safely stop the drug altogether.

Given your unfortunate experience, I suggest that you search out another practitioner in your community who will be more conscientious.

30

Gentlemen Only

Spotting symptoms of prostate cancer

Q. About a year ago you ran a column on the symptoms of prostate cancer. Since I had similar symptoms, I saw my doctor and found I had an elevated PSA reading. There was a hard spot on one side of my prostate that ultimately revealed cancer cells. I had the gland removed, the cancer had not yet reached the lymph glands, and there is no evidence of a need for future treatment. I really owe my thanks to you for this column. I'm truly fortunate I took the time to read what you had to say.

A. As your generous compliments attest, prostate cancer is a serious concern for men in their late middle age and beyond. In the past, physicians suspected such a disorder if they felt an irregular, overly firm or nodular prostate gland on rectal examination. Now the diagnosis has been refined by a series of tests.

The prostate specific antigen blood test is usually elevated in the presence of prostate cancer. Thus, it may confirm the doctor's suspicion. If the PSA is high, urologists ordinarily proceed to an ultrasound test with biopsy. If this next level of testing is abnormal, the physician and the patient have a tough decision to make: drug therapy or surgery, each of which has its own advantages and disadvantages.

You evidently were extremely fortunate that, at the time of diagnosis, your prostate cancer had not spread to the lymph glands, an ominous complication. Your cancer was appropriately treated and you can look forward to a long life. I am glad that I was able to play a role in such a favorable outcome.

Men over 50 should have rectal examinations as a part of any routine evaluation. Men with symptoms of prostate disease—for example, difficulty with (or frequency of) urination—should be examined by urologists.

There is ongoing disagreement in the medical community about whether the PSA test should be performed routinely on all men over 50, whether or not they have symptoms of a prostate disorder, because the test is not 100 percent predictive. I take a moderate approach by ordering the test, on a case-by-case basis, every one to five years on older men.

Congratulations on having received such a prompt therapy—and paying attention to the guy who writes the syndicated newspaper column.

Treatment for prostatic cancer

Q. In a recent article you seemed to favor ignoring an elevated PSA test, because prostate cancer is slow-growing. Were the thousands of men who have ignored the obvious problem and died from it given the same advice?

In my case, I had biopsy-proven prostatic cancer that my urologist believed could be "watched." He seemed uncomfortable when I questioned him about radioactive seed implantation. I had a fellow Navy pilot (circa WW II) who had the procedure and his PSA dropped to below 4! What do you think?

A. First of all, I am neither a urologist nor an oncologist; therefore, I would never intend to counsel my readers (or my private patients) to "ignore" a cancer anywhere in the body. That would not only be an irresponsible act, but a dumb one, to boot. I have, however, written in the past that in general, prostatic cancers do grow slowly, a feature that gives many victims (and their urologists) additional valuable time to make a sensible decision about how to address the problem.

Were you, for example, a 98-year-old nursing home resident with multiple medical problems, the chances are good that you would be better off monitoring the situation if your physician discovered a small area of cancer in your prostate gland.

On the other hand, if you were 46 and your biopsy indicated a high level of prostatic malignancy, I'd recommend aggressive therapy.

Also, if your exam (or blood test) showed unmistakable progression during the monitoring period, I would certainly address the situation in an active manner.

Finally, as I am sure you are aware, in some men prostatic cancer can be relentlessly malignant, the reverse of the rather indolent growth that is the general rule. In such cases, multiple therapies are indicated.

As to this last part of your question, radium-seed implants are a recognized and commonly used effective treatment for many types of prostate cancer. Although I have several patients who have successfully undergone this therapy, I would be overstepping my level of competency to endorse (or discourage) that option. Again, such decisions must involve specialists.

If you are concerned about the recommendations given you by your urologist, seek a second opinion. This tactic is always appropriate in the medical field, when confusion, conflict or communication problems may lead to patients who feel abandoned and uncertain about how to proceed.

I suggest that you sit down with your urologist for a strategy session that should include the following:

• How extensive is your prostatic cancer? Is it confined only to the gland itself or does it involve adjacent structures, such as lymph nodes?

• How malignant is it? If the biopsy showed a few scattered cancer cells, your approach would be different than in the situation where sheets of highly malignant cells literally fill the biopsy specimen.

• What therapy would be appropriate? At present, there are five basic approaches to this problem:

a. Do nothing and monitor the situation. We've discussed this.

b. Consider antihormone therapy, such as Lupron. These regular injections, although expensive, appear to stop certain prostatic cancers in their tracks.

c. Use radiation. Administered in a variety of ways, radiotherapy (including radium seeds) is basically painless and safe. It is, however, a nuisance (because of the daily or weekly commutation to a medical center), a discomfort (if seeds are used) and a common cause of side effects, such as colitis and bladder irritation from the radiation itself.

d. Weigh the possibility of chemotherapy. Although, in my limited experience, this option is not especially successful, it does seem to help some patients.

e. Resort to surgery. There are several procedures to be considered, ranging from a limited removal of the prostate gland to full excision.

Your urologist should be able to advise you about which therapeutic option would be appropriate. If not, as I indicated (or if I've answered an alternative), seek a second opinion.

Numerous choices today

Q. After having been diagnosed with prostate cancer, I was given therapy by my urologist. However, I have a friend with the same condition who underwent orchiectomy. Which therapy is superior?

A. Probably the most significant advance in treating cancer has been the enormous increase in various treatment strategies. Patients now have many more choices than were available a generation ago.

Prostate cancer is an excellent example.

While most cases of this malignancy do not require therapy because patients are often very elderly and have a slow-growing tumor, other men with this affliction can now choose between radiation, chemotherapy or surgery.

Your doctor chose chemotherapy with hormones. Because prostate cancer grows more aggressively in the presence of male hormone (testosterone), some specialists recommend treatment with female hormones or with drugs that block testosterone. Although these medicines virtually eliminate the sex drive (and sexual ability), they often arrest the growth of prostate cancer or even shrink the tumor.

The testicles are a major source of testosterone. Therefore, an operation to remove them (orchiectomy) accomplishes the same goal: less testosterone to feed the cancer.

Many men are understandably reluctant to be castrated. However, the operation is quick, painless and safe. After orchiectomy, men do not have to take hormones. As with the chemotherapy, sex drive and ability are diminished.

For all practical purposes, the two methods produce the same beneficial results (and complications). I am not aware that one is superior to the other.

If you are considering orchiectomy, ask your urologist to comment on this option, which may be appropriate for you. On the other hand, you'll probably achieve the same results with hormone therapy, so the decision comes down to personal preferences.

In either case, you should have close follow-up with regular exams and determination of the PSA (prostate specific antigen) blood test, the standard procedure for monitoring men under treatment for prostate cancer.

If the orchiectomy/hormone option fails to retard the growth of cancer, you may have to consider radiation or more extensive surgery.

Changing PSA levels need attention

Q. Two years ago, my PSA test was 27 and I had a prostate biopsy that did not reveal cancer. Now my PSA has risen to 41, but my HMO refuses to allow me to see a urologist because my biopsy was negative. They do, however, permit a follow-up with a nurse practitioner. Am I correct in insisting to see a urologist?

A. The prostate specific antigen blood test is typically elevated (above the upper limit of 4) in the presence of prostatic cancer. The fact that yours has risen from 27 to 41 in two years is a major concern because the abnormal level is consistent with cancer that is growing.

In my opinion, you should be examined by a urologist without further delay. You and your primary care physician should work together, through the appeals board of your HMO, to obtain the medical coverage that you need.

PSA levels are age-related

Q. I am 88 years and was told by my new urologist that, based on an elevated PSA level, I have a 50 percent chance of having prostate cancer. He wants to do a biopsy. My former urologist (in another part of the country) had told me for years not to have the test; he forgoes PSA testing in any man over 75. Should I proceed with the biopsy?

A. The prostate specific antigen blood test is a help in identifying men with prostatic cancer. I say "is a help" because the test is not 100 percent accurate. The level will usually rise (above the normal limit of 4) as men grow older, and can rise from simple prostatic enlargement or can exceed the normal limit if there is prostatic infection.

Therefore, I cannot answer your question specifically. If your PSA is 8 or 10 and is stable from year to year, I would ignore it. On the other hand, if it is about 40 or 50, you have a tough decision to make. In this instance, a needle biopsy of the gland is certainly an option—and if cancer is discovered, you would have to consider surgery (a risky and uncomfortable procedure for someone your age) or hormone therapy.

Before subjecting yourself to a biopsy, you should get a second opinion from another urologist. By and large, prostatic cancer is very slow-growing in elderly men, so you do not have to rush your decision, which will depend on the actual PSA value, your feelings about biopsy and other factors, such as your general state of health and how your prostate feels to the examiner. (A rock hard, nodular gland is more likely to contain cancer than is a smooth and soft prostate.)

I believe that a second opinion would go a long way toward resolving the issue of how to proceed.

Infection can elevate the PSA

Q. I'm 70 and have a PSA (prostate specific antigen) of 13. It's been stable for more than a year. I have had a dozen needle biopsies that showed chronic infection, no cancer. My doctor says forget it and just keep monitoring the PSA every year. I am now on antibiotics. What do I do now?

A. Continue the course of antibiotics and monitor your PSA annually.

This test is helpful in diagnosing prostate cancer, but at the same time, it may be elevated (above 4.0) in the presence of other afflictions, including chronic prostate infection. Biopsies have failed to reveal malignant cells. Therefore, you can safely conclude that infection is the problem. Follow your physician's advice.

Difficult decisions about prostate

Q. I have a difficult decision to make, and I would value your advice. I am 66 and experience frequent urination, urgency, reduced stream and so forth. During an annual exam, my urologist performed an ultrasound that confirmed the presence of a prostatic tumor. He urged me to have a prostatic resection, even though my PSA is only 0.9.

I discussed this with my family physician, who was visibly disturbed by the urologist's urging. He said, in no uncertain terms, that he could not recommend such a drastic procedure, which is associated with potentially serious side effects, such as impotence and incontinence. I'm stuck in the middle. What should I do?

A. The most striking part of your description is your conclusion that you are "stuck in the middle." This should not be the case. Let's analyze your situation.

You have urological symptoms that are common in men as they age. These symptoms are not, by themselves, indicative of a prostatic malignancy, nor is your PSA of 0.9 (prostate specific antigen, 0 to 4 normal).

Therefore, I and your primary care physician quite properly question the necessity of an operation to remove your prostate gland. I agree that some other factor should be present to justify such an invasive procedure.

On the other hand, not having felt your prostate, I cannot judge whether a biopsy is necessary. If you had a rock-hard nodule in the prostate gland, I'd certainly recommend biopsy, or maybe even removal. In

Erectile Dysfunction

Almost every man, at one point or another in his life, will experience the most common form of erectile dysfunction—impotence, or difficulty in achieving and maintaining an erection. This is a completely normal aspect of human sexual functioning, so long as these are brief or isolated instances. Common causes for temporary impotence include stress, fatigue and excessive alcohol intake.

Persistent impotence, following a period of normal sexual function, warrants medical investigation and possible therapeutic intervention.

When should impotence be considered a problem? In general, a man should seek consultation if he has difficulty with erections more than one-quarter of the time and if the disorder does not resolve itself within two or three months.

The role aging plays

Because the peak of sexual activity occurs relatively early in life for men, many are programmed to believe that impotence invariably accompanies aging. It is true that erectile dysfunction is more common in men over age 65 and that there can be some loss in potency after the age of 50, with subtle and gradual changes. For example, erections may be less firm, take longer to achieve, require more stimulation, be less frequent, and may sometimes be lost before orgasm occurs. These changes are quite variable over time.

On the other hand, even though some physicians may respond to an older patient's concerns with, "Well, what do you expect at your age?," in most normal men the ability to have an erection should persist into the 70s. Therefore, any abrupt change in sexual function in an older man deserves investigation and should not be ascribed merely to age.

Various treatments available

There is good news for men facing this problem today. What used to be a subject that was so forbidden it was only whispered about is now discussed openly by everyone from former generals and politicians to sitting mayors and TV journalists. The proliferation of new drugs, hormone and implant therapies has made impotence itself much easier to treat.

There is a wide range of options: medications, surgery, mechanical devices and counseling. If a drug is suspected of being responsible for impotence, its use sometimes can be stopped to see if impotence is reversed. Often, another drug of equal effectiveness that does not cause impotence can be substituted, particularly if the drug is a high blood pressure medication.

For those who have a testosterone deficiency, hormone replacement therapy may be indicated.

Vascular surgery. For men whose blood flow has been blocked by an injury to the penis or pelvic area, surgery may be appropriate. The goal is to correct the blockage so that erections can naturally occur. However, the long-term success of this method is unclear.

Penile implants. This treatment consists of surgically placing a device into two sides of the penis. This allow erection to occur as often and for as long as desired. The implants can be an inflatable device or semirigid rods made from silicone or polyurethane. This is an expensive treatment usually reserved as a last resort. Realistic expectations about sexual function after implantation play a major role in patient satisfaction. For example, men who are unable to ejaculate because of an organic problem will still not be able to ejaculate after surgical implantation of these appliances. Physicians urge that a man's sex partner be consulted before selecting the type of prosthesis to be implanted.

Vacuum devices. As an alternative to surgery, a vacuum-constriction device is available (by prescription) that produces an erection by trapping blood in the penis. The procedure involves using a hollow plastic tube placed over the penis and the use of an external vacuum and one or more rubber bands. Results are generally good, although some patients have discontinued using it because they felt it was too artificial or their partners didn't like it.

Counseling. Once physiological causes have been ruled out and psychological factors appear to be causing the impotence, the physician may refer the patient and his sex partner to a psychiatrist, psychologist or sex therapist. Such counseling will almost always be directed to identifying factors in the couple's relations, such as misunderstanding or lack of communication, that may have adverse effects on sexual expression. These approaches also use self-help exercises, relaxation techniques and education about facts of sexual arousal. For example, erections are not maintained for the entire period of love-making, but tend alternately to increase and decrease. If a man is not aware that this is natural, anxiety over partial loss of an erection can produce impotence. Sometimes only a few sessions are needed to correct the problem. In other cases, many months of therapy may be required.

New drugs

New drugs have revolutionized the therapy for impotence. Called phosphodiesterase inhibitors, the drugs enhance the effects of nitrous oxide, a chemical that relaxes the smooth muscles of the penis, leading to an increase in the volume of blood reaching the penis.

Viagra (sildenafil) was the first to reach the market. Levitra (vardenafil) and Cialis (tadenafil) followed. Typically these drugs are taken an hour before anticipated sexual activity.

Phosphodiesterase inhibitor must be avoided by people who take nitrates for cardiovascular conditions. See the chapter "Sex" starting on page 161 in this book for more information.

contrast, if your prostate gland is diffusely enlarged without specific, troublesome masses, I'd hold off further invasive investigation.

All of this brings me to an inescapable conclusion: A second opinion is mandatory. In my view, this situation can be resolved with such a step. Ask your primary care physician to refer you to another urologist. If the specialist advises surgery, so be it; if he suggests monitoring the situation, I would agree. A prostate exam and a PSA in about a year or six months could certainly resolve the disagreement.

Drug therapy for prostate cancer

Q. My doctor has prescribed Lupron injections for my prostate cancer. What is your opinion of this therapy? What side effects might I encounter?

A. Prostate cancer, a common affliction of older men, is ordinarily treated with surgery or by drugs to neutralize testosterone (male hormone). Lupron blocks the production and effects of testosterone, thereby reducing stimulation of the cancer cells.

Because this medication (and others like it) cause male menopause, it has predictable side effects: weakness, hot flashes, loss of libido (sex drive), erectile dysfunction and breast swelling. Other complications (because of fluid retention) include heart failure, ankle swelling, muscle aches, high blood pressure, stomach upset, diarrhea and insomnia.

Although Lupron and others are associated with a high incidence of side effects, these may be the price patients have to pay in order to suppress the growth of the cancer. As one of my patients remarked: "I don't like taking this drug, but considering the alternatives, I'll do it."

In your case, the prescribed treatment is standard and appropriate. However, you should discuss your concerns with your urologist, who may be able to alter or reduce the dosage to minimize side effects.

Antibiotics for prostatitis

Q. What is the most successful way to treat prostatitis?

A. Antibiotics. Most types of prostate infection are caused by low-level bacterial inflammation that can be cured by a prolonged course of drug therapy, sometimes lasting a month or more, administered by a urologist.

Some cases of prostatitis seem to be related to noninfectious congestion of the gland, which may be relieved by prostate massage. However, in the main, antibiotics offer the most consistent cure for most cases of prostatitis.

About testosterone supplements

Q. Please discuss the male hormone testosterone. I understand that it prevents bone weakness, but may also be a cause of prostate cancer. Would calcium tablets provide the proper nutrition for bones in the absence of testosterone?

A. Testosterone is a naturally occurring male hormone, manufactured primarily by the testicles but also, to a lesser extent, by the adrenal glands. Aside from the obvious consequences of testosterone (such as facial hair, deep voice and increased sex drive), the hormone also strengthens bones and muscles by its so-called anabolic effect. Testosterone is probably the primary reason that men do not develop osteoporosis as early and as rapidly as do their female counterparts.

Regrettably, as men age, their testosterone levels fall, leading to predictable results called "feminization"—sparse beards, less interest in sex (and more difficulty performing), loss of muscle mass and reduction in bone calcium.

(As a side note, women also produce testosterone in their adrenal glands. But, during the reproductive years, this is neutralized by the much larger quantities of female hormone secreted by the ovaries. After menopause, when the ovaries shut off, the small amounts of testosterone are no longer balanced and begin to make a difference. Thus, old women often grow facial hair and have deep gravelly voices. Now, where was I?)

Ideally, were old men to take supplemental testosterone, their health would probably improve. For one thing, their tendency to osteoporosis could be slowed or even arrested; some of their earlier strength would be maintained; their sex lives would not necessarily grind to a halt; they might feel better.

However, as you pointed out, such hormone supplements appear to be associated with an increased risk of prostatic cancer, an unacceptable trade-off.

Therefore, I assert that most men my age will have to be content with maintaining an active exercise schedule, take 1,500 to 2,000 milligrams of extra calcium a day, stopping smoking and losing weight (if necessary). Viagra, now and then, may also help such gentlemen retain the misperception that they are still young and virile. A low cholesterol diet may be in order. Other than that for healthy seniors, good luck.

31

Sleeping Well

Benadryl effective, safe for insomnia

Q. After reading in your column that 100 milligrams of Benadryl is an effective therapy for insomnia, I went to my pharmacist and was told that anything over 25 milligrams requires a prescription. Please clarify. I anticipate taking four 25-milligram capsules but hesitate until I hear from you.

A. Your pharmacist's reaction is one of the reasons that I sometimes get crazy. Nonprescription Benadryl is available in 25-milligram pills. My intention, in writing the column, was to indicate that four 25-mg tablets was an appropriate sleep aid. Case closed. Forget the need for a prescription.

Although there are many effective prescription medications to overcome insomnia, Benadryl is one of the safest. It is not habit-forming and is OK even for children in smaller doses; also, it is frequently used intravenously to neutralize serious allergic reactions. Here is a personal anecdote that proves my point about safety.

When I was an intern in a large teaching hospital, a man arrived in the emergency room. He was in bad shape from an unusual hypersensitivity to a tranquilizer he had taken at home. His face was frozen in a horrible grimace; he couldn't move his jaw—in fact, I actually thought he had lockjaw. He couldn't breathe and I was sure he was going to die.

The resident physician, who was more experienced than I, immediately ascertained what had happened by talking to family members who were present. The doctor quickly drew up 200 mg of Benadryl in a syringe and injected it by IV push, straight into the vein, undiluted. Even before the injection was completed, the patient returned completely to normal.

Since that experience, I, too, have used IV Benadryl in identical situations, always with good results, never with side effects.

Therefore, I believe you're safe to use the drug as a mild sleep-enhancer. All it really does is make you somewhat drowsy. And it's OK to take four 25 mg pills at one time. I might add that no sleep medication is appropriate for daily, sustained use; such medicine should be used only for short periods, when necessary.

Let's straighten out the Benadryl issue

Q. You have recommended taking Benadryl as a sleep aid. According to published reports, it should not be used because it can cause sedation and difficulty operating a motor vehicle. What gives?

A. What gives is that you need to review the issue. Diphenhydramine (generic Benadryl) is an antihistamine. One of its major side effects is sedation and sleepiness. This makes it an ideal first-step therapy for insomnia. Neither I nor any health care professional would recommend this drug for daytime use, despite manufacturer's claims that, at low doses, the medicine is safe for such use.

The fact that Benadryl causes sedation is precisely the reason that I recommend it as therapy for insomnia. Fifty to 100 milligrams at bedtime should result in a restful sleep. But I discourage patients from using Benadryl during awake hours. There are more appropriate antihistamines for this purpose, including (nonprescription) Actifed and Dimetapp, and (prescription) medications, such as Clarinex, Allegra and Zyrtec.

Benadryl has fewer side effects than other drugs

Q. I'm a nurse. Many years ago, my husband began using Benadryl, on occasion, to help him sleep. Because the generic equivalent, diphenhydramine, is so much cheaper than the trade-name product, he switched over without incident. The over-the-counter drug works fine, with no side effects, including hangover. I'm not ordinarily a proponent of generics, but I just wanted you to know.

A. Thank you for writing. I've had several letters from other readers who confirm that the generic brand, although cheaper than Benadryl, works just as well.

Sleeping pills can lead to forgetfulness and impaired judgment

Q. My doctor says I have "cerebral disease." I'm 80, in good health but have insomnia, for which I take one Halcion at bedtime. What's my problem? Am I getting Alzheimer's?

A. Cerebral disease is really too broad a term. It means that you are

Snoring

Snoring is caused by obstruction of the airway during sleep—the result of blocked nasal passages, lax muscles or excess tissue in the throat. It's most common among older people—especially older men—who are overweight or have poor muscle tone.

Snoring can be dangerous, since it taxes the cardiovascular system, can trigger hypertension or stroke and may cause irregular heartbeat and sleep apnea (a total interruption of breathing, mentioned earlier).

Treatment

Snoring may be managed by weight loss and exercise to reduce and tone tissues. It also may help to sleep on your stomach, since the back-sleeping position is most likely to obstruct the airway.

Snorers should seek treatment for allergies that cause nasal blockage and should avoid alcohol and antihistamines (including sleep medications), which over-relax the throat.

In extreme cases, orthodontic devices can keep the jaw from blocking nasal passages; and—as in sleep apnea—surgery can remove excess tissue that causes snoring.

experiencing symptoms because of a disorder in the part of your brain (cerebral cortex) that controls higher thought processes. Such symptoms often include forgetfulness, emotional outbursts and loss of judgment.

Although cerebral problems can certainly be related to Alzheimer's disease they have other causes as well, including mini-strokes, vitamin deficiencies, thyroid disorders, alcohol use and the effects of mind-altering drugs, such as sleeping pills. As I'm sure you are aware, the normal aging process can affect cognitive function. Insomnia is a common complaint in the over-70 set and does not necessarily reflect a physical malady.

However, Halcion and other types of sleeping pills can lead to forgetfulness and impaired judgment, particularly if used regularly and for long periods.

I believe you need a more specific diagnosis. Ask your primary care physician to refer you to a neurologist for testing. For instance, magnetic

Sleep-Wake Disorders

Normal sleep patterns vary widely: Most healthy people require six to eight hours of sleep, but some may need as little as four or as much as 10 in order to feel rested. Therefore, rather than a deviation from a "norm," most sleep problems consist of troublesome changes in one's personal sleep pattern.

For example, insomnia and restless sleep may be temporary reactions to stress, medication or a change of schedule. Concern about this loss of sleep can cause further sleeplessness—and an ongoing sleep problem. About 35 percent of U.S. adults have some degree of insomnia, but most people overestimate their problem. (Even chronic insomniacs get some sleep: More than a few days of total sleeplessness would cause physical collapse, a condition resembling psychosis and a complete inability to function.) In fact, studies show that people with insomnia actually lose very little sleep—but anxiety about sleeplessness makes them misperceive the problem or feel unrested.

Other disorders—such as sleepwalking, sleep apnea (interrupted breathing) and narcolepsy (an inappropriate urge to sleep)—aren't matters of perception: They're concrete problems that can pose health risks or indicate an underlying physical disorder.

Finally, some chronic sleep problems are caused by a disordered "internal clock"—the body's way of regulating hormones, sleep/wake cycles and biological functioning. People with a disordered "internal clock" may need treatment to help them readjust their biorhythms and adopt more satisfying sleep patterns.

resonance imaging (MRI) would provide more important information about your condition.

Sleeping too much can cause grogginess

Q. When I fail to get enough sleep during the week, I will occasionally sleep more than 12 hours a night on weekends. Why do I have difficulty waking up and then feel groggy all day? I would think I should awake rested, refreshed and feeling great. I don't.

A. Your experience is not unique. "Catching up" on sleep can often lead to the very symptoms you mention, which are normal. The reason for this is that each of us has a biological clock that is more or less set to accommodate our individual daily schedules.

When we don't sleep enough—or on the occasion when we obtain more sleep than usual—the biological clock becomes desynchronized. This is the basis of jet lag, when we cross from one time zone to another and have to readapt. Also, changing work shifts can cause grogginess, irritability, insomnia and headache until the biological clock becomes adjusted to the changed sleep pattern.

Try sleeping no more than 10 hours at a time on weekends. This may be enough, and you should feel more refreshed.

Sleep apnea and snoring may be related

Q. My husband snores loudly enough to awaken me. Then I poke him in the ribs and he is OK for several minutes. I believe that, during his snoring episodes, he may actually stop breathing for what seems like an eternity. This frightens me. What can I do?

A. As I have mentioned before, snoring often appears in middle age, when the tissues at the back of the throat become flaccid, sag and close off the airway. This may lead to sleep apnea, a potentially serious disorder during which the snorer ceases to breathe effectively. Aside from causing daytime exhaustion (in both patient and spouse!), sleep apnea may be associated with hypertension, heart disease and other problems.

This common condition is worsened by obesity and the use of alcohol and/or sedatives.

I can understand why you're frightened. I suggest that you encourage your husband to be examined by an otolaryngologist, who will perform a detailed exam and advise your husband if surgery to remove the offending, lax tissue is appropriate. Addressing any aggravating factors, such as a weight problem or alcohol use, may also help to resolve the situation. If surgery is not indicated, I recommend that the ear-nose-and-throat specialist refer your husband to a sleep laboratory.

In such a monitoring environment, doctors will observe your husband's sleep pattern overnight and then suggest therapy, such as continuous positive airway pressure (CPAP) treatments. I recommend that your husband address this issue sooner rather than later, before dangerous health consequences appear.

Ways to overcome insomnia

Q. What is a good sleeping pill for insomnia?

A. As a general rule, it's better not to rely on sleeping pills, which can affect judgment and mental functioning. Also, many are habit forming.

Insomniacs often have success by modifying their lives rather than taking pills. Here are some suggestions:

• Go to bed at the same time each night in a room that is quiet and dark. Listen to your biological clock. If you're a night owl, stay up longer and sleep later.

• Avoid stimulating activity, such as certain TV programs, at bedtime. (Sex doesn't count; it's OK.)

• Disdain caffeine and other stimulants in the evening. Drink a glass of warm milk before retiring.

• Try over-the-counter Benadryl (100 milligrams at bedtime) to make you sleepy.

If these strategies don't work, see your family physician. Depression can cause insomnia, so if that is a problem, it should be addressed. Also, the doctor may choose to prescribe limited quantities of prescription sleeping pills—such as Ambien or Sonata, both of which are safe in the recommended dosage.

Hallucinations and sleep disorders

Q. Your comments about a young man who sees ghostly figures may have fallen short. You indicated that he probably has a psychiatric disorder with secondary hallucinations. I would like to suggest that he may have a physical basis: "hypnagogic hallucinations," which may be a symptom of narcolepsy or other sleep disorders. It consists of vivid or scary visions and sounds, usually experienced while falling asleep or awakening. You might want to mention this as part of the differential diagnosis.

A. Hypnagogic perceptions may, as you point out, occur in the presence of sleep disorders and are experienced as "jumping" extremities or surrealistic dream sequences. People who do not have sleep disorders may occasionally experience such phenomena, too.

However, in the column you read, the man's mother was clearly concerned about "ghostly figure" hallucinations that were not associated with falling asleep or awakening. Therefore, I chose to address an alternative explanation for his problem.

Nonetheless, I appreciate your comments about sleep disorders, which are a valid concern for those people who have them.

32

Oral Hygiene

Kissing prevents tooth decay?

Q. I've read about various ways of fighting tooth decay, other than simply brushing. Examples are: drinking green tea, kissing, eating nuts, drinking through a straw, munching on Gouda cheeses, and chewing on an Indian evergreen tree leaf. Is there truth to this?

A. Wow. If kissing retards tooth decay, this is the best news since Napoleon's defeat at Waterloo. I don't believe it. Nor do I believe that the other methods you mention will help much, either.

You should ask your dentist about this, but it's my understanding that tooth decay can best be conquered by fluoridation (or using fluoride toothpaste), brushing after every meal, flossing regularly, going easy on sweets, and following a program of regular dental checkups and hygiene, such as that promulgated by the American Dental Association.

If your dentist endorses kissing as a decay preventive, let me know. But I must say that it hasn't particularly helped me—yet. Does it matter whom you kiss?

Is halitosis contagious?

Q. Is it possible to catch bad breath? Our of loneliness, I began an unfortunate relationship with a horrible older woman whose teeth were loose and whose breath was unbelievable. Inconceivably, I often kissed her. Now I find that my own breath stinks in the same way hers did. No kidding. Is it possible she had some unique bacteria that she passed on to me?

A. Absolutely. I just received a letter from an elderly woman who just terminated an affair with an unattractive younger man with terrible halitosis. Could this be…? (I'm just kidding and wanted to pull your chain.)

Most cases of bad breath are caused by bacterial action on food particles wedged between teeth. It is entirely possible that your former partner transmitted large number of bacteria to your mouth during your periods of intimacy.

I suggest that you see a dentist to discover if you have 1) a dental abscess unrelated to your past fling, 2) signs of pyorrhea ("trench mouth"), a serious disorder, or 3) a problem with food particles between your own teeth.

In any case, your problem might be solved by a course of antibiotics, coupled with renewed attention to dental hygiene. A dentist can advise you.

Respiratory infection can cause halitosis

Q. Is it possible for bacteria to invade the lungs and cause bad breath? Dentists cannot find a problem in my mouth, but my life is literally in shambles because of halitosis.

A. Although most cases of bad breath are caused by bacterial action on food particles between teeth, there is no doubt that infection anywhere in the respiratory tree—including the lungs—can lead to halitosis. If your mouth and teeth check out and you aren't regularly consuming food, such as garlic, that can affect your breath, you need further testing to rule out sinus or lung infections, both of which can be associated with halitosis without other symptoms, such as sinus tenderness or cough.

I suggest that you be examined by your family physician who will, I suspect, X-ray your chest and sinuses to make certain that you don't have a hidden abscess.

Burning mouth syndrome

Q. I had the pleasure of reading your recent column about a person who described a burning sensation in the mouth and throat. You listed several possible causes, but understandably did not mention "burning mouth syndrome," a tricky diagnosis for even the most experienced dentist.

I had the opportunity to pursue a doctoral degree in education and pain management at the UCLA School of Dentistry. During our training, we became familiar with "burning mouth syndrome" as a distinct phenomenon. Most commonly, it affects postmenopausal females. The cause is unknown but is suspected to be a neuropathy; consequently, there are several treatment plans built around the control of inappropriate peripheral nerve hyperactivity.

A. Thank you for being so polite about my lack of knowledge concerning burning mouth syndrome. Not all professionals are as forgiving and gracious.

I am printing your letter, in abbreviated form, because this syndrome needs to be addressed. Judging from my mail, it is not a rare phenomenon.

I am publishing specific information about your facial pain center in hopes that readers who need your expertise can receive it. This act is in no way meant to punish you; it is a compliment!

So, readers, if you have maxillofacial pain, please contact Dr. Bradley Eli, Director, San Diego Headache and Facial Pain Center, 9850 Genesee Ave., Suite 220, La Jolla, CA 92037.

Self-induced vomiting bad on teeth

Q. I'm experiencing cavities and dental problems. My dentist informed me that part of the cause could be related stomach acidity. I do have irritable bowel syndrome and am curious if there is a connection.

A. Ordinarily, there is no association between dental disease and IBS, a chronic intestinal condition marked by poor digestion, gas, constipation and/or diarrhea.

There is, however, a relation between dental problems and eating disorders, especially bulimia, which is characterized by binge-eating followed by self-induced vomiting. The gastric acid in the vomit will lead to deterioration of dental enamel, resulting in cavities.

Therefore, unless you vomit periodically (in which case you need medical attention), follow your dentist's advice about suitable oral hygiene and the use of fluoride to strengthen your teeth.

Peroxide for mouthwash?

Q. What is the proper solution strength for hydrogen peroxide used as a mouthwash? My dental technician says the 3 percent solution will kill good bacteria. Should I dilute the peroxide and rinse afterward with plain water?

A. Hydrogen peroxide is an antiseptic. As such, it kills "good" germs as well as "bad." The manufacturer recommends it for external use only. However, some consumers use it as a mouthwash.

To answer your question, as you dilute the solution to save beneficial bacteria, you are simultaneously reducing its effectiveness against harmful microorganisms. However, because the mouth is a fertile ground for bacteria of all kinds, the daily use of even a 3 percent mixture is not likely to make much of a dent in the total bacterial count.

Although I believe you can safely use the product as you described, avoid swallowing it—and ask your dental professional for advice and comments.

33

Substance Abuse

Inhaled tobacco tars may be permanent

Q. How long does it take for the lungs to become completely clear of nicotine and tar once smoking has stopped in a 20-year user of cigarettes? I say it takes five years; my friend says three weeks.

A. Nicotine is cleared from the lungs in a matter of days. Tobacco tars are a different matter, however, because these dangerous substances are retained in pulmonary tissue for years, perhaps indefinitely.

Most smokers are addicted to nicotine. Therefore, after stopping smoking, their physical craving for cigarettes usually disappears in about two weeks. (Any continuing craving is probably the result of emotional factors—such as, the act of smoking tends to reduce tension and stress.)

In contrast, the harmful effects of the tars, such as emphysema and lung cancer, persist much longer.

Stop smoking regardless of symptoms from abstinence

Q. My friend has been a heavy smoker for over 30 years. She has attempted to quit smoking but develops asthma each time. Her doctor cannot explain this phenomenon. Can you?

A. I've been told by ex-smokers that they felt worse, coughed more and viewed life with less optimism when they gave up cigarettes. Other former smokers experience increased appetite, constipation, insomnia, nervousness and a host of other complaints that—fortunately—tend to disappear as the period of tobacco abstinence continues. I have never heard of asthma worsening in a new nonsmoker.

I've read that some asthmatics wheeze under stress; their breathing is worsened by anxiety and emotional pressure. Perhaps this is why your friend complains of asthma in the absence of tobacco smoke; the stress that was once relieved by nicotine now has "nowhere to go."

Regardless of the cause of this unusual reaction, your friend made an appropriate choice to stop smoking. Her doctor should be able to get the asthma under control with minimal effort, using sprays, pills or special nebulizer breathing treatments. In this case, the physician needn't explain the no smoking/asthma idiosyncrasy; all he must do is treat the asthma so that your friend won't have an excuse to return to cigarettes.

The role of nicotine in disease

Q. I was somewhat shocked by your position when a woman wrote you about her husband's cigar smoking, and you implied that only smoke that is purposely inhaled is dangerous. You failed to inform the public of the link between cigars, pipes and oral cancer. In fact, nicotine absorbed through the gums and cheeks is just as damaging to the heart and vascular system as nicotine that is absorbed through the lungs. Please be more consistent in your analysis of the harmful effects of tobacco smoke.

A. I certainly did not intend to imply that inhaling tobacco smoke is anything but harmful, be it from cigarette, pipe or cigar. However, I challenge you on two points.

First, until recently there have been no reputable studies of cigar or pipe smokers. By a process of extension, we all assume that the risks of these habits approximate those of cigarette smokers—but there is no proof of this. In fact, one report revealed the pipe smoker's risk of lung cancer falls between nonsmokers and cigarette smokers, closer to the former than to the latter. Therefore, while cigar smoke may be objectionable to those in the vicinity, and cigar smokers may develop mouth cancer, there are no scientific data indicating cigars to be as dangerous as cigarettes.

Second, cigar smokers do not, as a rule, inhale. Therefore, the amount of nicotine and tars absorbed through the lining of the mouth is imperceptible compared to the amount absorbed through the lungs, organs with enormously more surface area. Moreover, even were a cigar smoker to inhale (or possibly breathe in environmental smoke), he would have less exposure than the cigarette smokers who partake more often and inhale more deeply.

While I endorse the laudable sentiments in your letter, we have to remember that our blanket prejudices against pipes and cigars may be biased and improperly extrapolated from the wealth of information on cigarette smokers.

Now, permit me to editorialize on a recent finding: Nicotine has been shown to increase the risk of cancer. For those people who for decades have been blaming tobacco tars (or the increased incidence of lung cancer in cigarette smokers), this finding was a bombshell, because it cast serious doubt on the universal practice of using nicotine gum and patches for those people who are committed to giving up smoking.

Here is the rationale. The body ordinarily maintains an active immune vigilance against cancer cells. Once one abnormal cell is identified, the immune system destroys it. This event happens billions of times a year, because in the process of cell division, abnormal cells are going to form (and do) with statistical regularity. Therefore, our primary defense against cancer is a normal immune system that obliterates malignant cells in their infancy, before they have had time to grow, mature and spread.

I've always had difficult understanding why smoking leads to cancer. If the tars in smoke cause malignant changes in lung cells, so what? The immune system should take care of the problem by destroying these cells—as they do untold numbers of times in all of us, repeatedly, decade after decade.

The new study gives the answer. Apparently, nicotine interferes with the immune system's identification of malignant cells. So, it's not that tobacco tars cause lung cancer; it's a more subtle arrangement. Components of the tars (and, possibly, nicotine itself) reduce the body's watchfulness in ferreting out malignancy, so that—instead of being wiped out at an early stage—cancer cells hide, unidentified and unaffected, until they can grow and strengthen. In a sense, this is cellular terrorism, a perfect parallel to the world situation. These cancer cells, escaping recognition, are free to produce destruction and death. They are hidden, disguised, dedicated and committed to an unrealistic goal. (Can the body's malignant cells survive once the host has died? No.) This is identical to the perverted agendum of religious fundamentalists who believe that a program of destruction will somehow improve the quality of life for those who are left.

To return to the mundane, studies have yet to decipher whether nicotine supplements—even those used for short periods—do, in fact, increase the risk of consequences from smoking.

Stay tuned. I'll keep you posted.

P.S. Don't smoke.

Decision to quit crucial for success

Q. What's the latest word on methods to kick a nicotine habit? I'm especially interested in the patches, gum and inhaler. Do support groups help?

A. Nicotine addiction can be a difficult problem to overcome. But, studies show, the main consideration for smokers is not the nicotine, but the habit of smoking—the relaxing quality, the social applications, the smoke lazily rising to the ceiling, the taste. You who smoke know what I mean. No wonder, then, the nicotine patches, gums and inhalers have been far from outstanding cures for smokers who want to quit. The most crucial factor in breaking any habit is the desire to stop and the commitment to do so. Each of us has the power to decide to do something—or not to do it.

While this view may sound somewhat heretical, there is a profound truth to it. Once people make the decision to alter their behavior, they've achieved a major potential for recover.

In the case of smoking, nicotine craving can certainly be controlled by a variety of products. Self-help support groups are useful to many ex-smokers. Hypnosis and similar alternative options assist some individuals. But the real success stories concern the smokers who say: "I'm tired of this nonsense and I'm not going to do it anymore. Period." And they don't.

How to handle a tobacco-chewing husband

Q. My diabetic husband finally stopped smoking about two years ago and changed to chewing tobacco—which, in some respects, is worse for the family. I now have "spit cups" in every room. He spits in sinks and toilets. I think he sleeps with a wad in his mouth. He claims that chewing isn't as dangerous as smoking. Please set him straight.

A. Although chewing tobacco is statistically associated with an increased risk of mouth and throat cancer, it is safer than smoking, both to the user and to those in his environment. Nonetheless, it is an unattractive habit. I believe that the issue here is one of moderation. From your description, your spouse appears to be severely overdoing his habit. I think that he should limit his "chew" to a few hours a day and use nicotine gum or a nicotine patch as a supplement. Perhaps he will discover that his craving can be relieved by a safer and more acceptable substitute. Once he has had success with the gum/patch option, he might be inclined to discontinue tobacco products altogether. This would certainly be a welcome change from the standpoint of health and family acceptance. Show him my response to your letter and encourage him to consider the settlement I suggested.

Health risks of cigars

Q. Several months ago, my 42-year-old son gave up cigarettes—only to take up cigars. He smokes only one a day, after dinner. What are the differences in health risks between cigarettes and cigars?

A. The issue here is two-pronged—the length of exposure to tobacco smoke and the concentration of smoke reaching the lungs.

Heavy cigarette smokers (on the order of a pack or more a day) have a much more intensive and chronic exposure to tobacco smoke. This increased "dosage" clearly leads to illnesses, such as heart disease, lung cancer and various pulmonary disorders. This is unlike the pattern that pipe and cigar smokers exhibit. They typically smoke far less, and the health data confirm that there is a corresponding reduction in serious health consequences.

Also, such smokers are not inclined to inhale as deeply as do cigarette smokers.

While it's true that people who smoke cigars or pipes (or who "dip" or chew tobacco) have a higher incidence of mouth and throat cancer, this risk is surprisingly quite low.

Therefore, I am not inclined to indict your son or make an issue out of his daily cigar. Would he be better off stopping altogether? Yes, without a doubt. But I believe that he has chosen a slightly dangerous practice that is far less hazardous than using life-threatening cigarettes.

Having said this, I will now light up my second pipe of the day and enjoy something I know I shouldn't.

Excess alcohol not good for the heart

Q. My husband underwent coronary bypass surgery last year. Although he has been an alcoholic for years, he has never stopped drinking, and actually consumes more alcohol now than he did before the operation. He has a tendency to high blood pressure. I am concerned that his excessive drinking will lead to health problems.

A. As indeed it may. Excess alcohol consumption will adversely affect people in a number of ways.

Alcohol often raises blood pressure in hypertensive patients. Because this excess pressure causes dangerous heart strain, it must be brought under control. Therefore, people with hypertension must discontinue heavy drinking.

More important, alcohol itself is a cardiac depressant, meaning that it poisons heart muscle, leading to heart failure and various forms of irregular pulse. Alcohol also affects the brain and may eventually result in permanent brain damage, similar to Alzheimer's disease.

Both the liver and the pancreas can be harmed by too much alcohol, which can be doubly serious in people with underlying heart disease.

Finally, alcohol may increase serum cholesterol levels. This fat is the purported culprit in the age-related arteriosclerotic narrowing of arteries. This is precisely the complication your husband should be trying to avoid; his grafted coronary arteries have to stay open in order to supply oxygen to the heart muscle.

In short, your husband has many compelling reasons for moderating his alcohol consumption.

One last comment. Alcohol is damaging to the body only when consumed in large quantities. A modest daily allowance (3 ounces of spirits, two glasses of wine or about three beers) is not harmful. Unfortunately, alcoholics cannot moderate their drinking. Consequently, the disease of alcoholism is best treated with abstinence.

From your description, I gather that your husband is unable to control his drinking. The reasons for this are probably complex, but the end result—multiple organ damage—should motivate him to alter his behavior. He may need help stopping the booze.

To that end, you and his doctor may want to set up an intervention to address the drinking problem head on, steer your husband to the proper resources (detox and/or Alcoholics Anonymous) and provide the emotional support that he will need. Also, you might consider attending Al-Anon meetings, a worldwide group that gives guidance to people who have alcoholics in their lives.

Alcohol abuse in the elderly

Q. My 70-year-old father has been retired for five years. He admits to me that he is lonely and bored. He also reluctantly admits that instead of his traditional two cocktails before dinner, he may have three—plus a nightcap at bedtime. Sometimes, when I telephone him in the evening, he seems forgetful and vague. I'm worried that the alcohol may be to blame. How can I address this issue without precipitating a family crisis?

A. This is a difficult question about a potentially serious disorder.

Drinking problems in senior citizens are, by all accounts, under-diagnosed. After retirement, many seniors begin to consume more alcohol—as a function of depression, loneliness, boredom or a feeling of liberation—at precisely the time in their lives when they are least able to handle it.

For example, alcohol has a much great impact on older adults than it does on the younger, because of physiological changes. An enzyme in the stomach (gastric alcohol dehydrogenase) is reduced. This enzyme begins the metabolic breakdown of alcohol; if it is deficient, more alcohol enters the bloodstream and will affect the nervous system. Also, the liver is less able to detoxify alcohol as we age. Finally, women at all ages are less tolerant of alcohol.

The National Institute of Alcohol Abuse and Alcoholism (NIAAA) has defined moderate and acceptable drinking in adults over 65 as no more than one drink a day. One drink is equivalent to 1.5 ounces of spirits, a 12-ounce beer, or a 5-ounce glass of wine. While this guideline may be conservative, experts agree that the elderly should not exceed 14 drinks a week for men, seven for women, and no more than four drinks on one occasion for men (three for women). Finally, researchers have estimated that the prevalence of alcoholism is 10 percent to 14 percent in the general population. Alcohol abuse is up to six times more common in elderly men than in their female counterparts.

To a large extent, the effects of alcohol consumption depend on a person's health profile and the use of medications. A healthy 70-year-old man without hypertension, heart disease, liver disorders or prescription medicines can safely consume up to two standard drinks a day without adverse consequences. In contrast, a senior in poor health should markedly moderate his intake.

As a general screening test, many physicians use the CAGE questionnaire:

- Have you ever thought you should *cut down* on drinking?
- Have people *annoyed* you by complaining about your drinking?
- Have your felt *guilty* about your drinking?
- Have you ever had an *eye-opener* to get going in the morning?

Two or more positive answers raise suspicion of alcohol abuse.

The issue is further complicated by the difficulty of clarifying drinking patterns. One drink may lead to subjective interpretations. (I once had an alcoholic patients who admitted to "one" drink a day—an 8-ounce glass of vodka.) A pint of beer is more than 12 ounces and a "refreshed" glass of wine is closer to two glasses than one.

Finally, many heavy (or "problem") drinkers are either in a state of denial or object to being questioned about their consumption, believing that this is a "personal matter" which is no one else's business.

All of this discussion, although interesting and (I hope) informative, is a long-winded way of answering your question. With respect to your father, I suggest a low-key initial approach. Talk to him (during the day) about your concerns. Emphasize that you love him but are concerned about the health consequences of his habit. Involve your siblings if necessary. Discuss the situation with your father's physician, who should be informed of the problem and will be able to offer immeasurable assistance. In addition, the doctor can perform liver tests, define moderate drinking and—if necessary—intervene in a treatment program, such as Alcoholics Anonymous.

If your father did not have a drinking problem before retirement, he may simply have slipped into an unhealthful habit that the doctor can correct by educating him. On the other hand, if alcoholism is to blame, a more structured rehab plan may be necessary.

The relationship between reflux and alcohol

Q. My 62-year-old son has suffered with acid reflux for many years. Now, since he has taken Nexium for two years, he has been fine. However, his doctor has not arranged for any follow-up visits. My son takes his pills with beer and drinks all evening when he gets home from work. Is this dangerous? Should he recheck with his doctor?

A. First an editorial comment.

While I well understand your concern about your son's health, he is at an age where he has endorsed and followed a lifestyle over which you have no control. Maybe it's time to back off and stop making "mother noises." Let him finally make his own choices.

I am glad the Nexium cured his symptoms of acid reflux. I agree with you that he should have, at his age, a complete examination every year or two. And I believe that he could appropriately make a suitable appointment with his physician. If he chooses not to do so, it's his busi-

Learning More on the Web

As with so many health and medical issues, there is an abundance of information on the Web. However, use caution. Many Web sites for illnesses and diseases are commercial sites advocating specific medications or dietary supplements. The best Web sites are those recommended by your doctor. (An excellent one, for example, is the American Diabetes Association's Web site, www.diabetes.org.) No course of treatment should be started without consulting your own doctor.

ness (hence my comment about "mother noises.") It is not necessarily the role of his doctor to follow up, in the absence of continuing symptoms, if the patient fails to take responsibility for his own health issues. (Having said this, I am prepared for the certain criticism that it's the physician's obligation to "get patients in" for follow up. However, I maintain that intelligent adults need to take responsibility for their own health.)

Most pharmacies will not permit automatic refills of medicine if the prescription is more than a year old. Because your son is continuing the Nexium, the doctor will have to refill the prescription annually. This is an ideal opportunity for the physician (and your son) to be reminded that some doctor/patient interaction is needed.

The problem of the beer is more troublesome. Your son may be drinking excessively. (Perhaps this is the reason he avoids his physician.) Alcohol can worsen acid reflux and, as you know, damage many organs in the body. If he is consuming more than three or four cans of beer a day, he needs to cut back. This can be a daunting task for which he may require help and support. (Again, his physician is the logical resource to provide such assistance.)

Having pondered your situation, I believe that I have finally arrived at a solution that—although unusual—may solve your problem in a simple and direct fashion, without placing you in the role of the interfering mom. Call your son's doctor and tell him that 1) your son hasn't been examined in two years; 2) he is continuing the Nexium without the physician's direct input; 3) he is consuming an unacceptably large quantity of alcohol; and 4) "Don't tell him I called."

Yes, I know that this is funny business, but, under the present circumstances, it may be required. Then you can cut down on the "mother noises." Meanwhile, you've placed the problem directly where it belongs: between your son and his doctor.

Dealing with an alcoholic spouse

Q. I believe my husband has a severe drinking problem. He drinks more than a half-gallon of wine a day, indicating that it's good for his heart. During his "drinking time," he is verbally abusive, swears and is generally unpleasant. At other times, he looks and acts pretty good. How can I protect my family from his outbursts?

A. Your husband's drinking has progressed to the point where it is affecting your family. Therefore, I think it is fair to assume that he is an alcoholic. Once you are able to accept this probability, you are in a position to make important choices—and obtain needed help.

No person should have to live with an abusive spouse, whether the form of abuse is mental, emotional or physical. Many alcoholics behave normally when they are sober; however, after a few drinks, they may turn from a Mr. Jekyll to a Dr. Hyde, the literary character created by Robert Louis Stevenson—one minute a responsible citizen, the next a malevolent monster. Eventually, your husband may come to realize that his problem drinking needs to be addressed, and he will seek help.

Meanwhile, you don't have to put up with his antics.

First off, don't confront him when he has been drinking. Wait for a calm time, when he is sober and in a "normal" phase. Then quietly explain your concerns and indicate to him that although he is the only one who can take steps to deal with his overindulgence, you no longer feel obligated to ignore it. Do not—I repeat, do not—verbally label him an alcoholic to his face. This is a conclusion that he will make when he comes to grips with his problem. Begin the process of taking care of yourself and your family.

During such a (sober) give-and-take, you and your husband may be able to achieve an understanding. In my opinion, an avowal on his part to moderate his alcohol consumption is fruitless; he needs professional help and, probably, a 12-step program to begin and maintain sobriety. This is where your family physician would come in handy, both by assessing whether your spouse needs detoxification and putting him in touch with appropriate outpatient resources.

Now, to you. Check the yellow pages for an Al-Anon group in or near your community. This support group is composed of adults whose spouses or loved one abuse alcohol. You will gain tremendous support, encouragement and knowledge by attending Al-Anon meetings. Most important, you will learn ways to avoid "enabling" your husband to drink.

You do not need to be part of the problem.

Finally, if your husband is really abusive to you and/or your children, you can obtain necessary assistance from police, a counselor or a women's shelter. Or, if necessary, you could leave your residence and stay with a friend or family member until the situation has been resolved.

In your discussions with your husband, you can point out that alcohol is NOT good for his heart. In fact, it poisons the cardiac muscle when consumed in excess.

Alcoholism: a treatable disease

Q. Please define alcohol addiction. Our family has a history of alcoholism from grandparents to parents to my husband and now my children. My daughter doesn't believe alcoholism is inherited, since she claims she can go without a drink for two or three weeks at a time. Your comments?

A. Alcoholism comes in many shapes and sizes, all of which add up to an inescapable conclusion: dependence on the drug. The cause of alcoholism is unknown, although recent studies have suggested a genetic disposition. Alcoholics run the gamut, ranging from terminal skid row bums to successful and outstanding community leaders.

To a large degree, alcoholism is a disease of attitude and intent. Binge drinkers may only imbibe once in a while—but when they do, they drink to get drunk. Other alcoholics drink heavily and consistently, even though they manage (for varying periods) to keep their jobs and hold their families together. It may sound trite, but alcohol is vital to the alcoholic. He or she thinks about it—a lot. The alcoholic's life is more or less tuned to alcohol: when to drink and how much, how to get it and control it. Abstainers and social drinkers don't think twice about such issues; they can take alcohol or leave it.

Alcoholics often believe they are "entitled" to drink and that they don't have a "problem." However, sooner or later, the alcohol catches up to them, in the form of lapses in judgment, absenteeism, driving under the influence—or, eventually, physical consequences, such as liver inflammation, cirrhosis, pancreatic disease and intestinal bleeding. Alcoholics are judged not so much by the amount they consume as how they drink. I know an alcoholic who drinks only once a year—but alcoholically—to blackout.

Therefore, I disagree with your daughter. If, after two or three weeks of abstinence, she begins to "need" a drink, if drinking is a vital issue, she may be an undiagnosed alcoholic. This concerns me more so in light of the strong history of alcoholism in your family. In fact, given the high incidence of alcoholism in your family, I'd be amazed if your daughter weren't an alcoholic.

The only treatment for this disorder is sobriety. This can be tough, but there is ample help available. Twelve-step support groups such as Alcoholics Anonymous can be invaluable. Because I sense from your comments that there may be unrest in your family from issues pertaining to alcohol, I'm wondering if you and your daughter might consider trying Al-Anon, a program for people whose loved ones or families have a drinking problem. In such a nurturing and supportive environment, your daughter may be able to learn ways to deal with her father's (and sibling's) alcohol abuse, as well as to begin to confront her possible dependency. Support groups for alcoholics (AA), their families (Al-Anon) and their children (Alateen) are listed in the yellow pages of your telephone directory.

Rather than assuming the role of "bad guy" because of your concern about the family's drinking pattern, get your daughter to a meeting where she'll meet other people like her, and learn to come to grips with a common, mysterious and dangerous disease.

Addiction? Maybe not

Q. My 60-year-old mother has been addicted to tranquilizers for many years. Early on, her physician readily supplied her with prescription medications if she requested them over the telephone. He retired 10 years ago. Soon she found another doctor who also supplied her with unrestrained prescriptions. Eventually, he retired as well. Currently, my mother is seeing yet another doctor who continues the pattern of unrestricted prescriptions. At present, she is taking about 100 pills a week in the form of Percodan, Paxil and Elavil. The physician mails her prescriptions with the refill line left blank, upon receipt of her money. To avoid detection, she uses different pharmacies.

Dr. Gott, my mother lives on Social Security, does not work, has battled depression all her life and recently underwent brain surgery to remove a tumor. She and her impoverished current boyfriend, age 65, live on the third floor of a dilapidated office building in another state, a six-hour drive from me. He knows that my mother has a problem and has tried to regulate her habit and pill intake, but this practice has proved to be dangerous, because she becomes panic-stricken, uncontrollable and deceitful when her consumption falls below 50 pills a week. Today, she called my sister (who lives in the same city) and begged her to ask her own doctor for prescriptions. My sister refused, fortunately.

As you can see, the problem is distressing. Although the family wants desperately to help, we don't have a clue how to proceed. Of major concern are the legal implications concerning prescription fraud. We do not wish to see our poor, frail mother sitting in a jail cell because she illegally tempered with prescriptions in order to supply her narcotics habit. On the other hand, she is clearly out of control; her habit is affecting her health, her mental stability, her social well being and her financial status. What are our options?

A. This is, indeed, a complex and tragic situation and, while I have no ready answers, I would like to offer some suggestions.

Your mother is taking at least three powerful medications. (There may be others that you don't know about.) One of these—Percodan—is a narcotic. In most states, doctors cannot authorize refills of narcotics without actually writing out new prescriptions. Therefore, I doubt that her use of narcotics is excessive unless she 1) obtains such prescriptions or 2) forges old ones. To get to the bottom of this, I urge you to call her current primary care physician and explain your concerns. Perhaps your mother is suffering postoperative pain and really needs pain relief. If, on the other hand, she is obtaining narcotics illegally, the doctor needs to know so that he can work with the family (and other sources) to correct the problem.

The other two medicines—Paxil and Elavil—are antidepressants, not tranquilizers. Patients vary widely in their responses to these drugs; some folks need more than others do. Maybe, given your mother's long history of depression, she needs more than the average dose. For the purposes of discussion, let's assume that she should ideally be prescribed three Paxil tablets a day and two Elavil pills at bedtime. That's five pills.

Assuming that she follows the minimal regular Percodan schedule (one tablet every four hours), she could be taking at least six tablets a day; in severe pain syndromes, that figure could easily be doubled. Let's take a middle ground: nine tablets a day.

In your letter, you express concern that your mother is abusing her prescription drugs, because she is taking 100 pills a week. Divide that by seven. I get about 14 a day. Seems like a lot, but let's do the arithmetic: three Paxil, plus two Elavil plus nine Percodan equals 14 pills a day. This is high, but not excessive.

One could argue that your mother's health problems amply justify the use of these medications; in fact, she is not even exceeding a maximum limit. Possibly, when the dosages are reduced by family members and live-ins, she becomes panicky, uncontrollable and deceitful, because she is having to deal with pain and distressing depression. In short, the family's position vis-a-vis her ailments and drugs may be totally unfair; you may, in fact, be worsening the problem, not addressing or relieving it.

In contrast, if your mother is really abusing drugs, her doctor needs to know this and initiate the complex procedure of detoxification and long-term therapy.

A final comment: No one in his or her right mind would dismiss family concerns about an unhealthy member. We care about our loved ones and want the best for them. But, at times, we must also step back and obtain better perspectives. My analysis of your mother's "addiction" was not meant to trivialize her position or yours. But I did want to play "the devil's advocate," if you will, and I hope that my position will give you better understanding and insight. For a depressed, lonely, angry, panicky, financially-strapped woman with a previous brain tumor, 100 pills a week seems like a small price to pay for, at least, the perception of good health. Again, her physician is the resource to which you should turn to resolve your concerns. Doctors are, by and large, pretty good at this kind of thing.

Other Issues, Mundane & Not So Mundane

Choose properly fitted footwear to avoid corns and calluses

Q. I suffer from corns and calluses. Can you help me deal with this problem?

A. Corns and calluses are simply the accumulated buildup of hard, dry, dead skin that appears over pressure points between the bones of the feet and footwear. Calluses form in locations where the skin is irritated, usually from shoes that are too tight.

As the layers of dead skin enlarge, they exert pressure on the underlying tissue (usually the toe bones), leading to pain. Corns can also form between toes from ill-fitting shoes that squeeze the toe bones together.

These common afflictions are easy to cure.

Use fine sandpaper, an emery board or a pumice stone to reduce the size of the callus or corn. Sand away the dead skin until the soft, healthy skin appears. This will take care of the discomfort.

However, to prevent a re-accumulation, you'll have to modify your footwear. Choose shoes that are comfortable and don't pinch your feet. Using a combination of prudent sanding and appropriate shoes, you should be able to avoid the discomfort and nuisance of corns and calluses.

Ankle and lower leg swelling may be caused by medication

Q. Could Dilantin cause edema in my ankles and legs? I've been treated with Lasix, but the problem remains.

A. Many drugs cause fluid retention (edema), which can be seen as ankle and lower leg swelling. Although this is not a recognized complication of Dilantin (a medicine used to prevent seizures), it is a remote possibility. Dilantin can affect the skin (rash) and other organs, such as the bone marrow and liver; this could lead to edema in unusual cases.

I suggest that you bring this symptom to your doctor's attention. He or she may choose to discontinue your Dilantin (as a trial) or substitute another drug. I don't believe it makes much sense to use a powerful diuretic like Lasix to counteract the presumed effects of Dilantin. Moreover, you might be interested to learn that Dilantin reduces the effectiveness of many medications, Lasix included. Therefore, if your edema is, in fact, caused by Dilantin, Lasix is not a particularly suitable antidote. Ask your doctor about this.

Lipomas safe to ignore

Q. I'm a 43-year-old man who had a dozen lipomas removed from my abdomen a few years ago. Since then, about 35 more have appeared on my arms, back and chest. Is liposuction an option I should consider, and how do I prevent them from occurring in the future?

A. Lipomas are soft, painless, movable nodules of fat under the skin. They commonly form on the trunk, forearms and back of the neck, more frequently in men than in women. The cause is unknown, and there is no preventive therapy.

These benign, fatty tumors rarely cause symptoms and do not have to be removed unless they are cosmetically unsightly or become inflamed because of their location—under belt-lines or bra straps, for example. In very rare instances, lipomas can undergo malignant change; therefore, rapidly growing lesions should be biopsied or surgically excised.

Liposuction, a technique to vacuum out fatty material through a hollow needle, is a method frequently used to remove lipomas that are large or annoying, enabling patients to avoid major surgery. However, most people with lipomas prefer to leave them alone and forgo the discomfort and expense of surgical treatment. Follow your primary care physician's advice about whether you need surgery or liposuction.

Ninety-six-degree apartment okay with elderly friend

Q. I have a 76-year-old friend who refuses to use her air conditioner in order to save money. The temperature was 96 in her apartment last summer. She claims the heat doesn't bother her. I cannot convince her otherwise. Is she at risk?

A. Possibly. Elderly people can be intolerant to heat because of sluggish metabolism or physical inability to recognize that a problem exists. If, for example, she tends to be somewhat vague and occasionally confused, she may not be able to take the necessary steps—such as turning on the air conditioner—to avoid overheating.

On the other hand, people for centuries have survived without air conditioning. In hot climates, they reduce activity, wear light clothing, use fans and utilize a variety of techniques to remain relatively cool.

Consequently, I do not necessarily believe that your elderly friend is at risk. That decision is one more properly made by someone who is very familiar with her general health and living arrangements. My own prejudice would be to leave her alone, providing she is a reliable judge of whether or not the environmental temperature is a problem.

Of course, you may be dealing with a potential disaster if your friend is unable to compensate for the difficulties of living, such as adequate nutrition, appropriate hydration and ability to obtain help. In such a case, the cold winter weather would also be a problem.

Perhaps your best approach would be to enlist the aid of your friend's doctor or close family members. These resources could be very helpful. I agree with you that appropriate monitoring and supervision are necessary. My advice is: Get some help with this situation if you feel that your elderly friend is truly at risk living alone.

Fibromyalgia somewhat mysterious

Q. Can you define fibromyalgia and its prognosis?

A. Fibromyalgia, a poorly understood disorder of unknown cause, is characterized by muscular pain, stiffness and tenderness. The condition frequently affects anxious, tense and depressed young women. It may be related to stress and physical strain.

The diagnosis is made by excluding other, similar diseases, such as rheumatoid arthritis.

Fibromyalgia may suddenly disappear without treatment. Or it may become chronic, requiring long-term use of anti-inflammatory drugs, such as Motrin. Nonetheless, the prognosis is favorable because fibromyalgia does not affect vital organs and is not a hazard to health.

Liver cysts often benign

Q. I was found, on an ultrasound exam, to have three cysts in my liver. My doctor assures me they are benign and require no therapy. What steps should I take now? Could these cysts turn cancerous?

A. In general, liver cysts are benign and need no treatment. Providing they are filled with fluid and do not dramatically increase in size (as judged by serial ultrasound examinations), you can safely ignore them. They will not undergo malignant change. This is a broad answer to your question, however. You should follow your physician's advice with respect to further testing and monitoring.

Some liver cysts coexist with kidney cysts, which can become infected and cause renal damage. Again, follow your doctor's advice if he or she suggests that you have a kidney ultrasound.

Temperatures commonly run below "normal" in elderly

Q. I'm 78 and frequently take my temperature. In the morning, it ranges between 96 F and 97 F. In the evening, it is 98.1 F to 98.5 F. Is this pattern of concern?

A. Many people, especially the elderly, tend to run body temperatures a degree or so below "normal" (98.6 F). This is completely innocuous and does not reflect a health problem. (Also, the temperature tends to rise slightly as the day wears on and a person increases his or her activity.)

You don't say why you feel a need to check your temperature on a daily basis. Unless you are feeling ill and achy, you can forgo this practice and use your time for more enjoyable pursuits.

Clarify conflicting instructions with your doctor

Q. I have a skin problem for which my doctor suggested a nonprescription ointment, which works fine. However, he said to use it twice a day for two weeks; the instructions with the package say once a day for one week.

When there is a conflict between the instructions of a physician and the recommendations of a manufacturer, how does a patient resolve this inconsistency?

A. By checking with the doctor.

For perfectly valid reasons, a physician may choose to revise the instructions in the package insert. In your case, for example, the skin condition may be severe enough to justify an alteration in dosage. When it comes to over-the-counter skin creams, such a modification should not lead to any health problems. Nonetheless, when similar situations develop, a physician is the most reliable resource to resolve the apparent disagreement.

Staph infections all too common complications of surgery

Q. My husband had heart surgery last autumn and contracted a staph infection. How long will it take to clear? He has had a second operation to clean out the infection, yet it persists.

A. One of the most common complications of any surgery is infection, and one of the most common causes of infection is staphylococcus bacteria. These microorganisms are plentiful in our environment and reside on our skins. Fortunately, most types of staph are killed by modern antibiotics.

After certain surgical procedures, however, infection can be a real problem, because foreign substances—such as artificial joints, suture material and synthetic tissues—act as a focus from which bacteria spread. Once the foreign material becomes contaminated in the body, it is extremely difficult to sterilize.

Therefore, infections have to be drained, as in your husband's case. In particularly resistant infections, the prosthetic substance may have to be surgically removed and the remaining bacterial infection aggressively treated with intravenous antibiotics before a new, sterile prosthetic component can be implanted.

In simple terms, foreign material acts like a splinter: Once it is infected, it causes problems until it is removed.

I do not know how long your husband may experience difficulty; this depends on the extent of his infection, which antibiotics are used and what foreign substances were used in his surgery. For instance, if he had a valve replaced in his heart, he may well need another operation to remove it and replace it with a new one. On the other hand, the infection on wire sutures behaves in a somewhat different manner: It will eventually disappear with extended antibiotic therapy. Ask your husband's surgeon to review the case with you and to indicate what lies ahead.

Grapefruit, alone of citrus, may react with medications

Q. I'm having a running argument with a friend. I maintain that orange juice, unlike grapefruit juice, will not react with medications. She thinks I am crazy. Who is correct?

A. You are. Because grapefruit juice and many medicines are metabolized by a certain enzyme system in the body, the combination can set the stage for an interaction that can include drug toxicity. Other citrus products, including orange juice, do not cause such reactions.

Gallbladder patient only looks pregnant

Q. As a result of gallbladder surgery, my stomach is so big that I look eight months pregnant. My surgeon says to be patient; the situation will resolve over time. What's your advice?

A. Be patient, the situation will resolve over time. The effects of gallbladder surgery may take up to six months to return to normal.

Fungus infection commonly trivial, but not always

Q. I have an acquaintance who suffers from histoplasmosis. His therapy consists of IV's lasting several hours, several times a week. Since this causes inconvenience and hardship, is there any other method to treat this disease?

A. Histoplasmosis is a chronic infectious disease caused by a type of fungus. It can affect any organ, most commonly the lungs, liver, intestine and lymph nodes.

In many instances, the infection is trivial and patients recover completely without therapy. For example, in certain parts of the country (chiefly the Ohio and Mississippi river valleys), inactive histoplasmosis is often discovered by accident on routine chest X-rays.

However, the disease is not universally benign. It can be fatal in persons with immune deficiencies, such as AIDS. In these cases, the infection leads to disabling lung disease and other serious consequences.

The generally accepted therapy for histoplasmosis is the intravenous antifungus drug amphotericin B. If your acquaintance has so-called "disseminated" (advanced) infection, IV amphotericin B treatment, although expensive and inconvenient, will offer the best chance of cure.

Interferon drug of choice for liver inflammation

Q. What is the prognosis of someone with cirrhosis from hepatitis C? He cannot take interferon therapy.

A. Liver inflammation from the hepatitis C virus often progresses to cirrhosis (liver scarring) and eventual liver failure. The treatment of choice to prevent this serious eventuality is interferon, an anti-virus drug.

If a person cannot tolerate this therapy (because of an allergy to the drug, for instance), and the cirrhosis progresses, the prognosis is grim. Ultimately, such a person would be a candidate for a liver transplant.

Cause of essential tremor unknown

Q. Please explain essential tremor and outline what can either cure it or give relief. So far, my mother's doctor is puzzled and has only recommended sleeping pills to let her get some needed rest. I think she needs more.

A. I think she needs less.

Benign essential tremor is a fine-to-coarse slow tremor that affects the hands, head and voice. The cause is unknown, but the tremor is ordinarily worsened by stress, anxiety and the performance of skilled acts. It may be virtually absent at rest. Therefore, I'm confused about why your mother has difficulty sleeping.

I wonder if, in fact, she may have Parkinson's disease, which causes a similar tremor that is *worse* at rest and disappears during purposeful movements. I suggest that you take your mother to a neurologist for a diagnosis.

Essential tremor is incurable and common. It is usually treated with beta-blockers or mild antianxiety drugs, such as Xanax, whereas Parkinson's disease requires different, stronger medicine, such as Sinemet. Sleeping pills are, in my opinion, inappropriate therapy for benign essential tremor.

Vertigo cause for concern

Q. For the past few months, I have experienced attacks of sudden and prolonged vertigo that occur without warning or pattern. My doctor ordered a stress test and a cardiac ultrasound exam, both normal. Last week, I had a normal CT scan of my head. What is my next step? My life is totally disrupted. I no longer can drive.

A. Your doctor has appropriately addressed this serious problem by testing you for a cardiac disorder and a brain tumor. At this point, you need to be examined by an ear, nose and throat specialist. Most cases of vertigo result from tiny flakes of calcium that float in the fluid of the inner ear and occasionally irritate the nerves in that area, leading to vertigo. The otolaryngologist may be able to help you control your attacks by using head-repositioning maneuvers, or you may need to take medicine, such as Antivert, for relief.

Peripheral neuropathy has many causes

Q. Please provide information on peripheral neuropathy.

A. Peripheral neuropathy simply means that nerves in the upper or lower extremities are not functioning normally. Initially, this causes numbness and tingling of the hands or feet, which progress to pain and, finally, to weakness. Any factor affecting a nerve can lead to neuropathy. Thus, common causes include:

• Direct pressure—from carpal tunnel syndrome, herniated discs or a tightly fitting cast, for example.

• Exposure to cold or radiation, with attendant nerve damage.

• Poor circulation from blood clots, diabetes or nerve trauma.

• Drug reactions, especially to barbiturates and sulfa.

• Toxic reactions to lead, arsenic and other heavy metals.

• Carbon monoxide poisoning.

• Nutritional disturbances, particularly deficiency of the B vitamins.

• Malignancies, which can affect blood proteins, leading to nerve damage.

As you can see from this partial list, the diagnosis of peripheral neuropathy is a challenge that usually involves several medical specialists, such as internists and neurologists.

Treatment depends on the cause. There is no single "generic" therapy for everybody; each case requires individual attention.

Why do lupus symptoms worsen?

Q. Please clarify the difference between discoid lupus and systemic lupus. I was diagnosed in 1992 with discoid lupus but my symptoms have gotten worse, to the point of having seizures. I even ended up in intensive care.

A. Lupus is an autoimmune disease that causes chronic inflammation of many of the body's organs.

When it is confined to the skin, it is called "discoid" lupus. This affliction is associated with little more than recurring reddish, scaly patches that eventually scar, becoming a cosmetic problem. Internal organs are not affected. Discoid lupus is not a hazard to health.

On the other hand, lupus can affect the body as a whole. Called "systemic" lupus, this disorder often leads to arthritis, heart disorders, lung inflammation, kidney failure—and a rash resembling discoid lupus.

Because systemic lupus can be fatal if untreated (with cortisone and other drugs), doctors always must assume it is present when skin lesions appear.

Therefore, discoid lupus is a "diagnosis of exclusion": Once blood tests and biopsies fail to reveal internal, widespread disease, physicians can conclude that discoid, not systemic, lupus is the culprit. Discoid lupus is treated with steroid creams.

Ordinarily, discoid lupus does not progress to systemic lupus. Thus, because of your troubling comments about seizures, I am concerned that the lupus may have affected your brain, a consequence of protein abnormalities in the blood stream that are common in systemic lupus.

The worst scenario is that your doctors missed the diagnosis of systemic lupus years ago by not testing you. They may have incorrectly assumed you had discoid lupus, when—in fact—you didn't. Now, you're left with some serious consequences of a late diagnosis.

The best scenario is that the discoid lupus and seizures are unrelated. Of course, seizures are a serious affliction that require treatment with anticonvulsant medications, such as Dilantin.

In my opinion, you need a thorough examination and testing, under the supervision of an internist and a neurologist. At the very lest, you need a CT or MRI scan of your brain and blood tests to check for abnormal proteins and internal damage. Ask you doctor about this.

Balance problems common in the elderly

Q. Please comment on the distressing phenomenon of imbalance and poor equilibrium in the elderly. I'm age 85 and in reasonably good health, but I often find myself off balance when I suddenly turn, walk on an uneven surface, look over my shoulder when I ride a bicycle or get out of bed in the dark. Is there anything I can do to reduce my risk of falls?

A. Poor balance is often an inescapable consequence of the aging process. There are many reasons for this—and, as the medical profession terms it, the disorder is "multifactorial."

For instance, vision is a factor—especially in dim light—because we don't see as well as we did as youngsters. Also, our reflexes slow down. Watch a child walk a balance beam. His or her proprioceptive reflexes are astonishing. You can barely perceive any effort to maintain balance, unlike an elderly subject who, by the time he senses an imbalance, is already on his way to falling or stumbling. In addition, the connections between brain and muscles slow with age, so we seniors have difficulty responding actively when the brain tells us to do so. Finally, there are other considerations, such as weakness from stroke or deconditioning, poor brain perception of motion and body position, distractibility, underestimation of risk (when walking on slippery surfaces, for example) and poor hand-eye coordination.

Needless to say, my brief review barely covers the basics. The long and short of it is that senior citizens lose balance skills, the degree of which depends on age, underlying illnesses and a complicated interplay of several factors.

The bad news is that, unlike a young person who falls, the elderly are far more likely to fracture a hip, a leg or a spine. So, improving balance (or leaning to live with a deficiency) is paramount. Here's what I counsel my elderly patients to do:

1) Remain active. Any physical exercises that are carried out regularly will not only aid the cardiovascular system, but will also keep muscles and nerves in shape.

2) Check with your doctor if your balance suddenly deteriorates. This phenomenon could reflect an underlying disorder, such as Parkinson's disease or mini-strokes, which should be addressed.

3) Regularly stress yourself with balance challenges. Using appropriate safety measures (such as being next to the bed), stand on one foot while putting on your hose or trousers. At times, for no particular reason, see how long you can stand on one leg; try to improve the length of the interval.

4) Anticipate. Look where you are walking. Learn to judge (and avoid) risky area, such as ice, puddles and ruts. Let your eyes tell you what path to follow. Ask your doctor to prescribe medication if you have arthritis, and the pain disrupts your balance.

5) Accident-proof your home. This means ridding the house of scatter rugs and waxed surfaces. Use ample night lights. Make sure that you have railings (on stairs), grab-bars (in bathrooms) and no trash (or "collectibles") that could cause you to trip. Use a cane for balance, if necessary.

6) Consider a lifeline. Known by other names, this is basically a telephone service that connects you to a responsible resource, such as a hospital. You wear an activator on a necklace. If and when you need help, you push a button to activate the system. Such a device, if used properly, will virtually guarantee that, should you fall, you will receive prompt treatment, rather than lying in your kitchen or driveway for hours on end after a fall.

7) Sign up for any formal balance programs in your community. In

my town, the hospital physical therapy department offers an extensive program, using a computer and other techniques, which my patients have highly recommended. If approved by a physician, Medicare will usually cover a balance program.

In summary, balance problems are common in the elderly, who may suffer dangerous consequences. Help is available. An integrated approach (self-help plus balance program) is often necessary to compensate for this common, even universal disorder.

Dealing with a mother's stress

Q. My mother, 78, is taking care of my father who has serious heart problems. The help she gives him—and the constant criticism he returns—are stressing her out. I suggested having a care worker come relieve her of some responsibilities but—being a workaholic—she is dedicated to my father, come what may.

> 66 The long and short of it is that senior citizens lose balance skills, the degree of which depends on age, underlying illnesses and a complicated interplay of several factors. 99

Unfortunately, she also has medical problems. These include insomnia, crying spells, earaches, nausea, blurry vision, and exhaustion. She has had a comprehensive medical work-up and was told of temporomandibular joint syndrome (TMJ). Everything else checked out. She has not responded to over-the-counter remedies. How can she get relief?

A. From the comments in your letter, which I have shortened for practical purposes, I am convinced that your mother is suffering from symptoms that are the immediate result of the stress she is experiencing. Workaholic or not, nobody can provide 24-hour ongoing medical care to a loved one who constantly grouses and complains.

Therefore, your mother needs help, whether or not she is willing to accept it. This issue should be taken up by your family physician, but I'd be surprised if he didn't echo my sentiments, meet with your mother, and say something like: "You are doing a fabulous job taking care of your husband. However, all humans have their limits. You have exceeded yours. Consequently, I insist that you allow us to obtain additional help in the home. This will enable you to have valuable time for yourself, while

Changes in the Normal Ranges

Q. I am a victim of what I call the "changing playing field." More people (and I) are being diagnosed with diabetes, high cholesterol and hypertension. Twenty years ago, a normal fasting blood sugar was considered to be 120 milligrams or less (the limit is now 110 mg), a normal cholesterol was 250 mg (now the limit is 200 mg), a normal blood pressure was 150/90 (now the limit is 120/80). These shifts mean that more people are falling out of the "normal" range, require prescription drugs and have their lives upset. And the drug companies are laughing all the way to the bank. What do you think?

A. I can certainly appreciate your frustration. To be judged suddenly as abnormal based on new limits is off-putting to say the least, not only to patients but to doctors as well.

Years ago, I was grateful if my diabetics had fasting blood sugars in the 120s, relieved when my patients' cholesterols dropped to 225, ecstatic when my hypertensives maintained blood pressure of 140/90.

Now, as you confirm, profound changes are taking place. I do not believe that these alterations are driven by the pharmaceutical industry, however. Rather, these new guidelines are the result of careful medical studies geared to answer the question: Are our recommendations for sugar, cholesterol and blood pressure valid and appropriate? This new information was developed to help patients maintain good health and avoid unnecessary consequences, not to anger and frustrate the public. The normal limits of behavior and lab testing constantly undergo change and will continue to do so. Let me give you an outrageous example of this.

I grew up in Westchester County, a suburb of New York City. In those days, many men commuted to the city by train. It was common practice to have a "two martini" lunch. Then, at day's end, they would fill the trains' cars for a "couple of pops." Upon returning home, they would enjoy cocktails before dinner (to "unwind"), followed by wine at dinner and a nightcap at bedtime.

This was considered to be normal, "social" drinking.

We now realize that this level of alcohol consumption was more than dangerous: It was a first-class ticket to permanent liver damage and other significant health problems. Thanks to many medical studies, we now know that the limit for healthful drinking is four ounces of spirits (or the equivalent in wine or beer) per day. Did this new criterion upset the commuting businessmen? Without a doubt. But, as a result, many adults have drastically modified their alcohol intakes. Now, thanks to these studies, the incidence of "suburban cirrhosis" has fallen.

Therefore, I believe that as limits are lowered—even for sugar, cholesterol and blood pressure—we all profit. Do the drug companies profit as well? Surely. But the real object of the new guidelines is to improve the longevity and quality of life for the public. So, my advice to you is: Don't view yourself as a victim; consider yourself fortunate. Follow your doctor's advice and—above all—be ready for future changes in the definition of what is "normal" and acceptable.

knowing that your husband is well cared for. In addition, such a health professional will be able to carry out mundane everyday tasks, permitting you to provide more personal and intensive support. In short, supplemental assistance will reduce your stress level and enable you to be more effective doing what you do best. I'll make the necessary telephone calls right now, to authorize home health care."

In my experience, such an approach—if endorsed by the family—could have phenomenal results. In particular, your mother must be told that as she becomes more stressed as sole caregiver, the quality of her life—and her care—will deteriorate, turning a difficult situation into a life-and-death crisis.

Treatment of schizophrenia

Q. Last year my wife's doctor told me she was schizophrenic. It's making me a nervous wreck, because—among other symptoms—she's become fixated on finances: Everything she talks about relates to money, money, money. Her mother is like that, too. Is this disease inherited? Is lying a lot typical? What can I do to keep my own sanity?

A. Schizophrenia is a serious mental disorder characterized by extreme disorganization of thoughts and feelings, resulting in delusions, lack of concentration, loss of touch with reality and inability to think or act normally. Although "schizophrenia" means "split personality," this description is inaccurate; despite popular belief, such "splits" are extremely rare. No one knows the precise cause of this disease although research suggests that both a biochemical factor and heredity may be involved. What is known is that schizophrenia is an illness and is not caused by outside events, although it can be triggered or worsened by stress. Schizophrenia can be helped with medicine administered under the supervision of a psychiatrist; psychotherapy also can be helpful. Hospitalization may be necessary if the person can't function, resists needed treatment or requires comprehensive care. Before release from a hospital, patients enter a rehabilitation program that reacquaints them with the everyday skills, tasks and pressures they may face outside.

Spouses and other relatives of schizophrenics often can cope more easily with the disease by joining local support groups, in which members discuss problems and offer emotional support and practical advice.

Spousal abuse is inexcusable

Q. After only three years of marriage, my 60-year-old retired husband chose to cheat on me with a younger woman. I won't bore you with the details of anonymous phone calls, his staying out late, the fact that I am depressed and angry or that I have repeatedly broached the subject with him—to no avail. He claims that he has every right to "fool around" and has, more than once, threatened me physically. Our marriage is in shambles, and I fear he may harm me. What can I do?

A. Although I am not a trained social worker, I am compelled to respond to your question with some common sense. You have many options that range from leaving him immediately to staying married and learning to accept his infidelity. I am especially concerned about the real chance of physical abuse and strongly suggest that you obtain professional help.

First, if your husband threatens you, call the police. Spousal abuse is totally inappropriate; no woman or man should put up with it. Second, hook up with a marriage therapist who will be your advocate and help you decide how best to proceed, at the same time assisting you in handling your depression and anger. Third, make an appointment to see a good divorce lawyer who can analyze this unfortunate situation and advise you about your legal rights.

Part of your psychological upheaval may be due to your feelings of abandonment and helplessness. But this needn't be. There are resources out there—such as women's support groups—to help you explore all your options, keep you safe and get your life back on track. In my view, the worst thing you could do is nothing, an unrealistic choice, given your marriage situation. Getting all your ducks in a row will empower you, increase your self-confidence and prove to your wandering and abusive husband that you are to be taken seriously. Regardless of what action you eventually choose, there is no excuse for abuse. He needs to learn that.

35

Managing Health Care Costs

The problems with American health care

Q. I have had experiences that give me new insight into this country's health care industry.

I frequently suffered from shoulder dislocations during my childhood and teens. Although the situation was painful, I soon learned that if treated immediately—by "popping" it back into place—I could avoid serious discomfort. Consequently, my dislocations in those days were successfully reduced by simple traction.

It happened again when I was 42. Unfortunately, I was alone and couldn't correct the problem, so I drove one-handed to the nearest emergency room. First, the doctor examined me, then obtained an X-ray. Satisfied that no fracture was present, he applied traction and the shoulder returned to normal. The bill was a few hundred dollars.

This year, at age 60, the dislocation happened again. My wife drove me to a nearby hospital ER, where I had to wait while insurance information was filed. I was examined by two nurses and, eventually, had X-rays. While I was waiting (by then about three hours), the shoulder went into spasm, causing the most discomfort I have ever experienced. I was given narcotics, hooked up to an oxygen saturation monitor and given an injection that put me out. I woke up with my shoulder in place but with a bill for $2,500.

This experience scandalizes me, yet I know where it comes from: health care providers' potential liability, the need to justify every step and procedure in the treatment program, and the use of anesthesia. Americans want no pain. If it hurts, they look for someone to sue. Americans demand complete healing. Never mind if a transplant costs half a million dollars and staves off death only for weeks.

As an attorney, I can understand trial lawyers' horror at legislation that caps malpractice pay-outs, but no one should use an injury to get rich—not the injured, and certainly not their lawyers. Also, I'm concerned about the public's perception of death. Actually, this is merely a "graduation" to the next level of eternal life, a form of ultimate healing, if you will. I don't want to join a society—our society—that says "do whatever it takes; just keep me alive."

I really worry about this because it doesn't make sense to spend, say, hundreds of thousands of dollars on myself just to keep me half-alive in a hospital bed for a few months. I blame physicians for not having the sense to say "enough is enough."

We need our elected representatives to act with sensible, evenhanded laws; judgment awards could return to reasonable levels, malpractice rates would substantially diminish, and experimental or heroic end-of-life treatments must be subsidized in some say (without all of us paying through increased health insurance premiums).

I don't have all the answers to these issues. I wish I did.

A. You raise several crucial points in your letter, which I have had to edit because of space restrictions. I agree with you about capping malpractice awards, helping the public to accept death as an unavoidable part of life, and reorienting doctors in finding a better way to integrate new and experimental surgical and medical therapies into health coverage.

Thank you for writing. I don't have any easy answers either.

Getting care when money is tight

Q. I read a column of yours today with disbelief and some amusement. Do you really think people can take you seriously when you make statements such as "most physicians and hospitals are willing to accept patients who are financially in trouble"? You've got to be kidding!

A. In my experience, most reputable hospitals and physicians are willing to provide a certain amount of free work to those patients who cannot pay and who are not covered by Medicare or welfare programs.

The trick here is to be up-front right from the beginning. Doctors and hospitals must be informed of patients' financial problems early on, so that the health-care providers aren't stuck holding onto a big, unexpected bill after the fact. This is, I can assure you, a frustrating and maddening experience.

In addition, once medical personnel are aware of the situation, they can certainly enlist the aid of social workers, who can often obtain federal or state financial assistance.

OK, I know that there are exceptions to this scenario. And, obviously, there are limits. Public charity hospitals are becoming relics of the past, and no hospital or doctor can afford to take care of nonpaying patients exclusively. But I stand fast.

What's more, I'll go one step further by stating that any doctor of hospital that doesn't perform at least some pro bono work ought to be drummed out of the corps.

Look, I wouldn't want my son to be deprived of necessary medical attention if he were in a far-off, uncaring city. So, if someone in need of help in my community comes to the office for medical care—and tells me he can't pay—what am I going to do, kick him out? Is that what medical practice is all about? I'll tell you, my friend, when that time comes, I'll take down my shingle.

In my view, doctors and hospitals have a humanitarian responsibility to care for those in need; when we stop providing this service, the health care industry will not only lose its luster but will cease attracting qualified and dedicated workers. The very purpose of doctoring will evaporate. The end.

Medical rationing here to stay

Q. I believe that today's medicine is based solely on the almighty dollar. Before restrictions on expenditures, patients could be thoroughly tested in advance of prescribing or operating. Now, with HMOs, tests are avoided at all costs because they mean a smaller bottom line and smaller year-end bonuses for the administrators. Better to treat a presumed problem, hoping for success. If it doesn't succeed, the patient is dubbed a hypochondriac and will just go away.

A. Backward step or not, health maintenance organizations are not only here to stay, but will probably become more important in whatever health plan is ultimately adopted by Congress. Although some of your viewpoint (e.g. testing versus profits) is correct, you need to realize that the true "bottom line" is a primary concern that has far-reaching—and unnerving—consequences. It seems that everybody running HMOs is intent on designing a system that will cost less and enable the CEOs to collect enormous and undeserved profits.

Proposed Insurance Lets Patient Do the Rationing

After having been shot in the head by a legless man whom she was attempting to rob, a pregnant 28-year-old woman and mother of four was rushed to Highland General Hospital in Oakland, Calif., where she was declared brain dead. Doctors decided, through advanced life support, to keep the woman "alive" until her baby was mature enough to be delivered. Experts anticipated this would be approximately 15 weeks, until the fetus reached 32 weeks gestation. The financial cost was estimated to be $3,200 a day; the emotional cost is incalculable. Such a bizarre medical case highlights the many complex medical and ethical problems burdening the American health-care system.

In the April 25, 1993, issue of the *New York Times*, Dr. Robert Levine, a Connecticut neurologist, began his "Viewpoint" essay as follows: "Whatever health reforms come out of Washington, they won't succeed unless they recognize that our resources are finite and rationing of care is necessary. One powerful way to do that is a new kind of insurance allowing policyholders to choose in advance the medical services they want and do not want."

Levine then described the concept of "discretionary insurance," in which each citizen is offered a wide variety of insurance programs from which he or she picks a plan that is highly individualized.

For example, one patient might choose to exclude certain cancer treatments, whereas another person could define what coverage would be available for a major stroke. Age would certainly be a factor— for instance, the inappropriateness of coverage for renal dialysis in the elderly.

Although it appears to be a cumbersome and complicated solution to the problem, discretionary insurance does have one striking advantage: It gives each of us choices.

Of course, patients who sign living wills and insist on "Do Not Resuscitate" orders are making choices, too. But Levine's system transcends such generic options because particular decisions about specific situations would be mandatory. Thus, the patient becomes the rationer of his or her own health care. Those who refuse respirator treatment or feeding tubes—or even intravenous fluids—would get what they want, with a corresponding reduction in their insurance premiums.

Discretionary insurance would be an administrative nightmare, no doubt. It's probably not practical. And, really, how many people could possibly be sophisticated enough to be able to define exactly which treatment they want and which they don't? Nonetheless, Levine concludes that the idea is workable. I'm not sure, but I agree that it must be seriously considered. Because any federal program of health insurance is bound to include arbitrary rules and regulations (thereby virtually rationing health care by fiat anyway), a privately funded system based on consumer preferences may be the smart choice. As an example, if coronary bypass surgery after 75 were excluded, the enormous savings could be directed toward covering more promising therapy of other diseases in younger subscribers.

Personally, I'd have a hard time deciding the precise circumstances under which I'd accept—or reject—high-tech treatment. I know I don't want to be kept alive artificially without a reasonable likelihood of survival, but I might want a chance to live if temporary life support could tide me over an acute illness. Of one thing I'm certain, however. I'm willing to exclude this life support if I were brain dead from a head wound suffered in a botched burglary.

I cannot predict what effect this mentality will ultimately have on the medical system as a whole—but, I suspect, the effect will not be positive, because patients are going to have to learn to live with medical rationing of one kind or another.

Welcome to health care in the 21st century.

Non-MD assistants offer good care, save money

Q. When I called my gynecologist for an annual Pap test, I was told that all such tests are now being performed by a nurse practitioner, not the physician. This upset me. My doctor is now "too busy" to see me.

A. Don't take it personally. More and more routine testing is being carried out by well-trained non-MD personnel such as nurse practitioners and physicians' assistants. Blood tests, cardiograms, Pap tests, sigmoidoscopies and minor surgical procedures are now performed routinely in some practices by professionals who are not physicians. The doctors can then devote their attention to more serious issues, such as sick patients and challenging health matters. I encourage you to have your annual Pap test by the nurse practitioner; you might be quite surprised and delighted at how gentle and efficient she is.

Doctors need to address the issue of drug costs

Q. Are physicians ever aware of the retail prices of the drugs they prescribe? My doctor is always astounded at the cost of my medications.

A. Doctors rarely discover the retail costs of medicines because—until recently, when this became a national problem—they seldom asked. Also, there is considerable variation in price from one pharmacy to another. Thus, physicians may be genuinely surprised when patients complain bitterly about how expensive medications are to purchase.

Patients need to address the issue by asking their doctors to be mindful of price. For those patients whose insurance plans do not cover the costs of drugs, the financial burden may be fearsome unless their practitioners are alerted to this potential problem.

Although substituting a less expensive drug may not always be appropriate, the use of cheaper equivalents or generics is usually advisable. For example, when it comes to antibiotics, the less expensive amoxicillin (or just plain penicillin) may be just as effective as the new synthetics, which can cost as much as $8 a pill.

Therefore, I urge patients to work with their doctors to achieve a suitable balance between price and effectiveness.

Make lifestyle changes to save on prescriptions

Q. Did you catch the "60 Minutes" segment about senior citizens having to travel to Canada to purchase affordable medications? This seems to be an outrageous example of intimidation by the pharmaceutical industry. Your comments?

A. I, too, was appalled to learn that the prescription bills for some senior citizens are so high that these patients have chosen to travel to

Canada just to obtain affordable medication. Surely, this difficult problem must be addressed by the appropriate legislative authority.

However, as in any troublesome issue, there are two sides. The woman interviewed by Mike Wallace admitted to taking several medications, some of which were prescribed for her high blood pressure, another for stomach upset and yet another drug for anxiety. Moreover, the woman was grossly overweight.

Most physicians are aware that some of their colleagues overprescribe to beat the band. Not only is this practice harmful (because many drugs interact adversely and often cause serious side effects), but it is unnecessarily expensive, too. Perhaps if patients saddled with huge medication bills were to discuss the situation with their doctors, the total amount of prescriptions could be substantially reduced, leading to less of a financial burden.

For example, the Mike Wallace interviewee had been prescribed relatively expensive Prilosec for her stomach. Would a cheaper over-the-counter substitute, such as Zantac or Pepcid, be just as effective at a fraction of the cost? Moreover, I don't prescribe antianxiety medicine to the elderly to be used daily. A much safer program would include using such a drug only on occasion.

Finally, we need to ask the obvious question: Can seniors contribute significantly to their health by making lifestyle changes, in contrast to relying on the pharmaceutical industry for a quick fix? As I mentioned, the woman interviewed was morbidly obese. Most lay people know that obesity contributes to hypertension and heart disease. Why, then, did the woman choose to avoid exercise and a weight-loss diet? If she shed 40 or 50 pounds under medical guidance, her blood pressure would probably drop like a stone; she could reduce or eliminate some of her prescription drugs, leading to a significant reduction in her bills.

Medication is occasionally lifesaving; certainly, it frequently improves quality of life and independence. But despite the wonders of modern pharmacology, each of us has a vital role to play in maintaining our own level of health. The woman on "60 Minutes" should work harder on her health and complain less about the cost of drugs to counteract the consequences of her bad habits.

For their part, doctors have an obligation to prescribe sensibly and stop engaging in what some experts have dubbed "polypharmacy."

As far as the drug companies are concerned, they ought to market medicines in the United States at prices similar to those in other countries.

Doctors set fees in obscure ways

Q. How does a doctor figure out what to charge? Has someone made up a chart of fees? Is there any way to contest a doctor's fee? We were charged over $1,000 for 10 stitches in our daughter's lip and eyelid. When we told the clinic we thought $600 was a more reasonable charge, they said OK—as long as we paid it in one lump sum. There was no way we could do that, so now we have to pay them $5 a month for the next 18 years.

A. Although there is no "chart of fees" for doctors, there are customary and prevailing charges for each part of the country. These vary from speciality to speciality.

If you believe that you have been overcharged by a doctor, consider the following steps:

• First, find out from other doctors in your community (or from the county medical society) if the fee exceeded the customary charge.

• If it did, request that the doctor reduce his fee, accept insurance reimbursement as full payment or accept Medicare assignment for full payment.

• If the doctor refuses, make a formal written complaint to the ethics committee or board of censors of your county medical society.

The committee will investigate your complaint and, if the doctor's fee was excessive, pressure the doctor to reduce the fee. This usually works.

However, if you are still dissatisfied, your final step is to seek legal counsel.

As a general rule, a doctor sets fees according to his or her evaluation of what a service is worth (based on time spent and skill required) and what his colleagues charge for similar services. The process if a mystical one, and I'm not sure that I myself understand it completely.

Malpractice insurance issues

Q. What is malpractice insurance and why do doctors and hospitals have to pay such high premiums for coverage?

A. Malpractice insurance, a necessity in today's litigious society, is purchased by doctors, nurses, hospitals and health-care facilities—as well as increasing numbers of attorneys and other professionals. If a patient (or a client) claims that the services he or she received were wrongful, deficient or below a certain standard of care, a lawsuit may result.

The plaintiff can sue for millions of dollars to cover pain, loss of income, damages, ill health and so forth.

Once presented with a lawsuit, the defendant turns to his malpractice insurer to protect him and—if necessary—pay all or part of a court-ordered judgment (or, as is commonly the case, a settlement). Without such insurance, the defendant would have to pay all legal expenses and awards out of pocket, a devastating and ruinous blow.

Malpractice insurance is like homeowners'

> 66 As a general rule, a doctor sets fees according to his or her evaluation of what a service is worth (based on time spent and skill required) and what his colleagues charge for similar services. 99

insurance: You may never need it, but when you do, it's nice to have.

To a large degree, insurance companies set their premiums in relation to risk. For example, obstetricians/gynecologists who deal with high-risk pregnancies pay much more (tens of thousands of dollars) than do general medical practitioners (several thousand dollars). This pattern is changing, however. As you have probably read, Ob/Gyn specialists in some states, notably Pennsylvania, are being charged hundreds of thousands of dollars in premiums, causing many of them to leave the state or trim their practices. Also, family physicians' premiums have more than quadrupled in the past two years, while HMOs and Medicare annually reduce allowable fees.

Doctors and hospitals now pay more in insurance premiums because patients are more likely to sue, and dollar judgments have increased over the years. As you might expect, these added costs are, when possible, passed on to patients, thereby inflating the cost of an already burdensome system of medical care.

There are no easy answers to this increasingly troublesome problem. However, to control burgeoning insurance costs, some experts have urged that legislators pass laws to cap malpractice awards—primarily the "pain and suffering" provisions. (California has had such a statute on the books for years and it works well.) However, this and other solutions seem a long way off to the physicians, surgeons and hospitals who live in constant dread of being sued.

It's about service, not wealth

Q. I recently received a bill from a doctor for a "telephone consultation." My insurance won't pay for it. What gives?

A. "What's in it for me?" seems to have become the rallying cry of the new millennium. Fewer people are willing to perform services for others, unless doing so might help them get money or power.

I recently received a bill from my attorney for various legal matters. The statement included charges for telephone calls that were billed in tenths of an hour. I calculate that to be six minutes. (Thanks, but I was never great at arithmetic.) I couldn't remember having spoken to the lawyer for as long as six minutes. But, of course, I didn't time our infrequent conversations with a stopwatch, either. Since legal counsel costs me $200 an hour, these damned telephone charges added up. In fact, they added up to a figure I calculated to have exceeded any practical benefits of legal consultation.

I wouldn't have objected to token charges—say, two or three dollars per call—for the type of informal advice given, but I objected to the senseless and pseudo-scientific ring of the transaction. A tenth of an hour. Really.

I object even more to this practice when I hear that some doctors, too, are doing it. True, physicians spend a lot of time on the telephone. At the end of a working day, I am deluged with a lengthy list of callbacks to make. In addition, I am in the habit of picking up the phone to inquire how a patient is faring, especially if she or he is elderly and lives alone. The telephone comes with the territory. It is (literally) a physician's lifeline. When it stops ringing, there's major trouble ahead.

However, I do not choose to demean myself by charging for telephone calls. I am convinced that practitioners who give into this penny-ante urge are doing themselves, their patients and their profession no favors. For lawyers, it may be ethical and routine; for doctors, it's just plain tacky.

There's talk these days about how medical practice has lost its allure and pleasure. Maybe it has. M.D.s worry about many problems and, unfortunately, (with the advent of managed care) these problems are often financial. Consequently, medicine has certainly lost much of its luster—if money is the purpose of doctoring. This is reflected by the fact that fewer medical school graduates are entering the field of solo practice, preferring large, multi-specialty groups instead. Solo practice is viewed by young doctors as being less financially rewarding.

However, the real luster of medicine isn't gold. It never has been. The basic and compelling attraction of medical practice has always been service—or should be. And a dedication to service is about as popular among many modern doctors as emptying bedpans.

This trend is a shame. Some time ago—certainly within my memory—practitioners expected and were willing to provide free care for needy patients. This was a principle upon which the great medical centers were based. Doctors examined and treated people for whom no fees were billed and none collected. Well-known practitioners routinely donated several days a month to working, without reimbursement, on the wards of city and charity hospitals. They did this for a variety of reasons: a sense of community responsibility, a willingness to pay back their mentors—most important, it felt good. Such service gave renewed meaning and significance to hard-earned skills.

Few, if any, doctors do it today.

In my opinion, a major portion of this new century's disillusioned doctors has lost interest because the service aspect of medical care has become a poor cousin to financial considerations. More practicing physicians need to justify their careers solely on the basis of income. It's a no-win situation. Wealth isn't what it's about; service is—or, as one of my colleagues succinctly concluded, "It ain't what you got, but what you give."

"What's in it for me?" is the insistent question asked by attorneys, teachers, businessmen, politicians, and money-minded yuppies. But such a question will not improve medical care, the status of the profession, the satisfaction of being a doctor. If, for a change, M.D.s could set an example, we might reverse a trend.

"What's in it for them?" would be a more crucial question for the physician with respect to his patients. Then, perhaps, the tenth-of-an-hour telephone charge would finally be exposed as an obscenity more in keeping with the pecuniary professions than with the healing arts.

Next, we can address the problem of uppity, pompous and reactionary medical writers who yearn to turn the clock back.

36

End of Life Issues

Wishes should be followed

Q. I am 88, a great-grandmother and a woman who has lived a long and productive life. Now my health is being brought down by advanced age and accompanying diseases.

I do not want drooling, incontinent and comatose "golden" years, mandated by mindless, overzealous medical intervention. I want to keep my appointment with eternity. I do not need counseling, spiritual guidance or antidepressants. I want and need to die, going gently into the last good night.

I view human existence as three stages: conception and birth, living, and dying. For all of the many wondrous things that doctors did for me during the first two stages, I am enormously grateful. For abandoning me in this third stage by forcing your cruel and unwanted "life at any price" mind-set upon me, shame on you.

A. I am publishing your provocative and touching letter because you express yourself so effectively—and, I believe, you speak for millions of adults whose end-of-life issues are a concern—a concern because their wishes are disregarded or trivialized by the medical profession. Thank you for writing.

Quality of life is most important

Q. My 97-year-old mother, with severe Alzheimer's disease, was recently transferred from a nursing home to the hospital because of difficulty breathing. Thank heaven her regular doctor was available and examined her. He diagnosed bronchitis and sent her back to the nursing home on antibiotics, where she is recovering.

Our family has repeatedly requested that she be kept comfortable and that no heroic measures be employed. I am afraid of what might have happened if her doctor, who knew of and accepted our wishes, had been off-duty.

All this is just a prelude to my question: How on earth can we justify keeping the elderly alive year after year—up to 110 or 120 in a few decades, if we believe the experts—when the quality of their lives will be so hideously compromised, even in the face of future medical advances?

A. Boy, you've asked a tough one.

People are, indeed, living longer. But, as you pointed out, their quality of life may suffer as a result.

I care for a large population of nursing home residents, many of whom are institutionalized because of dementia and other serious ailments. All of these people were once independent, responsible, productive adults, who raised children, had stunning careers, contributed to society, remained active through their 60s, left profound cultural legacies, and had loving and supportive families. Now, unfortunately, they may not be able to feed themselves, take care of the most essential hygiene or even recognize family members. In such cases, I am like the doctor that you described. My primary goal—with the families' approval and encouragement—is to provide comfort-care and to avoid doing anything to prolong life artificially. I often must let these dear old people die with dignity and without pain. While prolonging life is a doctor's first responsibility, prolonging death is a cruel and senseless act, in my opinion.

Consequently, I—like you—am deeply concerned about the present publicity surrounding the experts' pronouncements that the aged can, perhaps, be kept alive well into their second centuries. Is charming and frail Aunt Ella going to be better off living to 110, using heroic medical therapy, if she is bedridden, doesn't know she is on planet Earth and is hopelessly incontinent? Are the experts simply playing the numbers on this issue? Is this the reason that nursing homes are filled to overflowing? Is this what we want when we reach this stage of hopeless, dependent existence?

Not I.

Longevity may be a great goal, but it has to be accompanied by an equally important end-game, called quality of life. I don't know about you, but I don't want to be a burden to my family and heirs, no matter how much they love me. I have no intention of squandering what little inheritance I've set aside. I vote "No!" to being kept alive indefinitely because of someone's guilt feelings or a doctor's commitment to life at any cost.

So, my answer to you—and to the experts—is: Keeping us oldies alive until we pass 100 would be a great medical breakthrough, provided

we are cognitive enough to appreciate our surroundings and to partici-
pate in the vital decisions about our future and very existence. If not, I
pray we will be cared for by sensitive physicians who consider helpless,
irreconcilable, inhuman dependency a far greater enemy than death.

Significance of DNR

Q. What actually does a DNR order mean? Does it prohibit patients in
hospitals or nursing homes from receiving antibiotics or pain medication?

A. Do Not Resuscitate (DNR) is an expression of patients' wishes
to avoid undergoing resuscitative efforts at the end of life. For example,
a DNR patient who is found to be pulseless and not breathing would not
receive closed chest cardiac massage, artificial ventilation, machine life
support and other techniques used to revive a person who appears to
have died. DNR does not cover the use of medications (such as antibiotics), does not prohibit hospitalization (for heart attack or stroke, for instance) and does not mean that a person would be deprived of pain medication if this were needed.

Most patients who opt for DNR status do not want heroic efforts to
bring back life in situations where death appears to have occurred.

Other quality-of-life issues (such as tube feedings and advanced
life support) are best addressed in a document called a living will. Most
older adults should have living wills. The forms are available through a
variety of sources, including attorney's offices.

Living wills are appropriate

Q. My mother-in-law, age 91, has been in a nursing home for two
years. Although she recognizes family members, she doesn't know where
she is. She was recently hospitalized for pneumonia complicated by congestive heart failure. She is diabetic and has a pacemaker.

I've lost count of her hospitalizations over the past two years; she
continues to pray to die—but cannot. She is wheelchair-bound, tired, worn
out, sore and weary.

The nursing home staff does an excellent job of monitoring her. We
visit a couple of times a week. But it's extremely depressing to see the
residents and know that this is what we have to look forward to.

There are some things worse than death. This is one. Many of these
patients are overmedicated, because well-meaning doctors are simply out
of ideas. They prescribe one medication to counteract the side effects of
another.

I'm in pretty good health at 65, but when I get to the point where I cannot function mentally or physically, I'll be ready to move on. Sadly, we don't get that choice.

What do you think?

A. You raise a plethora of questions in your letter, which I have edited because of space restrictions.

Your mother-in-law, with advanced age and multiple medical problems, has expressed a wish to die. Yet her doctors (and family?) persist in admitting her to a hospital for various reasons.

First of all, she needs to sign a legal document that expresses her opinions about advanced life support or "Do Not Resuscitate." Such a form should be available through the office of your family attorney. In the event that she is mentally incapable of signing such a document, the family needs to appoint (through legal channels) a person who can make medical decisions regarding your mother-in-law's choices about medical care and quality-of-life decisions.

Second, your experiences should certainly act as a "wake-up call" for you to register your wishes vis-a-vis your own health. You must address topics such as resuscitation, advanced life support and terminal care when you are relatively healthy and free of ailments. If you believe that, at your age of 65, you need to define your wishes about medical care when you "cannot function mentally or physically," do so at once. Plan to meet with your family lawyer, who will lead you through the process. (Because each state has individual requirements, I cannot offer you a generic option.)

End-of-life issues call for legal counseling

Q. At the age of 84, I have seen many of my friends and relatives die unnecessarily slow, sad and expensive deaths at the hands of doctors and hospitals.

Although I do not wish to hasten my death, I am frightened at the prospect of my dear wife's assets being taken from her, when my time comes, by medical profiteers who lie in wait for such occasions. To me, the reason for this sad state of affairs is a combination of greed and religion. What can I do to reduce my fears, take control of my death and protect my wife?

A. The issues you raise are common, important and real. I have received many letters from elderly readers that express concerns identical to yours.

Although one might be tempted to conclude that these are strictly medical problems, the situation is, in fact, largely a legal one.

First, you may want to have a family conference, to share your beliefs and wishes with your wife, children and other relatives. Everyone has got to be on the same page in this issue.

Once the family has reached a consensus, you should meet with your attorney to put into pace the appropriate legal documents, such as a living will, power of attorney and health care proxy. States differ widely in how these goals are achieved, so you will want to involve an attorney who specializes in estate law and related issues.

If your children can (and are willing to) have the legal power to achieve your objectives (in the event you become incompetent), the whole process should proceed smoothly.

Once you have developed the basic documents that spell out your convictions, copies should be distributed to your family physician. Also, you should have copies readily available at home so that medical personnel (EMTs and so forth) will have access to them in an emergency situation.

In short, your attorney should be able to advise you and thereby reduce your apprehension.

Patient's preferences should be honored

Q. This letter concerns my late father and end-of-life issues. He was 87, did not enjoy life and suffered from dementia. Last year, he was found to have an aneurysm and told us: "no hospital, no operation." Despite this, my mother called 9-1-1 when he passed out—and he became a cog in the wheel of medical technology.

At the hospital, he was unable to alter the inevitable. After 24 days, he had been put on (and off) a respirator, defibrillator, a pacemaker, dialysis and a feeding tube. Eventually, the treatment was too much for him; we took him home on hospice, and he quietly died two days later.

Was the medical intervention a benefit? No. Did we have to allow it? Yes. Why? Because the doctors offered it, and my dad was unable to refuse.

I realize that it is human instinct to fight for life. Even if a person has a living will, it takes a clear mind, a strong constitution and great faith to stick with it. The best thing we did was to bring him home, tell him he did a good job with his life and give him permission to die. I wish the doctors hadn't given us all those medical choices.

A. There is certainly enough blame to go around.

First, although your father made clear his preferences (with a living will) before his demise, these wishes were not honored. I find this extraordinary. In my practice, when I see a terminally ill patient, the first thing I want to know about is his or her instructions about end-of-life issues. I will follow the instructions. So there was a serious glitch here: The meaning of the living will was ignored.

Second, your mother should not have called 9-1-1, because your father specifically forbade it.

Third, although emergency medical technicians should follow the patient's expressed wishes, many EMTs don't. When called to action, they respond aggressively. Nonetheless, the hospital doctors should have honored your father's choices. Lord knows, there was certainly ample opportunity for them to back off during your dad's extensive hospitalization.

Fourth, some family member should have said: "Whoa! Let's have a conference here and develop a strategy that is in keeping with Dad's wishes." If these wishes were contradictory or confusing—or if your father was incompetent—a family member should have petitioned a probate court for a power of attorney and health care proxy, legal documents giving that family member the power to make life-and-death decisions.

Finally, I suggest that you ask for a hospital review of this case. Here was an elderly, demented man who had an aneurysm (and, obviously, other medical problems) and who had a living will. I'd like to know the reasons the attending physicians failed your father so miserably. In my opinion, when the extent of the disorders was recognized (and aggressive, invasive therapy was being considered), a caring physician should have approached the family and said something like: "I am very sorry that your father is so ill. His condition is extremely serious, but it may be helped by using techniques such as a pacemaker, dialysis and so forth. However, there is no guarantee of recovery. Judging from your father's living will, he does not want such efforts. Therefore, I would like your permission to give him palliative care: therapy to minimize pain and suffering. Rather than merely extending his life, these measures will dramatically improve the quality of the time he has left."

All of us in the over-50 set have strong and personal feelings about end-of-life care. Some folks want resuscitation and a "full-court medical press." Their choice should be honored. In contrast, others of us believe that we should be allowed to die gracefully, painlessly and with dignity when the time comes. Once we have made our preferences clear, we have to rely on other people—family members, spouses and children—to make sure that our instructions are followed. And that expectation can, as you have discovered, be ignored, resulting in precisely what we don't want to happen.

Making use of a living will

Q. I would like to know your opinion on living wills and power of attorney. I have also signed an ambulance form refusing heart compression, defibrillation, etc. How much actual power do my son and doctor have to see these carried out? Although my sister who recently died had the same requests, they were ignored until her blood pressure read 48/0 and, at that stage, treatment was stopped. I'm 80 years old and realize my own mortality may soon be in question.

How do I assure that my wishes will be carried out? This is a very pertinent issue.

A. We all can sign living wills until we are blue in the face, but our wishes may not be honored if, subsequently, we experience a life-threatening catastrophe.

If you do not want to be subjected to life support during an emergency, you must distribute copies of your living will to your doctor, next of kin, attorney, and local hospital. Hopefully, with everyone "on board," your wishes will be respected.

In my experience, it's the family members and the doctor who must really be instructed about your desire to avoid resuscitation. As part of that plan, make sure those who are involved in your care will not call an ambulance if you are unable to express your wishes at the time. Unless the ambulance personnel know your preferences, they are mandated—often by state law—to administer lifesaving measures.

A further consideration might be a MedicAlert bracelet or neck emblem, indicating that you have a living will on file. These devices will give emergency responders critical information regarding your life support wishes. Further details can be obtained by calling 1-800-432-5378.

In summary, discuss this with your attorney who, depending on your state's legal position, can advise you whom to notify and in what form.

Doctor's responsibility to dying patients

Q. Is it hard for doctors to take care of terminally ill patients?

A. One of a doctor's most difficult responsibilities is to help people through the process of dying. For the most part, this role is not taught in medical school or residency programs, where new practitioners are instructed, through formal academic training, to diagnose illness, treat disease and cheat death whenever possible.

Once out in the real world, however, most young doctors quickly learn that dealing with death is as much a part of medical practice as is the stethoscope. Death takes away the good, the innocent, the respected; it takes away patients who have become friends, and friends who are patients. It is not always welcome. It comes in the night, and in daylight, on holidays, in all seasons, sometimes unexpectedly, always with grim harshness.

Regardless of the circumstances, death also takes away a piece of us doctors when it happens to someone to whom we have committed time, interest, energy, effort—yes, even love. It constantly reminds us of how ineffectual—how really ineffectual—we are at preventing it. This realization and these feelings are, at best, hard for us to accept. We are forced to learn new skills and extraordinary talents to cope with our sense of loss and vulnerability.

Not all of us are capable of doing this. In the face of dull reality, it's easier to justify our omnipotence and deny that death is a part of our lives. It's far simpler to regard death as an enemy and, in the process, put emotional distance between us and our patients at the very time they most need us.

We look for excuses. The heart attack was too massive. We use magic: Although the cancer has spread, try chemotherapy anyway; it might work. We place blame: What can you expect from a pack-a-day smoker? Worst of all, we resist learning from terminal patients under our care. Out of a mistaken fantasy that we do harm by removing hope, we compulsively strive to keep people alive, when every humane instinct screams that this heroic enterprise is futile and dehumanizing.

This doesn't have to be. I recently learned an important lesson from a patient to whom I'd grown very close. A year ago, he was found to have inoperable lung cancer. Because he was pain-free and relatively independent, I encouraged him to have radiation therapy. The tumor shrunk and, except for weakness and weight loss, he seemed to rally. He wanted to know the prognosis. I told him. He put his affairs in order and attempted to lead as normal a life as he could. In this effort, he was moderately successful—until unmistakable signs of recurring cancer appeared. We struck a bargain at that point, under which I agreed to no lifesaving procedures and promised to keep him as comfortable as possible.

Near the end, he required hospitalization for jaundice and dehydration. He lingered for two weeks. During this time, I gave him as much morphine as he wanted. At the end, he refused the narcotic because it made his thinking "too fuzzy." On the day of his death, he was lucid and serene. His family was with him. I held his hand and asked him how he felt. "Peaceful," he replied. "I no longer have to struggle. I can surrender."

If, as the writer/philosopher Joseph Campbell suggested, heaven is really within us, at death the energy of life ultimately joins with itself; peace comes when the struggle to maintain individuality ends.

This knowledge is not part of the standard medical school curriculum. Perhaps it should be, because I believe that when all is said and done, when the machines and the medicines are deemed insufficient, once patients have entered the final phase of life, doctors have a duty to help the terminally ill surrender with peace. We must take away fear and provide a real service to those who desperately need it. This emotional bond serves to strengthen both the doctor and his dying patient.

Why is this relationship so important to me? For obvious reasons, of course. Also, I selfishly hope that my doctor will honor me, when the time comes, with the same respect and kindness I try to give my patients today.

Pain control is vital in the terminally ill

Q. I just read your column about the importance of pain relief in terminal patients, and I heartily agree. I suffer from advanced cancer and pain, and accept the inevitable reality of my death. However, I really do need relief during this terminal illness. Some physicians are strangely reluctant to prescribe narcotics. When I am lucky enough to receive a supply of opioid pain pills, the medicine causes nausea and vomiting. What can I do?

A. Terminal patients requiring narcotics for pain relief are often sensitive to these medicines in pill or liquid form. In such instances, a medication to control nausea should be administered simultaneously. There are many such drugs available including Compazine, Phenergan, Tigan, Zofran and others.

Also, while these patients may react adversely to oral pain relievers, they can tolerate opioids in the form of patches or injections. The reason for this isn't known. But it is certainly another option you might consider. Ask your oncologist about this. In my opinion, you should not have to live out your last days with uncontrollable pain, nausea and vomiting.

Is euthanasia really a solution?

Q. What is your feeling about the possibility of Medicare paying for euthanasia and the government legalizing it?

A. Once you have government-sanctioned killing, there is enormous potential for abuse. Therefore, I'm against the system you mentioned.

As I see it, the real issue isn't euthanasia. Rather, it's that the health care industry just can't bring itself to let terminally ill patients die natural deaths.

We're always interfering, prolonging, dehumanizing. In my view, we could—as a society—accomplish much good if we simply let some people die when they are ready. This is a far cry from assisted death, however, which I think should not be institutionalized.

Because this whole topic is so pertinent, I urge people—of any age—to discuss it with their personal physicians. The issue of living wills and health directives is only part of the picture. Each person needs to inform his or her doctor about the circumstances under which a comfort-only, non-heroic approach to serious infirmity is appropriate.

Pancreatic cancer patient says suicide would be a thoughtless and selfish choice

Q. I was horrified by your response to the woman considering suicide.

Possibly facing incurable cancer, you said she should probably commit suicide if she so desired.

Her attitude seemed to me to exhibit a lack of caring for others and a total absorption in self. What about the loved ones who are left behind to deal with the carnage and guilt?

I am sad for this woman; she sounded so alone and lost.

I am comfortable offering my opinion because I am dying of incurable pancreatic cancer that has spread to my lymph nodes and liver.

At the time of my diagnosis, I allied myself with a wonderful and caring oncologist who is the person I have chosen to direct my final plan for life and eventual death.

Also, I have ongoing discussions with my exceptional family physician who has offered more help and hugs than anyone is entitled to expect.

In addition, I have been directed to a wonderful hospice that gives unlimited support for both my mind and body.

Thanks to medical professionals, I am virtually free of pain and nausea and will remain so until the end.

Perhaps the most positive attribute of this whole process is the time my family and I have to draw together and strengthen our bond of love.

I hope that after I'm gone, my family and friends will feel good about the experience and, I hope, will never have a shred of regret, remorse or guilt.

I am convinced that it is more important to include those I love in this difficult process of dying than to think only of myself and thereby ruin the lives of others, perhaps forever, because of an irreversible act of selfishness and thoughtlessness.

A. I am printing an edited version of your touching and powerful letter because it reinforces my belief that the issue of suicide is an extremely personal matter that each of us must address.

It would be imprudent, in my view, to limit one's options across the board because this virtually removes the right of an individual to make appropriate choices about a subject as vital as end-of-life decisions.

Thank you for writing and sharing your opinion.

Assisted suicide unethical

Q. Thank you for writing about terminally ill patients being allowed to die naturally. Hopefully, your column appeared in many newspapers, informing people so eloquently with your medical expertise and ethical consideration. I support your statements and am grateful.

A. Thank you for the compliment.

The column, in which I argues that patients' wishes should be followed when a terminal illness if present, prompted a lot of reader response, almost all of which was favorable. I'd like to emphasize, however, that my position is not the same as assisted suicide, nor am I suggesting that the terminally ill should simply be left alone to die.

On the contrary, it is precisely in such situations that the physician must commit himself to a comfort-oriented approach, in conjunction with an enormous amount of support and empathy. Dr. Jack Kevorkian (and others like him) do behave unethically, in my opinion, by publicizing the fact that they assist patients in committing suicide.

Most caring doctors draw the line at actually killing someone; rather, we let nature take its course and attempt to make the final hours or days as comfortable as possible for the patient who is fatally afflicted and welcomes a painless death. This usually takes the form of skilled nursing care, as well as the judicious use of narcotics. Most important, we don't interfere by relying on high-tech medicine, antibiotics and lifesaving drugs.

As I have written before, patients must enlist their physicians as allies before death is imminent, by using various legal documents (such as living wills) and heart-to-heart discussions.

Terminal starvation does not appear to be painful

Q. My 90-year-old grandmother is terminally ill with dementia and cancer. She currently resides in a skilled nursing facility, refuses to eat and has an advanced directive indicating that she doesn't want heroic measures, including a feeding tube, when the time comes for her to die.

I and the family have every intention of following her instructions, but we are concerned that a program of starvation would give her pain and discomfort. Can you help us in this predicament?

A. You raise several crucial issues—not the least of which is self-imposed starvation—that families have to deal with, as loved ones reach terminal status. We all want to exert some control over our lives and wish to have our end-of-life decisions honored. Nonetheless, such decisions can be traumatic for family and loved ones. Unfortunately, decisions about life support are easily made in the beginning (do we start artificial nutrition?), but are much more difficult later (when do we stop?).

I recommend that you and your family read the article "Withholding Nutrition at the End of Life: Clinical and Ethical Issues" from the Cleveland Clinic Journal of Medicine, June 2003. I was surprised to learn that starvation in terminally ill patients can actually be more comfortable than force-feeding. Numerous case reports confirm that withholding nutrition and hydration near the end of life "leads to greater patient comfort, while providing it may increase edema (congestion), secretions and dyspnea (difficulty breathing)." In addition, many terminally ill patients require only small amounts of food or liquid; those who "ate to please their families experienced nausea and abdominal discomfort."

Therefore, I recommend that you allow your grandmother to choose her own course. If she is thirsty, she will drink; if hungry, she will eat. More aggressive therapy may serve only to increase her level of discomfort. She has had a long and, I suspect, interesting life. While many well-meaning physicians may disagree with me, I urge you to let your grandmother make her own choices.

At this stage, were I her doctor, I would do whatever it takes to keep her comfortable: encouraging family members and friends to visit her, ensuring competent nursing care, and prescribing whatever medications are necessary to reduce pain and suffering.

This is exactly what I would choose when my time comes. And, I suspect, most people would agree.

How best to handle terminal illness

Q. My father is 76. Four years ago, he had a resection for colon cancer. Two years ago, he had part of his liver removed, because the cancer had spread there. Now tests show that the colon malignancy has spread to his lungs. He has not responded to chemotherapy. The doctors give him nine months to live, but operated on his lungs anyway. The operation nearly killed him because he has a bad heart. The doctors say nothing more can be done.

What is his best hope for a cure? He has extensive cancer in both lungs, had not responded to chemotherapy and would not survive another operation.

I can't see my daddy not doing anything. He clearly believes in his doctors and refuses to try experimental treatment. He is weakening and is bedridden. I can't stand this.

A. One of the most difficult challenges a person has to face is how to deal with terminal illness in a loved one. I know, because I struggled with this issue when my mother developed lung cancer and, later, my father was diagnosed with multiple myeloma. Both my parents died, but the process was agonizing because of the very reasons to which you alluded. The question here is relatively simple. What do you do when a parent (or spouse or child) develops a serious illness, such as cancer, and the options for therapy have been exhausted? The answer, unfortunately, is also simple: Accept reality.

At this stage—after the surgery, the chemotherapy and possibly, the radiation—the patient needs to be kept comfortable. This involves sensitive caretakers (such as hospice), pain medication and a world of love and support from caring family and friends.

While it is difficult for the living to accept death as an inevitability, we must try to do so and to detach with love when someone we care about is in the terminal stages of a serious affliction. Your father is going to die. From your brief description, I predict that he has, at best, weeks to live. Therefore, you must accept this, shower him with attention and affection (until he reaches the phase when he feels uncomfortable with this), and make sure—absolutely sure—that he is pain-free. (Here is where his doctor can be of real help by prescribing large doses of narcotics and other medications.)

Your father knows he is going to die, but he may feel an obligation to keep on fighting, even when this activity is exhausting and futile. Therefore, as difficult as the task may be, you have to permit him to give in and let go. When my mother was on her death-bed, I whispered in her ear: "It's all right, Mom. It's time. Just relax and give in. We love you." She smiled, squeezed my hand, closed her eyes and died by mid-afternoon, pain-free and in peace.

> 66 One of a doctor's most difficult responsibilities is to help people through the process of dying. For the most part, this role is not taught in medical school or residency programs... 99

I sense from your question that you are frantically searching for some last miracle, a hope. Call an end to your search. Fixate on hope. Not the hope that your father can somehow be cured, but the conviction that although he will die, you have done what you can, been supportive, value him and paid him the highest compliment: letting him die with dignity. At this stage, cure is not as important as acceptance. And, when you think of it, what a relief acceptance is! Your father will no longer have to suffer the indignities of medical testing and treatment, the fatigue of keeping your spirit up and the whole, harsh world of pretending that nothing has happened.

In my opinion, you could—during one of your frequent visits—speak to him about this. Here's what I would say: "Daddy, I love you. But both you and I know that there is no cure for your problem. I respect your reluctance to consider experimental therapy, so maybe the best we can do is to accept the situation. I will continue to visit you regularly and be of what help I can. I've instructed your doctor to relieve whatever pain you have. The family is here for you. I accept whatever decision you make about your life. I'll see you tomorrow."

I wouldn't feel comfortable advising you in such a detailed manner if I hadn't experienced the same situation—twice. My prayers are with you.

Index

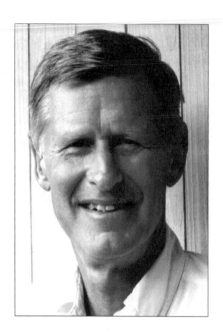

About the Author

Peter H. Gott, M. D. is America's most popular medical columnist. His column appears in more than 350 newspapers worldwide. Dr. Gott has had a solo family/general practice in rural Connecticut since 1966 and is the medical director of the Hotchkiss School, a coed preparatory boarding school in his community.

Dr. Gott has been published in the *New England Journal of Medicine, USA Today, Saturday Review, Working Mother, Lancet, Patient Care,* and a host of other periodicals. His other books include *No House Calls: Irreverent Notes on the Practice of Medicine* and *Summer Windows of 'Sconset.*

Other Great Books in

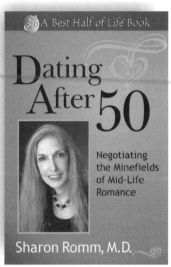

A Best Half of Life® Book

ISBN 1-884956-39-4

Dating After 50
Negotiating the Minefields of Mid-Life Romance
by Sharon Romm, M.D.

$12.95 *($19.95 Canada)*

Dating is especially scary if you haven't dated in a long time. But it *can* be fun and rewarding.

Psychiatrist Sharon Romm helps the reader negotiate the many aspects of dating. Expect sound advice on the safest and easiest way to find dates, who pays for what, if and when to have sex, how to deal with jealousy, second families, former spouses, and myriad other issues common to later-life romances.

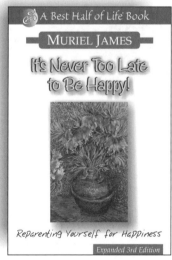

A Best Half of Life® Book

MURIEL JAMES

ISBN 1-884956-26-2

It's Never Too Late to Be Happy
Reparenting Yourself for Happiness
by Muriel James

$12.95 *($19.95 Canada)*

Muriel James, coauthor of the 4-million-copy best-seller *Born to Win*, presents a clear, layman-friendly self-reparenting program through which the reader can actually create a new internal parent—one which is fully functional, supporting, encouraging, and loving—to replace the old parent figure, whose negative psychological messages consistently thwart one's hopes for happiness.

Other Great Books in

The Best Half of Life® Series

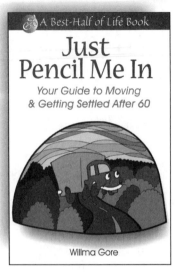

A Best-Half of Life Book

Just Pencil Me In

Your Guide to Moving & Getting Settled After 60

Willma Gore

ISBN 1-884956-21-1

Just Pencil Me In

Your Guide to Moving & Getting Settled After 60

by Willma Willis Gore

$12.95 ($19.95 Canada)

While moving never is simple, moving after one has reached the age of 60 often presents its own special challenges. Yet, it also offers its own special rewards— it's a chance to simplify one's life, to kind of clear out the cellar, both literally and figuratively. It's an opportunity to meet new people, to visit new places, and to learn new things. In fact, with proper planning and execution, moving can and will be an enjoyable adventure.

Just Pencil Me In addresses the unique, distinct concerns encountered by those of us over 60 when faced with relocating. Smooths the way to making your move uncomplicated and enjoyable.

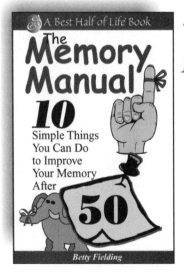

A Best Half of Life Book

The Memory Manual

10

Simple Things You Can Do to Improve Your Memory After *50*

Betty Fielding

ISBN 1-884956-15-7

The Memory Manual

10 Simple Things You Can Do to Improve Your Memory After *50*

By Betty Fielding

$14.95 ($21.95 Canada)

- Tired of looking for where you left your car keys?
- Embarrassed when you forget the name of someone you've just met?
- Wish you could remember more details about what you read?

Then *The Memory Manual* is the book for you! No gimmicks, no long codes or systems to study and memorize, just a simple, holistic program that will get you or a loved one on track to a better memory and a fuller life!